Clinical Procedures in
Small Animal
Veterinary Practice

Content Strategist: Robert Edwards
Content Development Specialist: Veronika Watkins
Project Manager: Beula Christopher
Designer/Design Direction: Christian Bilbow
Illustration Manager: Jennifer Rose
Illustrator: Antbits

Clinical Procedures in
Small Animal
Veterinary Practice

Victoria Aspinall
BVSc, MRCVS

Senior Lecturer, Veterinary Nursing, Hartpury College, Gloucester and Director, AAS Veterinary Services Ltd, Abbeydale, Gloucester, UK

Richard Aspinall
BVSc, Cert. VR, MRCVS

Director/Practice Principal, AAS Veterinary Services Ltd, Abbeydale, Gloucester, UK

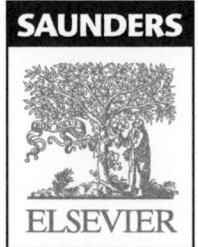

SAUNDERS

ELSEVIER

EDINBURGH   LONDON   NEW YORK   OXFORD   PHILADELPHIA   ST LOUIS   SYDNEY   TORONTO   2013

ELSEVIER
SAUNDERS

© 2013 Elsevier Ltd. All rights reserved.

ISBN 978-0-7020-4770-1

British Library Cataloguing in Publication Data
A catalogue record for this book is available from the British Library

Library of Congress Cataloging in Publication Data
A catalog record for this book is available from the Library of Congress

Notices
Knowledge and best practice in this field are constantly changing. As new research and experience broaden our understanding, changes in research methods, professional practices, or medical treatment may become necessary.

Practitioners and researchers must always rely on their own experience and knowledge in evaluating and using any information, methods, compounds, or experiments described herein. In using such information or methods they should be mindful of their own safety and the safety of others, including parties for whom they have a professional responsibility.

With respect to any drug or pharmaceutical products identified, readers are advised to check the most current information provided (i) on procedures featured or (ii) by the manufacturer of each product to be administered, to verify the recommended dose or formula, the method and duration of administration, and contraindications. It is the responsibility of practitioners, relying on their own experience and knowledge of their patients, to make diagnoses, to determine dosages and the best treatment for each individual patient, and to take all appropriate safety precautions.

To the fullest extent of the law, neither the Publisher nor the authors, contributors, or editors, assume any liability for any injury and/or damage to persons or property as a matter of products liability, negligence or otherwise, or from any use or operation of any methods, products, instructions, or ideas contained in the material herein.

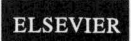

Contents

Preface

The inspiration for this book came from three sources: our memories of what it was like to be thrown in at the 'deep end' of veterinary practice, the employment over the years of several new graduates, and the introduction by the Royal College of Veterinary Surgeons (RCVS) of the Professional Development Phase (PDP) listing the 'Day One Skills' required by the new veterinary graduate. We have used this list as a basis for the clinical procedures covered within the book.

When you sit down to write a step-by-step guide to a procedure you are faced with an immediate dilemma: do you describe several methods as detailed in a wide variety of texts, or do you describe how we do it in our practice? In the majority of cases we have covered the most common method(s) in current use and / or taught at university, but have added in the occasional short cut or useful tip, and of course we have also referred to the accepted authorities on the subject. We have also used veterinary nursing textbooks because, aside from the obvious surgical procedures, veterinary nurses need a not dissimilar range of skills.

It is almost easier to say what this book does not do than what it does do. The book is not designed to cover every single type of procedure that can be performed on a body system or organ, nor does it discuss the constantly evolving new surgical techniques for the treatment of such areas as the stifle joint or the ear. Advancing knowledge in these areas is the responsibility of referral practices, specific training courses, conferences or the veterinary literature. What the book does aim to do is to describe the fundamental techniques that we would expect a new graduate to be able to do within a reasonable timescale. By the end of the first year in veterinary practice, we would hope that he / she would have become proficient in the subject, and prepared for encountering the conditions in practice. Some conditions, such as gastric dilatation and volvulus, are mercifully rare and competency in dealing with them may not happen for several years.

We hope that this book will be useful to both veterinary students in the clinical years of their training and to veterinary graduates in their first 2–3 years of practice. As well as a wide range of everyday clinical skills, it covers some aspects such as basic animal handling that may have been taught in the very first year of a university course and some more theoretical subjects such as parasitology and laboratory work that are taught later in the course, but the details tend to be forgotten once the relevant exams have been passed. We hope that this will become a useful reference book for everybody working in small animal practice and one that can be consulted when you are too frightened to ask a more senior member of the profession!

Victoria and Richard Aspinall
2013

Acknowledgements

So many people have helped with the writing of this book and many of them have been unaware of their contribution. I would particularly like to thank Kate Oldershaw, Laura Dobson, Suzanne Muirhead and Becky Benge who, as relatively new graduates, have all acted as 'guinea pigs' in reading through the text of the procedures and making suggestions as to how the wording could be improved. All the staff at AAS Veterinary Services Ltd have been unfailingly patient in allowing me to poke my camera into their operations whenever something noteworthy has been taking place and apparently not minding when a certain position had to be repeated. In particular, the contribution from Vic Evans, Nic Bullock, Rachael Ford, Michael Stevenson and Erika Jones should be acknowledged.

Finally I would like to thank the team at Elsevier, notably Robert Edwards and Veronika Watkins and the focus groups assembled by Elsevier, who showed great enthusiasm for the original idea of the book. I hope it lives up to their expectations.

ILLUSTRATIONS RESOURCES

The following figures have been reproduced with permission from various books published by Elsevier.

Figures 1.1A–E, 1.2AB, 1.3, 1.4 AB, 1.5 AB, 1.15, 1.16, 1.17A, 1.18, 1.21, 2.4, 2.5, 2.6, 2.7, 3.3, 3.4, 4.1A–D, 4.2 AB, 4.3B, 4.5 AB, 4.6A–C, 4.7A–C, 5.3, 5.4 AB, 5.8, 5.12A–C, 5.14, 5.16, 5.19, 6.2, 6.3, 6.4, 6.7, 6.11AB, 6.13, 6.14, 6.15AB, 6.22, 6.23, 7.2, 7.3, 9.2A–E, 9.4A–C, 9.5, 10.18A–C have been reproduced from Aspinall V 2008 Clinical Procedures in Veterinary Nursing. Butterworth-Heinemann, Oxford.

Figures 2.8A–G, 5.2, 5.5, 5.9, 5.17, 6.12, 8.2, 8.3, 8.4, 8.5, 8.6, 8.7, 8.8A–D, 8.9 AB, 8.10, 10.2 have been reproduced from Aspinall V 2011 The Complete Textbook of Veterinary Nursing. Butterworth-Heinemann, Oxford.

Figures 1.6AB, 1.20, 10.28 have been reproduced from O'Malley B 2005 Clinical Anatomy and Physiology of Exotic Species. Elsevier Saunders, Oxford.

Figures 3.1AB, 5.6, 5.15A–F, 5.18A–F, 6.18A have been reproduced with permission from Lane D, Cooper B 2003 Veterinary Nursing, 3rs edn. Butterworth-Heinemann, Oxford.

Figures 3.2 ABC, 10.1A–C, 10.11AB, 10.16, 10.17, 10.19, 10.20, 10.21 AB, 10.23BC, 10.24(1–3), 10.26A–H, 10.29A(1–4), 10.30(1–4) have been reproduced from Fossum TW 2007 Small Animal Surgery. Mosby, Missouri.

Figure 3.7 has been reproduced from Slatter D 2003 Textbook of Small Animal Surgery. Saunders, Philadelphia.

Figure 5.1 has been reproduced from Masters J, Bowden C 2001 Pre-Veterinary Nursing Textbook. Butterworth-Heinemann, Oxford, in association with BVNA.

Figure 5.7B has been reproduced from Samuelson D 2006 Textbook of Veterinary Histology. Saunders, Missouri.

Figure 6.21 has been reproduced from Aspinall V, Cappello M 2009 Introduction to Veterinary Anatomy and Physiology, 2nd edn. Butterworth-Heinemann, Oxford.

Figures 7.6, 7.7, 7.8, 7.11AB have been reproduced from Taylor SM 2010 Small Animal Clinical Techniques. Saunders, Missouri.

Figure 7.10 has been reproduced from Bowden C, Masters J 2003 Textbook of Veterinary Medical Nursing. Butterworth-Heinemann, Oxford.

Figures 8.11A and 8.12 have been reproduced from McKelvey and Hollingshead 2000 Small Animal Anesthesia and Analgesia. Mosby, Missouri.

Figures 9.6AB, 9.7A–G, 9.8A–E have been reproduced from Martin C, Masters J 2007 Textbook of Veterinary Surgical Nursing. Butterworth-Heinemann, Oxford.

CHAPTER 1

Restraint, handling and administration of medication

CHAPTER CONTENTS

Correct handling and restraint of the patient are essential if you are to perform any procedure effectively. If the animal is allowed to move it may hurt itself or you. An animal that is held firmly will feel much more secure and will be less inclined to struggle or to make an escape.

The majority of animals that are brought into the surgery are used to being handled, but this does not mean that they necessarily enjoy having things done to them, especially by a 'strange-smelling stranger'. There will also be a small proportion of animals that are wary of human contact and this includes stray dogs and feral cats. These animals may be unpredictable and potentially dangerous and you must protect your own safety and that of anyone around you.

When handling any species you must approach quietly and confidently; you must know exactly what you are going to do and get it right the first time – the more often you have to attempt a procedure the more frightened or aggressive an animal becomes and the more likely you or the animal are to get hurt. Animals become very upset by clumsy inept handling, but respond positively to someone with a calm, confident demeanour.

So, at the very least, before you start anything:

1. Know how to do the procedure correctly – this will give you confidence and affect your attitude to the animal.

2. Have all your equipment prepared and ready to hand – this may include restraint equipment such as dog catchers or cat bags.

3. Organize assistance if you think you are likely to need it – having a 'go', failing and then deciding you need help causes delay, upsets the patient and may upset the watching client.

Procedure: Muzzling a dog (Fig 1.1)

It will not be necessary to muzzle every canine patient, but it is essential to be able to perform this technique quickly and effectively when you need it. It is rarely necessary, and it is much more difficult, to muzzle cats. If you do need to muzzle a cat there are suitable commercial muzzles available.

1. **Action:** Place the dog in a sitting position on the floor or on a stable examination table covered with a non-slip mat.

   Rationale: In this position the dog will feel comfortable and will be less likely to wriggle.

2. **Action:** Ask an assistant to stand astride the dog, or if on a table to stand behind the dog, and grasp the scruff on either side of the head just below the ears.

   Rationale: The head must be held firmly to prevent it moving around, allowing the muzzle to be tied quickly.

3. **Action:** Using a length of cotton tape or bandage, you should tie a loop in it.

   Rationale: Any long strip of material can be used (e.g. a tie or even tights) but the material must be strong enough to hold the jaws together.

4. **Action:** Approach the dog slowly and deliberately, crouching down to its level if necessary.

   Rationale: Crouching low prevents fear aggression; standing over the dog may provoke it to jump up and bite.

5. **Action:** Place the looped tape over the dog's nose and tighten it quickly with the knot over its nose.

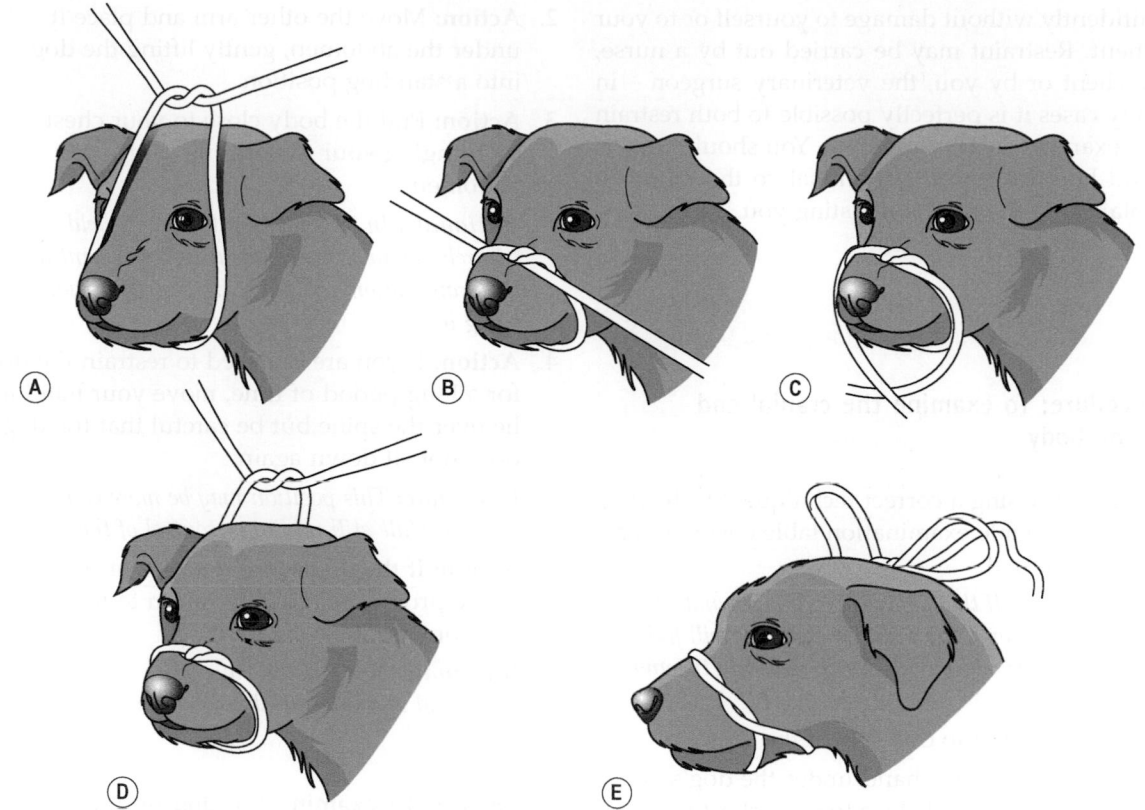

Figure 1.1 Tying a tape muzzle.

Rationale: Any delay in tightening the loop may give time for the dog to shake its head free.

6. **Action:** Bring the long ends of the tape downwards and cross over under the chin.

   Rationale: Further throws around the nose before finally crossing over will strengthen the muzzle.

7. Take the two ends of the tape backwards and tie them in a bow behind the ears.

   Rationale: A bow allows a quick release if the dog becomes distressed.

8. Ask the assistant holding the dog to keep the head pressed down.

   Rationale: This position prevents the dog from lifting its forefeet to pull the muzzle of its nose.

9. If the dog is a brachycephalic breed insert another length of tape under the loop on the nose and under the piece at the back of the head.

   Rationale: This prevents the muzzle from slipping off the short nose. This technique could be used for cats.

10. Bring the two ends of this piece of tape together and tie them into a bow on the bridge of the nose.

    Rationale: The dog must be carefully observed as pressure over the nose of a brachycephalic breed could lead to respiratory distress.

NB Never leave a muzzled animal unattended, as there is always a risk of asphyxiation by vomit or saliva. There are commercial muzzles available. These come in a range of sizes and may be quicker to put on, but they are much more expensive.

RESTRAINT FOR GENERAL EXAMINATION

When examining any animal it is important that it is restrained correctly. This allows you to complete the examination quickly, efficiently and confidently without damage to yourself or to your patient. Restraint may be carried out by a nurse, the client or by you, the veterinary surgeon – in many cases it is perfectly possible to both restrain and examine at the same time. You should understand how to restrain an animal so that you can explain it to the person assisting you.

DOGS

Procedure: To examine the cranial end of the body

1. **Action:** Using a correct technique, lift the dog on to a stable examination table covered in a non-slip mat.

    Rationale: If the table does not shake and the animal's paws do not slip, the animal will feel more secure and will be less inclined to try and escape.

2. **Action:** Stand to one side of the dog.

3. **Action:** Place one hand under the dog's neck and pull the head close to your chest with your hand.

    Rationale: If the head is held firmly against your chest the dog cannot move to bite you.

4. **Action:** Place the other arm over the dog's back with your elbow pointing towards the far side.

5. **Action:** Apply pressure with your elbow along the spine making the dog sit down.

    Rationale: In a sitting position the dog will feel secure.

NB Always remember that the closer you are to the animal the less able it will be to bite you!

Procedure: To examine the caudal end of the body or take the rectal temperature

(This continues from the previous procedure.)

1. **Action:** Keep one arm under the neck pulling the head close to your chest.

    Rationale: If the head is held firmly against your chest, the dog cannot move to bite you.

2. **Action:** Move the other arm and place it under the abdomen, gently lifting the dog into a standing position.

3. **Action:** Pull the body close to your chest by bringing your forearm up under the abdomen.

    Rationale: In this position the dog is held securely against you, preventing movement during the examination and reducing the risk of your being bitten.

4. **Action:** If you are required to restrain the dog for a long period of time, move your hand to lie over the spine but be careful that the dog does not sit down again.

    Rationale: This position may be more comfortable for you while still retaining control of the dog.

5. **Action:** If the dog starts to move or to object to the procedure, quickly return to the previous position.

    Rationale: You must always be aware of the dog's mood and respond quickly to prevent anyone being bitten.

Procedure: To examine the dog on its side or to provide stronger control (Fig. 1.2)

1. **Action:** Apply a tape muzzle if appropriate (Fig. 1.1).

    Rationale: This method is used to restrain more aggressive or more difficult dogs so you should be prepared for trouble.

2. Using correct lifting procedure, lift the dog on to a stable examination table covered in a non-slip mat.

    Rationale: If the table does not shake and the dog's paws do not slip, the dog will feel secure and less inclined to try and escape.

3. With the dog in a standing position, stand to one side of it.

4. Reach over the dog's back and grasp the foreleg and hindleg furthest away from you (Fig. 1.2) at the level of the radius and tibia.

    Rationale: It may be difficult to reach over the back of large dogs especially if you are short or the table is too high.

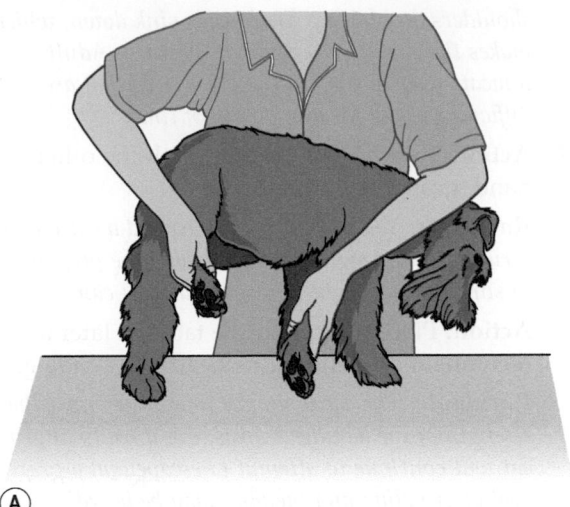
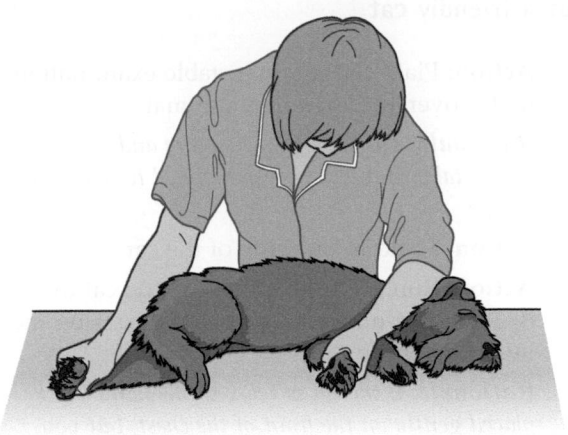

(A) (B)

Figure 1.2 Restraining a dog on its side.

5. As quickly and as firmly as possible, pull the dog's legs away from you supporting its spine against your chest.

   Rationale: This must be done quickly before the dog begins to struggle and change position.

6. **Action:** Gently lower the body down to the table.

   Rationale: Avoid letting the body drop to the table as it may frighten or injure the animal.

7. **Action:** Place your arm across the chest and neck and apply firm pressure to keep the dog's head on the table.

   Rationale: Most dogs will become submissive in this position, but some will try to stand up again and you must be prepared. With a large dog you may have to lean quite heavily on it, but you must always observe the condition of the animal.

Procedure: To examine or restrain a dog on its back

1. **Action:** Place the dog on its side as previously described.
2. **Action:** Ask an assistant to hold both the back legs while you hold the forelegs.

   Rationale: If the dog is small this manoeuvre can be performed by one person.

3. **Action:** Roll the dog over until it is lying on its back.
4. **Action:** Extend the forelegs and hindlegs presenting the ventral abdomen for examination.
5. **Action:** Greater restraint can be achieved by bringing each forelimb to lie on either side of the neck then grasping the scruff of the neck on each side with the same hands.

   Rationale: Most dogs will feel quite comfortable in this position and will struggle only if they feel insecure or in pain.

CATS

Most cats are used to being handled and will respond to being stroked and spoken to quietly. Examining these cats should not pose too much of a problem, but some, and particularly feral cats, can be very difficult to handle and you must be prepared to exercise varying degrees of restraint depending on the individual. Remember cats have five weapons of offence: one set of teeth and four sets of claws!

Cats that are used to being handled respond to minimal restraint, but you should be prepared to use firmer methods on more difficult cats, particularly if you are single-handed.

Procedure: Restraint for the examination of a friendly cat

1. **Action:** Place the cat on a stable examination table covered with a non-slip mat.

   Rationale: The cat will feel secure and comfortable and will be less inclined to make its escape.

2. **Action:** Stand to one side of the cat.

3. **Action:** Run the hand closest to the cat over its back and under the jaw, gently raising the head up a little.

   Rationale: If the cat is relaxed this hand can be placed gently on the front of the chest, but you should be ready to restrain the head if necessary.

4. **Action:** Place the other hand over the forelegs.

   Rationale: This prevents the cat from raising its forepaws to scratch.

5. **Action:** If the cat begins to struggle or object to the examination, move the hand from under the chin and grasp the scruff.

   Rationale: This controls the head allowing examination of the body.

6. **Action:** Use the elbow on this side to press the cat's body firmly against your side.

   Rationale: In this position the cat is unable to move or gain enough grip to make an escape. It may be more comfortable to lift the cat, supporting it against your body rather than leaning over the examination table.

7. **Action:** Use the other hand to hold the forelegs firmly down on the table.

   Rationale: This controls the forepaws and prevents scratching.

NB This position uses minimal restraint but will allow you to examine the whole body and take the rectal temperature.

Procedure: Restraint for examination of a fractious cat

1. **Action:** Firmly grasp the scruff of the cat with one hand.

   Rationale: Some fractious cats seem to have the ability to 'use up' their scruffs by hunching their

shoulders and letting their heads sink down, which makes the scruff very difficult to grasp. Adult tomcats also develop thickened scruffs that are difficult to hold for any length of time.

2. **Action:** Pick up the cat and, with the other hand, grasp its hindlegs.

   Rationale: You should never suspend a cat by its scruff for any length of time. Always be prepared to support its weight as quickly as you can.

3. **Action:** Place the cat on the table in lateral recumbency extending its head and hindlegs.

   Rationale: The cat is unable to move against the strength of the handler's arms, but a really angry cat will continue to attempt to escape and a great deal of growling and mewing may be heard!

4. **Action:** As the cat struggles, make sure that you keep your arms wide apart to maintain the position.

   Rationale: As the forelegs are not restrained you must be careful to avoid getting scratched.

NB This position allows examination of most of the body but it is inadvisable to use it to take the rectal temperature as the cat may struggle and injure itself. For the welfare of the cat, another method of restraint should be adopted as soon as possible.

Restraint equipment, which can be useful for more aggressive cats, includes crusher cages, cat grabbers and cat bags out of which the head or legs can be extended while the rest of the body is retained inside. Wrapping an aggressive cat in a towel is also a useful and cheaper means of restraint. Chemical restraint is widely used, principally by means of an intramuscular injection, but some form of contact with the cat is still required.

In the surgery when moving a cat from room to room it is important to ensure that it does not escape – cats are far more likely to try to escape than dogs. The procedure used depends very much on the nature of the cat.

Procedure: Lifting a friendly cat used to being handled

1. **Action:** Approach the cat calmly and confidently, talking to it quietly.

Rationale: Most cats are used to the sound of the human voice and will be reassured by a low quiet tone.

2. **Action:** Assess whether the cat is safe to stroke.

   Rationale: A frightened or aggressive cat will warn you by hissing or growling as you approach, while a friendly cat may rub itself against your hand and even purr!

3. **Action:** If safe, gently stroke the top of the head and run your hand along its back.

   Rationale: This will reassure the cat and may elicit a purr. If the cat hisses, use another method of lifting and restraint.

4. **Action:** Gently but firmly grasp the scruff of the neck with one hand and lift the cat.

   Rationale: Picking a cat up by the scruff mimics the way in which the queen carries her kittens. It initiates an innate relaxation response which in the wild would enable the queen to move her kittens safely from place to place without the risk of them struggling and escaping.

5. **Action:** Place the other hand under the sternum and support the cat.

   Rationale: Kittens and smaller cats may be lifted by the scruff, but heavier cats need added support.

6. **Action:** Place the cat on an examination table covered in a non-slip mat.

   Rationale: If the cat feels insecure, it may try to scratch bite or escape.

Procedure: Lifting a frightened or aggressive cat

1. **Action:** Grasp the scruff of the cat quickly and firmly.

   Rationale: If you do not take enough scruff or make any mistake in handling, you are likely to get bitten or scratched.

2. **Action:** Lift the cat by the scruff letting the body hang down.

   Rationale: Do not leave the cat 'hanging' for more than a few seconds, as this is unpleasant for the cat, particularly if it is large.

3. **Action:** Place the cat on a table and restrain in an appropriate way.

Rationale: Aggressive cats may have to be restrained using such equipment as a crusher cage or a cat bag.

Procedure: Carrying a cat (Fig. 1.3)

1. **Action:** Place the body of the cat under one elbow and forearm, holding it close to your side. Let the hindlegs dangle.

   Rationale: The body is supported by the angle of your arm, but the hindlegs are unable to push the cat's body up in order to make an escape. Watch out for the hindlegs getting caught in your side pockets.

2. **Action:** Hold the forepaws together between the fingers and thumb of the hand on that side.

   Rationale: This controls the forepaws and prevents them from scratching you.

3. **Action:** Hold the scruff of the cat firmly with your free hand.

   Rationale: In this position the cat feels secure and comfortable. If it tries to escape you have control of the head via the scruff and you can apply stronger pressure to the body with your elbow.

NB Avoid carrying aggressive or frightened cats around in your arms as such animals' movements are unpredictable. They should be carried in a wire cat basket, which allows them to see out whilst providing you with clear visibility to assess their condition.

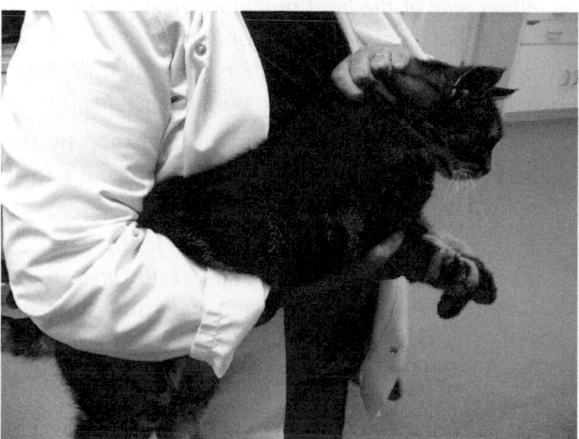

Figure 1.3 Carrying a cat.

RABBITS

The rabbit is the third most popular pet in the UK and it is the most difficult to handle correctly. The rabbit has thinner bones than either the dog or cat and this makes it more prone to fractures of the legs and spine. The domestic rabbit has developed from the wild rabbit *Oryctolagus cuniculus* and its reactions are much the same, in that its instinct is to run and hide when threatened. There are around 50 breeds of domestic rabbit and they vary in size from dwarf breeds weighing around 1 kg to breeds such as the Flemish Giant, which can weigh up to 8 kg. This may be a significant factor in restraint and handling.

Procedure: To restrain a rabbit (Fig. 1.4)

1. **Action:** Observe the rabbit before attempting to handle it.

    Rationale: This allows you to assess the nature of the patient – if it is aggressive you may need to ask for assistance. Restraint may cause respiratory distress.

2. **Action:** Rabbits should be handled gently but firmly.

    Rationale: Rabbits have an innate fear of humans whom they perceive as predators.

3. **Action:** Talk quietly to the rabbit and approach from behind its head.

    Rationale: The eyes of a rabbit are placed on either side of the head providing good lateral vision but very poor backwards vision. There is no need to offer a hand to sniff as you might do with a dog or cat and it may be mistaken for food!

4. **Action:** If the animal is fractious, grasp by the scruff and support the weight with one hand (Fig. 1.4) under the hindquarters.

    Rationale: Never pick a rabbit up by the ears! The hindlegs must be supported at all times. Rabbits have a fragile skeleton and strong lumbar muscles, so they can easily dislocate or break their legs and spines by struggling or kicking.

5. **Action:** More docile rabbits may be restrained by placing one hand under the thorax, gripping the forelegs between the thumb and

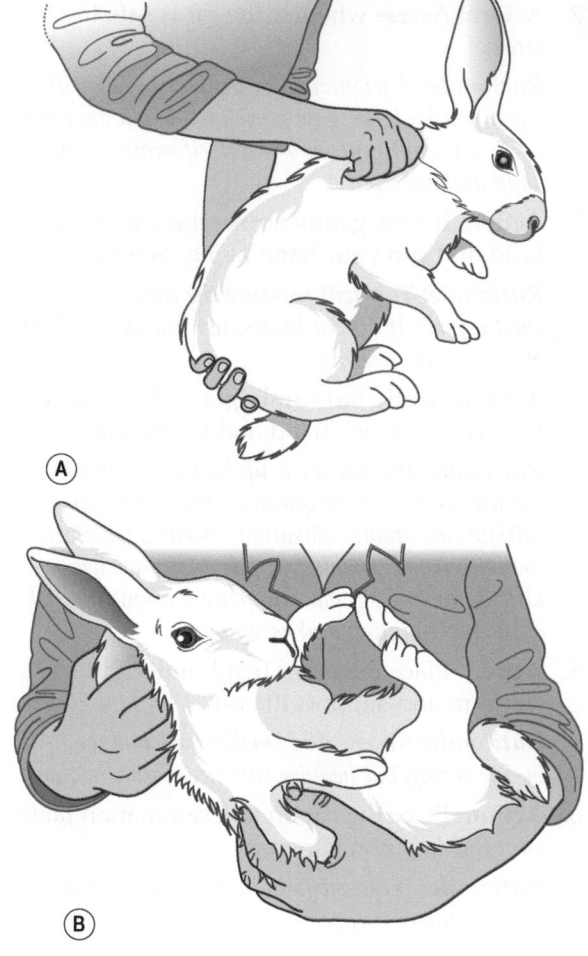

Figure 1.4 Restraining a rabbit (A) Male. (B) Female.

forefingers of that hand. Support the hind end with your other hand.

Rationale: Some rabbits may resent being scruffed. The back should be kept in a normal curved position to avoid spinal fracture.

6. **Action:** To carry the rabbit, tuck the head and front feet under your upper arm and support the body along your forearm (Fig. 1.5A).

    Rationale: Keeping the rabbit close to your body avoids the risk of it kicking and scratching you. Keeping its head in the dark makes the rabbit relax.

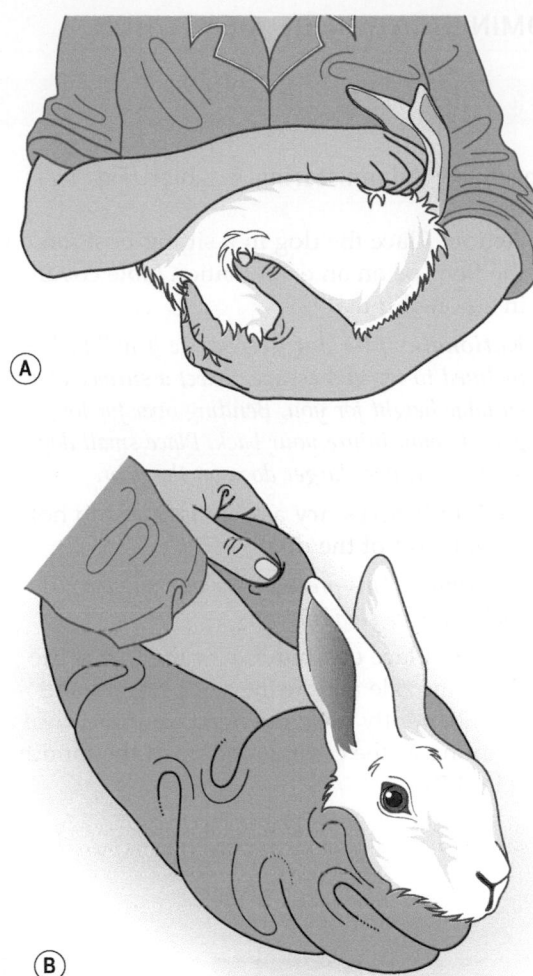

(A)

(B)

Figure 1.5 (A) Carrying a rabbit with the head tucked under your arm. (B) A large towel wrapped securely around the rabbit can be very helpful for restraint.

7. **Action:** A large towel can be used as an additional means of restraint. Unfold the towel on a table. Place the rabbit on the towel with its head projecting from one side. Wrap the towel around the body, covering the feet and leaving the head exposed (Fig. 1.5B).

   Rationale: Covering the feet protects the handler from injury while the head is available for examination and administration of medications.

8. **Action:** An excessively aggressive rabbit may be removed from a cage by throwing a towel over the animal and covering it completely. The rabbit can be unwrapped when it has been safely placed on an examination table.

   Rationale: Aggressive rabbits can come at you as you open the cage and may growl and hiss in fury! Being in the dark may help to reduce the rabbit's stress. Care must always be taken to prevent injury to you and to the rabbit.

Procedure: To differentiate the sex of rabbits (Fig. 1.6)

1. **Action:** Hold the scruff of the rabbit and support its weight by placing one hand under its hindquarters.

   Rationale: The rabbit must be held firmly to avoid possible injury to you or the rabbit.

2. **Action:** Gently lower the rabbit onto an examination table so that it lies in dorsal recumbency. Maintain your hold on the scruff and tilt the animal so that it is almost upside down.

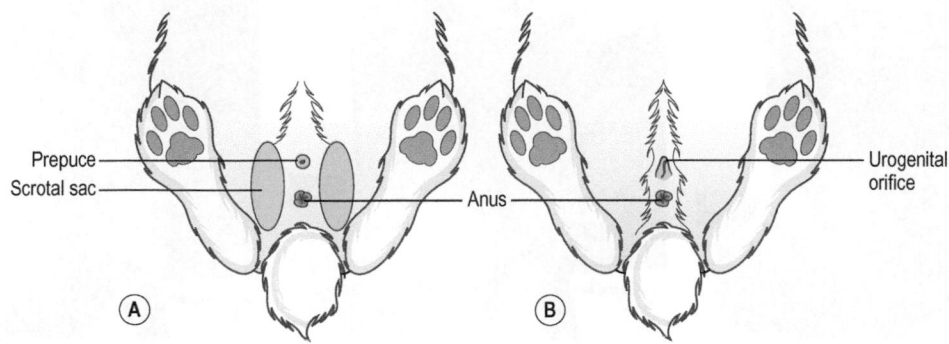

Prepuce
Scrotal sac
Anus
Urogenital orifice

(A)   (B)

Figure 1.6 Sexing a rabbit. (A) Male. (B) Female.

Rationale: In this position the rabbit is almost hypnotized and will then be easier to examine.

3. **Action:** Using your forefinger and middle finger, apply pressure to the vent area just in front of the anus. With some rabbits you may find it easier if the examination is carried out by you while an assistant restrains the rabbit as described above.

Rationale: In both sexes the area will protrude when pressure is applied. Bucks under 5 weeks will show a blunt white tube without a central line, whereas older bucks will show a pink tube with a pointed end that resembles a bullet. The doe has central slit-like opening to the vulva with a band of pink tissue on either side.

NB Young rabbits are notoriously difficult to sex up to the age of 3 weeks – you will not be the first to make a mistake! Adult bucks have large scrotal sacks that are visible lateral and cranial to the penis. The adult testes can be retracted into the abdominal cavity. Adult does have a prominent fur-covered dewlap under the chin from which hair is plucked to line the nest prior to giving birth.

ADMINISTRATION OF MEDICATION

DOGS

Procedure: Administering a tablet (Fig. 1.7)

1. **Action:** Place the dog in a sitting position on the floor or on an examination table covered in a non-slip mat.

   Rationale: If the dog feels secure it will be less inclined to try and escape. Select a surface of a suitable height for you. Bending over for long periods may injure your back. Place small dogs on a table, but dose larger dogs on the floor.

2. **Action:** If necessary ask an assistant to hold the tail end of the dog.

   Rationale: This prevents the dog moving backwards or standing up.

3. **Action:** Place one hand over the top of the dog's muzzle and, using your fingers and thumb, gently raise the head until the nose is pointing at the ceiling, and open the mouth (Fig. 1.7).

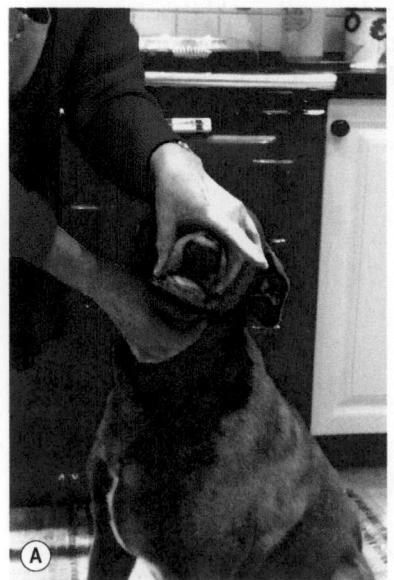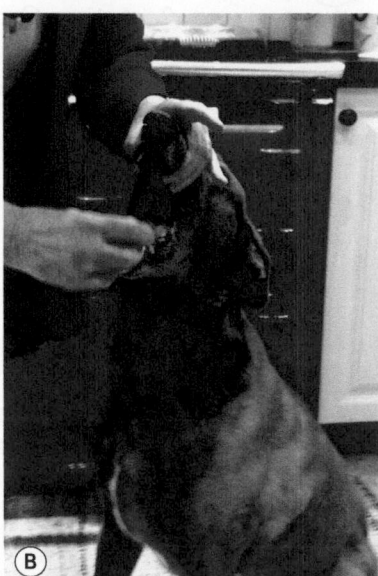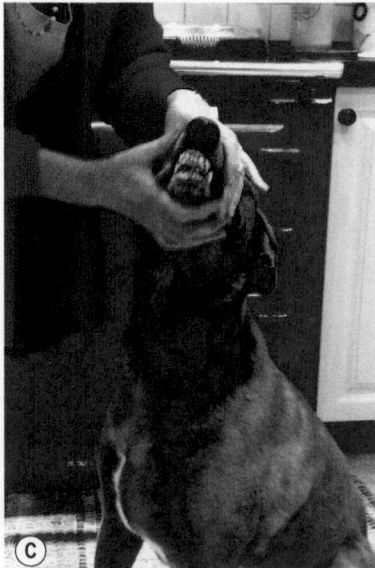

Figure 1.7 Administering a tablet to a dog.

Rationale: Raising the head to a vertical position causes the lower jaw to relax enabling the mouth to be opened more easily.

4. **Action:** Hold the tablet in the fingers of your other hand and with the forefinger of this hand pull down the lower jaw.

5. **Action:** Place the tablet on the back of the tongue.

 Rationale: If the tablet is placed as far back on the tongue as possible, the swallowing reflex is initiated and the dog cannot spit it out.

6. **Action:** Close the mouth and hold it closed with one hand.

 Rationale: This also prevents the dog from spitting it out.

7. **Action:** Stroke the dog's throat until you feel the dog swallow.

 Rationale: The dog may hold the tablet in the side of its mouth and spit it out as soon as you relax your grip. If you know that swallowing has occurred, the tablet should be passing down the oesophagus!

Procedure: Administering a liquid feed or medication

1. **Action:** Place the dog in a sitting position on the floor or on an examination table covered in a non-slip mat.

 Rationale: If the dog feels secure it will be less inclined to try and escape. Select a surface of a suitable height for you. Bending over for long periods may injure your back. Place small dogs on a table, but dose larger dogs on the floor.

2. **Action:** If necessary ask an assistant to hold the tail end of the dog.

 Rationale: This prevents the dog moving backwards or standing up.

3. **Action:** Place one hand over the top of the dog's muzzle and, using the fingers and thumb of one hand, gently tilt the head upwards and to one side.

 Rationale: This position restrains the head while encouraging the jaw to relax.

4. **Action:** Open the jaw slightly creating a pocket at the angle of the jaw.

Rationale: The pocket holds the liquid as it runs into the main part of the oral cavity.

5. **Action:** Using a syringe filled with the liquid, insert it into the side of the mouth.

 Rationale: Try to avoid scraping the syringe over the gums as you may damage the mucous membranes.

6. **Action:** Depress the plunger so that the liquid trickles into the back of the mouth.

 Rationale: If you depress the plunger too quickly the liquid will squirt out over both you and the dog.

7. **Action:** Continue until the syringe is empty and repeat as necessary.

8. **Action:** When the procedure is complete, wipe the mouth clean and wipe up any spillage on the dog's coat.

 Rationale: Never leave the dog covered in liquid as it will become wet and cold and, in summer, dried material may attract flies.

Procedure: Applying ear medication (Fig. 1.8)

1. **Action:** Place the dog in a sitting position on the floor or on an examination table covered in a non-slip mat.

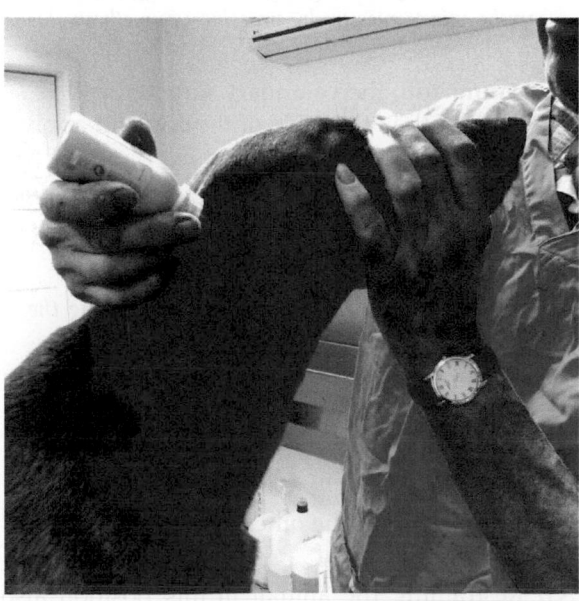

Figure 1.8 Applying ear medication to the ear of a dog.

Rationale: If the dog feels secure it will be less inclined to try and escape. Select a surface of a suitable height for you. Bending over for long periods may injure your back. Place small dogs on a table, but dose larger dogs on the floor.

2. **Action:** If necessary apply a muzzle.

   Rationale: Some dogs may object to the application of ear medication, especially if their ears are sore.

3. **Action:** Ask your assistant to stand to one side of the dog and follow the instructions for steps 4 and 5.

   Rationale: This method can be done single-handedly on an amenable dog and many clients have to do this by themselves; however, if help is available the procedure is better carried out with two people.

4. **Action:** Placing one arm under the dog's neck and over the muzzle, pull the head towards your chest.

   Rationale: This prevents the head from moving suddenly when the medication is applied. Avoid holding the head in the area of the ear as this will interfere with the treatment.

5. **Action:** Place the other arm over the dog's back with your elbow pointing towards the far side.

   Rationale: If the dog begins to struggle you can apply extra pressure by pressing your elbow closer to your side.

6. **Action:** You, the veterinary surgeon, will stand on the other side of the dog and apply the medication to the nearest ear.

   Rationale: The applicator is introduced down the vertical ear canal and squeezed.

7. **Action:** Massage the ear gently.

   Rationale: To disperse the medication along the ear canal.

8. **Action:** Wipe the surrounding area.

   Rationale: To remove any spilt medication. Never leave a dog in a messy state – it wastes medication and annoys the client.

9. **Action:** To treat the other ear, change places with your assistant.

NB Restraining the animal in this position also allows you to examine the ear with an auroscope.

Procedure: Applying eye medication

1. **Action:** Place the dog in a sitting position on the floor or on an examination table covered in a non-slip mat.

   Rationale: If the dog feels secure it will be less inclined to try and escape. Select a surface of a suitable height for you. Bending over for long periods may injure your back. Place small dogs on a table, but dose larger dogs on the floor.

2. **Action:** If necessary apply a muzzle.

   Rationale: Some dogs may object to the application of eye medication, especially if their eyes are sore.

3. **Action:** Ask your assistant to stand to one side of the dog and follow the instructions for steps 4 and 5.

   Rationale: This method can be done single-handedly on an amenable dog and many clients have to do this by themselves; however, if help is available the procedure is better carried out with two people.

4. **Action:** Placing one arm under the dog's neck and over the muzzle, pull the head towards your chest.

   Rationale: This prevents the head from moving suddenly when the medication is applied. Avoid holding the head in the area of the eye as this will interfere with the treatment.

5. **Action:** Place the other arm over the dog's back with your elbow pointing towards the far side.

   Rationale: If the dog begins to struggle you can apply extra pressure by pressing your elbow closer to your side.

6. **Action:** You, the veterinary surgeon, should stand in front of the dog and cup the head in both hands. Using the thumb of one hand the lower eyelid of one eye can be pulled down and the medication can be applied around the edge of the conjunctiva.

   Rationale: You must ensure that the head is held firmly as sudden movement may result in damage to the eye.

7. **Action:** Release the tension on the eyelid and close the eyelids over the medication.

Rationale: This enables the medication to spread over the tissues of the eye and the eyelid.

8. **Action:** If necessary repeat with the other eye.

9. **Action:** After the procedure is completed make sure that, as your assistant relaxes his / her hold, the dog does not rub at its eye with its paws or rub its face on the ground.

   Rationale: After about a minute most medication will have dispersed and will no longer cause any discomfort. If there is evidence of persisting pain, then consider using an Elizabethan collar to prevent self-trauma to the eye.

NB Restraining an animal in the position described also allows you to examine the eye.

Procedure: Administering a subcutaneous injection. Site: Scruff of the neck

1. **Action:** Place the dog in a sitting position or in sternal recumbency on an examination table covered in a non-slip mat.

   Rationale: If the dog feels secure and comfortable it will be less inclined to move or to try and escape.

2. **Action:** Apply a muzzle if necessary.

   Rationale: This procedure is usually quick and painless, but some dogs may object and should be muzzled to prevent injury to you.

3. **Action:** Make sure that your syringe is already filled and that a suitable-sized needle is attached.

   Rationale: To complete this procedure quickly and efficiently you must have your equipment prepared and ready to hand.

4. **Action:** Grasp the scruff firmly with one hand.

   Rationale: This restrains the head and tents the skin ready for injection.

5. **Action:** Using the other hand, insert the point of the needle with the bevel-side uppermost into the raised skin of the scruff.

   Rationale: The needle will go through the skin more smoothly if the bevel-side is uppermost. Be careful to avoid pushing the needle right through

the scruff to the other side, causing you to spray the contents over the dog's coat.

6. **Action:** Inject the contents of the syringe into the subcuticular space and withdraw the needle.

   Rationale: If you wish you may draw back on the syringe before injecting the contents to check that you have not penetrated a small blood capillary. This is good practice, but the blood supply to the area is relatively poor so the chances of penetrating a blood capillary are low.

7. **Action:** Gently massage the site of the injection.

   Rationale: To disperse the drug. Absorption from this site takes about 30–45 minutes.

NB If the dog is likely to object to this procedure, it may be safer to arrange for an assistant to restrain the dog.

Procedure: Administering an intramuscular injection. Site: Quadriceps femoris muscle (Fig. 1.9A)

1. **Action:** Place the dog in a sitting position or in sternal recumbency on an examination table covered in a non-slip mat.

   Rationale: If the dog feels secure and comfortable it will be less inclined to move or to try and escape.

2. **Action:** Apply a muzzle if necessary.

   Rationale: This injection may be slightly painful and some dogs may object.

3. **Action:** Make sure that your syringe is already filled and that a suitable-sized needle is attached.

   Rationale: To complete this procedure quickly and efficiently you must have your equipment prepared and ready to hand.

4. **Action:** Ask your assistant to stand to one side of the dog and then follow the instructions for steps 5, 6 and 7.

   Rationale: This procedure should never be done single-handedly as it can be painful. Lack of restraint may cause the dog to move suddenly, resulting in damage to the muscle tissues.

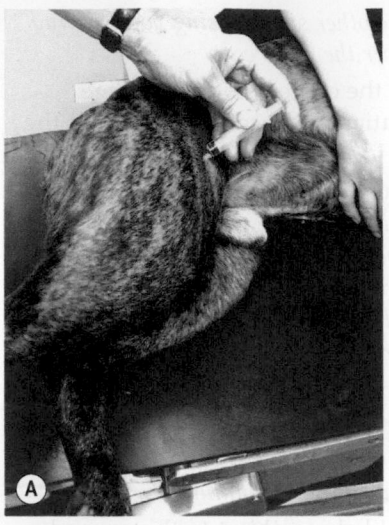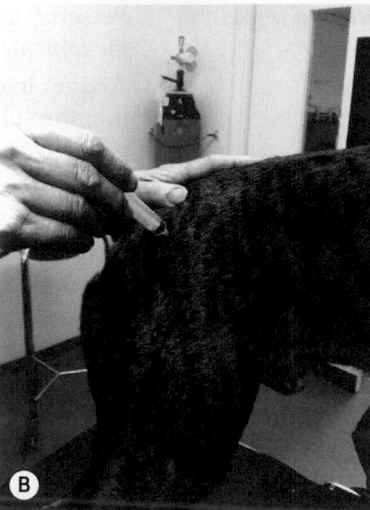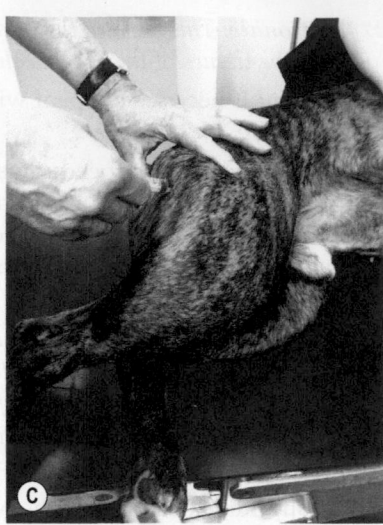

Figure 1.9 Administering an intramuscular injection to a dog: (A) to the quadriceps femoris muscle; (B) to the gluteals; (C) to the hamstring muscles.

5. **Action:** Place one arm under the dog's neck and pull the head close to your chest.

   Rationale: If the head is firmly restrained the dog cannot move suddenly or turn to bite.

6. **Action:** Place your other arm over the dog's chest.

   Rationale: Be prepared to restrain the dog in this position as sudden movement may cause damage and pain at the site of injection.

7. **Action:** You, the veterinary surgeon, should stand to one side of the dog and towards the hind end of the body.

   Rationale: The quadriceps femoris muscle is located on the cranial aspect of the femur.

8. **Action:** Pick up the hindlimb nearest to you. Fix the quadriceps femoris muscle between the thumb and fingers of the non-injecting hand.

   Rationale: The quadriceps femoris muscle is the most common site for intramuscular injections because it is easily reachable and because there are relatively few vital structures running through it (Fig. 1.9A).

9. **Action:** Using your other hand, introduce the needle, bevel-side uppermost, through

the skin and the muscle mass pointing towards the femur and almost at right angles to the lateral aspect of the thigh.

Rationale: At this angle the needle is unlikely to penetrate any major blood vessels or nerves.

10. **Action:** Draw back slightly on the plunger.

    Rationale: Muscle tissue has a good blood supply and there is a risk of vascular penetration. Drawing back also helps to free the needle tip of muscle fibres, which could impede the flow of the drug.

11. **Action:** If there is no blood in the syringe, inject the contents slowly.

    Rationale: Muscle tissue is very dense and rapid injections may be very painful. The density of muscle tissue also limits the volume that can be given. Avoid giving any more than 2 ml in one injection.

12. **Action:** Withdraw the needle and massage the site.

    Rationale: Gentle massage will help to disperse the drug into the blood stream. Absorption from this site takes about 10–15 minutes.

NB It is possible to use other muscle masses for intramuscular injections. The choice may be largely due to personal preference and the ability to restrain the animal appropriately. Other muscles used include:

- Lumbar – approximately midway between the last rib and the wing of the ilium.
- Gluteals – on the dorsal aspect of the pelvis (Fig. 1.9B).
- Hamstring group (semimembranosus / semitendinosus) – located on the caudal aspect of the hindlimb; insert the needle caudal to the femur and direct the tip caudally to avoid damaging the sciatic nerve, which runs along the line of and caudal to the femur (Fig. 1.9C).
- Triceps – runs on the caudal aspect of the humerus; direct the needle caudally away from the humerus.

Procedure: Administering an intravenous injection. Site: Cephalic vein (Fig. 1.10)

(Assume that the skin has been clipped and cleaned with a swab soaked in spirit prior to the procedure.) The cephalic vein is the most common site for venepuncture and runs down the dorsal aspect of the lower forelimb.

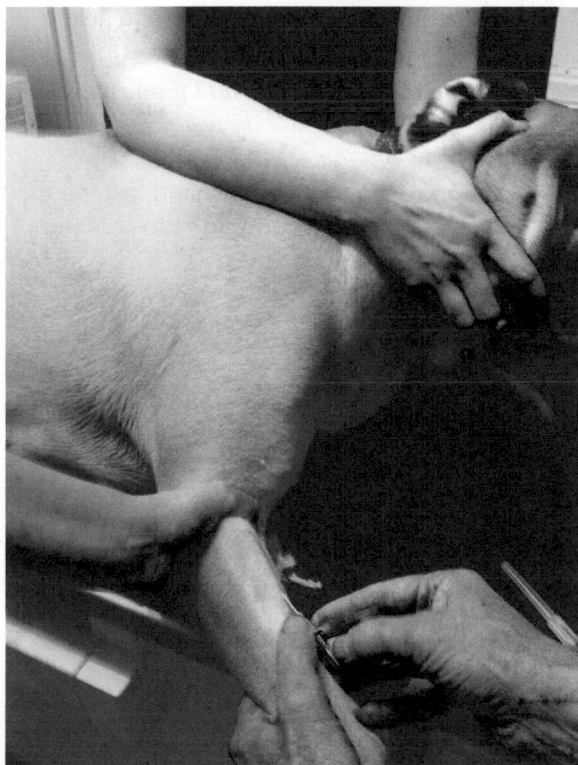

Figure 1.10 Restraining a large dog for an intravenous injection using the cephalic vein.

1. **Action:** Place the dog in sternal recumbency on a stable examination table covered in a non-slip mat.

   Rationale: If the dog feels secure it will be less likely to try and escape. Select a surface of a suitable height for you – bending over for long periods may injure your back.

2. **Action:** Apply a muzzle if necessary.

   Rationale: Some dogs may object to this procedure and a muzzle will protect you from being bitten.

3. **Action:** Make sure that your syringe is filled and that you have attached a suitable gauge and length of needle.

   Rationale: The syringe should be of a size to hold the appropriate volume of drug, but not too large as this will make it difficult to control. Gauge of needle depends on the thickness of the drug and the species of animal – usually 21G is suitable for dogs. The most common length is ⅝ inch (16 mm).

4. **Action:** Ask your assistant to stand to one side of the dog and then follow the instructions for steps 5, 6, 7, 8 and 9.

5. **Action:** Place one arm under the dog's chin and around the head, holding the head close to your chest.

   Rationale: If the head is held firmly and as close to you as possible the dog is less likely to be able to bite.

6. **Action:** Using your other hand, extend the foreleg on the opposite side towards the veterinary surgeon.

   Rationale: Your hand can rest on the table ensuring that the foreleg is supported and held firmly.

7. **Action:** Cup the elbow in the palm of your hand, bringing your thumb across the crook of the elbow.

8. **Action:** Apply gentle pressure with your thumb and rotate your hand slightly outwards.

   Rationale: This pressure acts as a tourniquet trapping blood passing up the foreleg towards the heart. The result is that the vein dilates – known as 'raising the vein' – and becomes more visible.

9. **Action:** The assistant should maintain this pressure while you, the veterinary surgeon, continue with the procedure.

 Rationale: The cephalic vein should clearly be seen under the skin.

10. **Action:** You should hold the leg firmly and insert the needle bevel-side uppermost into the cephalic vein (Fig. 1.10).

 Rationale: Inserting the needle bevel-side uppermost makes it easier to penetrate the wall of the blood vessel.

11. **Action:** Draw back on the plunger of the syringe to check that you have penetrated the vein.

 Rationale: If the vein has been correctly penetrated a small amount of blood will appear in the syringe. Perivascular injection may lead to tissue damage. Do NOT continue with the injection if you are not in the vein.

12. **Action:** If you are certain that the needle is in the vein, ask your assistant to raise his / her thumb a little, and slowly inject the contents of the syringe into the vein.

 Rationale: Releasing the pressure allows the drug to flow into the vein and around the circulation.

13. **Action:** When the procedure is complete, withdraw the needle slowly and apply gentle pressure to the entry point with a swab or small piece of cotton wool for about 30 seconds.

 Rationale: This prevents haemorrhage into the area around the vein.

Procedure: Collection of a blood sample from the cephalic vein

1. **Action:** Place the dog in sternal recumbency on a stable examination table covered in a non-slip mat.

 Rationale: If the dog feels secure it will be less likely to try and escape. Select a surface of a suitable height for you – bending over for long periods may injure your back.

2. **Action:** Apply a muzzle if necessary.

 Rationale: Some dogs may object to this procedure and a muzzle will protect you from being bitten.

3. **Action:** Make sure that you have a needle of an appropriate size attached to a 2 ml syringe close to hand. You will also need a suitable blood-collecting tube.

 Rationale: You should use a 21G needle to collect a blood sample from a dog. If the gauge is too narrow there is a risk that the blood cells will rupture as they pass into the syringe. Selection of the blood-collecting tube depends on the reason for sampling. The most common ones contain anti-clotting agents such as heparin or EDTA. An unclotted sample is required for the majority of blood tests.

4. **Action:** Ask your assistant to stand to one side of the dog and then follow the instructions for steps 5, 6, 7, 8 and 9.

5. **Action:** Place one arm under the dog's chin and around the head, holding the head close to your chest.

 Rationale: If the head is held firmly and as close to you as possible the dog is less likely to be able to bite.

6. **Action:** Using your other hand, extend the foreleg on the opposite side towards the veterinary surgeon.

 Rationale: Your hand can rest on the table ensuring that the foreleg is supported and held firmly.

7. **Action:** Cup the elbow in the palm of your hand, bringing your thumb across the crook of the elbow.

8. **Action:** Apply gentle pressure with your thumb and rotate your hand slightly outwards.

 Rationale: This pressure acts as a tourniquet trapping blood passing up the foreleg towards the heart. The result is that the vein dilates – known as 'raising the vein' – and becomes more visible.

9. **Action:** The assistant should maintain this pressure while you, the veterinary surgeon, continue with the procedure.

Rationale: The cephalic vein should clearly be seen under the skin.

10. **Action:** You should hold the leg firmly and insert the needle bevel-side uppermost into the cephalic vein.

    Rationale: Inserting the needle bevel-side uppermost makes it easier to penetrate the wall of the blood vessel.

11. **Action:** Draw back on the plunger of the syringe to check that you have penetrated the vein.

    Rationale: If the vein has been correctly penetrated a small amount of blood will appear in the syringe.

12. **Action:** If you are certain that the needle is in the vein, your assistant should maintain pressure on the vein while you continue to withdraw blood.

    Rationale: Maintaining the pressure ensures that blood flowing up the leg towards the heart is prevented from doing so and is easier to withdraw into the syringe.

13. **Action:** When the procedure is complete, withdraw the needle slowly and apply gentle pressure to the entry point with a swab or small piece of cotton wool for about 30 seconds.

    Rationale: This prevents haemorrhage into the area around the vein.

14. **Action:** As quickly as possible gently squirt the blood from the syringe into the collecting tube. Replace the lid and rotate the tube between your finger and thumb for at least 1 minute.

    Rationale: Do everything gently – blood cells can easily be damaged by rough treatment and this may affect the results of the blood analysis. Rotating the blood tube allows the blood to mix with the anticoagulant so preventing clotting.

Procedure: Administering an intravenous injection. Site: Jugular vein (Fig. 1.11)

(Assume that the skin has been clipped and cleaned with a swab soaked in spirit prior to the procedure.) The jugular vein runs in the jugular furrow, on either side of the trachea.

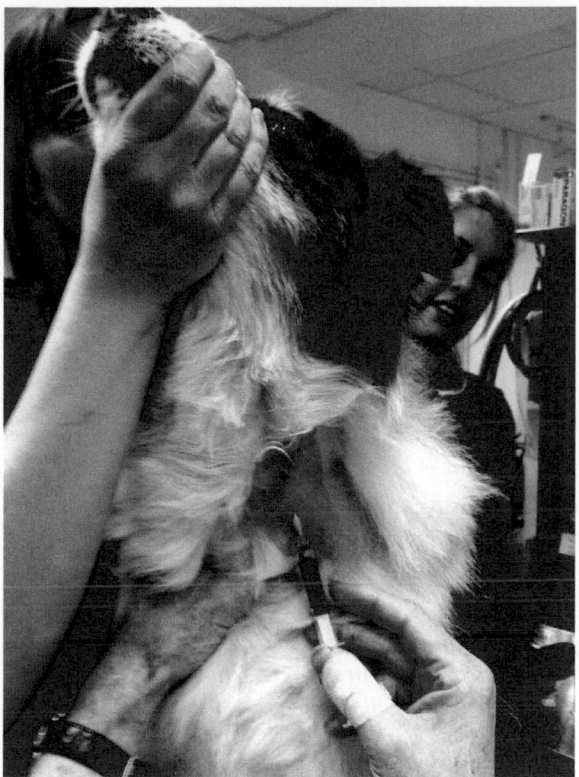

Figure 1.11 Raising the jugular vein of a dog by placing the thumb at the base of the jugular furrow.

1. **Action:** Small dogs – place the dog in a sitting position on a stable examination table covered in a non-slip mat. Large dogs may be placed in a sitting position on the floor.

    Rationale: The dog must feel secure and comfortable so that it will not try to move or to escape.

2. **Action:** Apply a muzzle if necessary.

    Rationale: Some dogs may object to this procedure.

3. **Action:** Make sure that your syringe is filled and that you have attached a suitable gauge and length of needle.

    Rationale: The syringe should be of a size to hold the appropriate volume of drug, but not too large as this will make it difficult to control. Gauge of needle depends on the thickness of the drug and the species of animal – usually 21G is suitable for dogs. The most common length is ⅝ inch (16 mm).

4. **Action:** Ask your assistant to stand to one side of the dog and then follow the instructions for steps 5 and 6.

5. **Action:** Place one hand under the dog's chin and raise the head, bringing it close to your chest.

   Rationale: Firm restraint is essential for this procedure to prevent the dog moving suddenly and causing injury to itself or to you.

6. **Action:** Place your other arm over the dog's back and round to the front of the chest, holding it close to your body.

   Rationale: The closer the dog is to you the less able it is to move or to bite.

7. **Action:** You, the veterinary surgeon, should stand in front of the dog and apply pressure at the base of the jugular furrow with the fingers of one hand (Fig 1.11).

   Rationale: The jugular vein on each side of the trachea runs in a groove known as the jugular furrow. It collects venous blood from the head and neck and returns it to the heart. Pressure applied at the base of the vein will prevent the flow of blood towards the heart causing the vein to dilate – known as 'raising the vein'.

8. **Action:** Using the other hand, insert the needle bevel-side uppermost through the skin and into the underlying vein.

   Rationale: The vein should be clearly visible. Positioning the needle with the bevel-side uppermost makes it easier to insert through the skin and wall of the blood vessel.

9. **Action:** Draw back on the plunger of the syringe to check that you have penetrated the vein.

   Rationale: If the vein has been correctly penetrated a small amount of blood will appear in the syringe. Perivascular injection may lead to tissue damage. Do NOT continue with the injection if you are not in the vein.

10. **Action:** If you are certain that the needle is in the vein, release the pressure exerted by your other hand and slowly inject the drug.

    Rationale: Releasing the pressure allows the drug to flow into the vein and around the circulation.

11. **Action:** When the procedure is complete, withdraw the needle slowly and apply gentle pressure to the entry point with a swab or small piece of cotton wool for about 30 seconds.

    Rationale: This prevents haemorrhage into the area around the vein.

NB Jugular puncture can also be used for collecting a blood sample and may be a better site than the cephalic vein for collecting large volumes. If a blood sample is to be collected maintain pressure on the vein until there is enough blood in the syringe (see procedure for the cephalic vein).

Procedure: Administering an intravenous injection. Site: Lateral saphenous vein (Fig. 1.12)

(Assume that the skin has been clipped and cleaned with a swab soaked in spirit prior to the procedure.) The lateral saphenous vein runs over the lateral aspect of the hock.

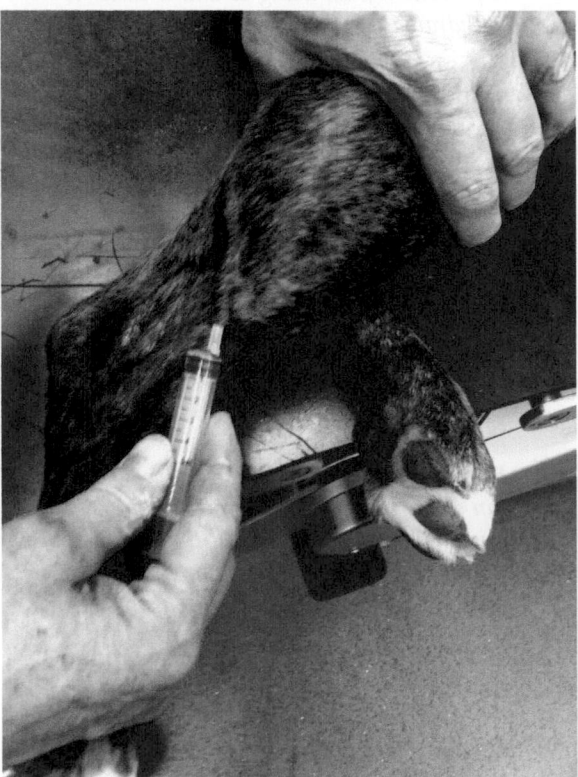

Figure 1.12 Raising the saphenous vein on the hindlimb for an intravenous injection.

1. **Action:** Apply a muzzle if necessary.

   Rationale: Some dogs may object to this procedure. It is easier to apply the muzzle before restraining the dog.

2. **Action:** Place the dog in lateral recumbency on a stable examination table covered in a non-slip mat.

   Rationale: If the dog feels secure it will be less likely to try and escape.

3. **Action:** Make sure that your syringe is filled and that you have attached a suitable gauge and length of needle.

   Rationale: The syringe should be of a size to hold the appropriate volume of drug, but not too large as this will make it difficult to control. Gauge of needle depends on the thickness of the drug and the species of animal – usually 21G is suitable for dogs. The most common length is ⅝ inch (16 mm).

4. **Action:** Ask your assistant to stand on the dorsal side of the dog with the legs directed away from him / her and follow steps 4–7.

5. **Action:** Using the arm closest to the head, place your forearm across the dog's neck and hold both forepaws.

   Rationale: In this position you can use the weight of your body to restrain the cranial end of the dog's body.

6. **Action:** Place the other hand around the uppermost hindleg at the level of the mid tibia / fibula.

   Rationale: The lateral saphenous vein collects blood from the hindpaw and runs superficially on the caudal aspect of the hock and distal tibia.

7. **Action:** Stretch out the leg and apply gentle pressure.

   Rationale: Pressure applied around the distal tibia acts as a tourniquet trapping venous blood and causing the vein to dilate – known as 'raising the vein' (Fig. 1.12).

8. **Action:** You, the veterinary surgeon, should hold the leg and insert the needle bevel-side uppermost through the skin and into the vein.

   Rationale: The vein should be clearly visible. Positioning the needle with the bevel-side uppermost makes it easier to insert through the skin and wall of the blood vessel.

9. **Action:** Draw back on the plunger of the syringe to check that you have penetrated the vein.

   Rationale: If the vein has been correctly penetrated a small amount of blood will appear in the syringe. Perivascular injection may lead to tissue damage. Do NOT continue with the injection if you are not in the vein.

10. **Action:** If you are certain that the needle is in the vein, ask your assistant to release the pressure on the vein and gently inject the drug.

    Rationale: Releasing the pressure allows the drug to flow into the vein and around the circulation.

11. **Action:** When the procedure is complete, withdraw the needle slowly and apply gentle pressure to the entry point with a swab or small piece of cotton wool for about 30 seconds.

    Rationale: This prevents haemorrhage into the area around the vein.

NB The saphenous vein may also be used to collect a blood sample. Your assistant should maintain pressure on the vein while the sample is being collected (see procedure for the cephalic vein).

Procedure: Placement of an intravenous catheter in a peripheral vein

Intravenous catheters may be used for fluid and drug administration and in situations where repeated blood samples are required. It is essential that the catheter is placed in as aseptic a manner as possible to prevent the introduction of infection.

For peripheral veins an over-the-needle catheter is recommended. This consists of a stylet (or needle) with a catheter that fits closely over it. Select the size and length of catheter to deliver as rapid a flow of fluid as possible and to reduce the chance of blockage – for dogs select 18–22G, for cats 22G, and for puppies and kittens 24G. The most common peripheral vein is the cephalic vein.

Figure 1.13 illustrates the procedure in a cat, but the technique is the same in all species.

1. **Action:** Ask an assistant to restrain the patient as described previously.

   Rationale: The patient must feel secure, and correct restraint will prevent injury to the patient and to you and your assistant.

2. **Action:** In some cases it may be necessary to muzzle the patient.

   Rationale: Some animals will object to the procedure.

3. **Action:** Clip an area of skin on the dorsal surface of the forelimb surrounding the intended point of entry (Fig. 1.13A).

   Rationale: This will make aseptic preparation more effective. Cutting any long hair away from the palmar surface of the forepaw will help to prevent contamination and to secure the catheter when it is in place.

4. **Action:** Prepare the site aseptically using an appropriate antiseptic solution.

   Rationale: To prevent introduction of infection into the site.

5. **Action:** Wear sterile gloves.

   Rationale: This may not be essential but, at the very least, your hands must be washed in an antiseptic solution prior to placing the catheter.

6. **Action:** Ask your assistant to raise the vein.

   Rationale: To visualize the vein.

7. **Action:** Make a small incision in the skin over the vein with a scalpel blade.

   Rationale: To facilitate introduction of the catheter. This may not always be necessary, but it may help in dehydrated patients or those with thick skin.

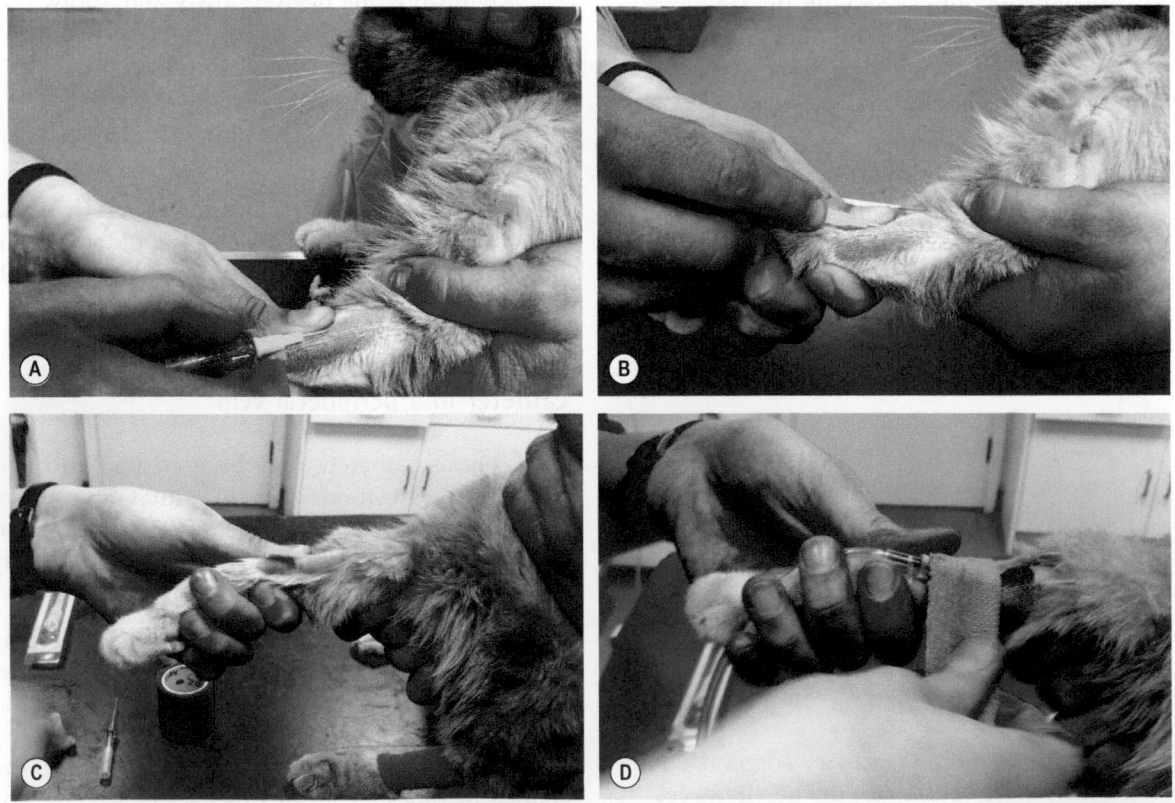

Figure 1.13 Placing an intravenous catheter in the cephalic vein of a cat. The catheter is placed in the vein, held in place using zinc oxide tape and the giving set is attached.

8. **Action:** Push the tip of the catheter, with the bevel of the stylet uppermost, through the incision at an angle of 30–40 degrees and advance it into the vein (Fig. 1.13A, B).

   Rationale: By pushing the catheter at this angle you reduce the risk of pushing it through the vein and out the other side.

9. **Action:** Watch for blood within the flash chamber of the catheter (Fig. 1.13C).

   Rationale: This indicates that you have penetrated the vein satisfactorily.

10. **Action:** Once blood has been seen, reduce the angle between the catheter and the leg by flattening the catheter.

    Rationale: This makes it easier to advance the catheter further up the vein without the danger of going right through the vein.

11. **Action:** Slowly advance the catheter and stylet a short distance into the vein.

    Rationale: To make sure that the catheter lies fully in the lumen.

12. **Action:** Hold the stylet in position and advance the catheter completely into the vein.

13. **Action:** Remove the stylet.

    Rationale: The catheter is now in position.

14. **Action:** Ask your assistant to apply pressure over the vein at the distal end of the catheter.

    Rationale: This occludes the vein preventing unnecessary spillage of blood.

15. **Action:** Secure the catheter in place with adhesive tape (Fig. 1.13D).

    Rationale: To prevent it slipping out of the vein.

16. **Action:** Flush with a small amount of heparin saline.

    Rationale: To make sure it is in place and to prevent the formation of clots.

17. **Action:** Depending on its intended use either attach to a giving set and fluid bag or close the end with an injection cap.

    Rationale: Never leave the end of the catheter open to the air as contaminants may get into the circulation.

Box 1.1 Care of peripheral venous catheters

- Check the catheter and replace the bandage at least twice a day.
- Check the site of insertion for heat, swelling, erythema, pain or leakage of fluid.
- If there are signs of phlebitis remove the catheter.
- Check for signs of swelling above the catheter site – this may indicate fluid leakage under the skin and may necessitate replacement of the catheter.
- Check the toes for signs of swelling – this may indicate that the bandage is too tight.
- If the catheter is used intermittently it may block up – check for patency and prevent clotting by flushing heparinized saline through it every 4 hours and before and after use.
- Remove the catheter if it becomes blocked.
- Always close a catheter port with a sterile injection cap when it is not in use. A port should never be left open to the air.

---

18. **Action:** Cover with a bandage and pack with swabs (Box 1.1).

    Rationale: This ensures that the area is comfortable, reduces the chance of slippage, self-mutilation and contamination.

Procedure: Placement of an intravenous catheter in the jugular vein using the modified Seldinger technique (Fig. 1.14)

This procedure is used when fluids are to be administered for longer than 5 days or when hypertonic fluids are to be given. It is also used for measuring central venous pressure and in some cases where the conformation or temperament of the patient makes use of a peripheral vein more difficult. It is not recommended where there may be a problem with blood clotting.

The patient may be conscious if it is weak or debilitated, but general anaesthesia or sedation will make placement of the catheter much easier. The patient should be attached to an ECG monitor.

1. **Action:** Place the animal in lateral recumbency.

   Rationale: This position provides the best access to the jugular vein.

2. **Action:** Place a sandbag under the neck.

   Rationale: This makes the neck bend over the sandbag, enabling the jugular vein to be accessed more easily.

3. **Action:** Prepare area over and around the jugular vein aseptically.

   Rationale: It is vital to ensure that infection is not introduced into the vein.

4. **Action:** Cover with a sterile fenestrated drape.

   Rationale: To prevent introduction of infection.

5. **Action:** Wear sterile gloves.

   Rationale: To prevent introduction of infection.

6. **Action:** Ask your assistant to raise the jugular vein by placing his / her hand under the drape and applying pressure to the base of the jugular furrow.

   Rationale: To visualize the jugular vein.

7. **Action:** Make a stab incision over the jugular vein.

   Rationale: To facilitate introduction of the catheter.

8. **Action:** Insert either the introducer needle from the Seldinger catheter pack or an over-the-needle catheter into the vein in a rostro-caudal direction (Fig. 1.14).

   Rationale: The needle or catheter is pushed towards the heart, i.e. away from the head.

9. **Action:** If using an over-the-needle catheter, remove the needle.

   Rationale: This clears the way for introduction of the guide wire.

10. **Action:** Ask your assistant to stop raising the vein.

11. **Action:** Insert the guide wire into the vein through the introducer or the catheter holding it within an adapter.

    Rationale: Holding the adapter helps placement of the guide wire. The guide wire may have a J-shaped tip and this should be straightened by withdrawing it into the adapter before it is inserted.

12. **Action:** Monitor the ECG for arrhythmias.

    Rationale: Over-long wires can enter the heart and cause arrhythmias.

13. **Action:** Do not let go of the guide wire at any time.

    Rationale: There is a risk of losing the wire in the vein if you let it go.

14. **Action:** Remove the introducer needle or catheter, leaving the guide wire in place.

15. **Action:** Advance the vessel dilator over the guide wire and into the vein.

    Rationale: To enlarge the subcutaneous tunnel.

16. **Action:** Remove the dilator.

17. **Action:** Advance the Seldinger catheter over the guide wire and into the vein and remove the wire.

    Rationale: The catheter is now in place.

18. **Action:** Put sterile injection caps over each port of the catheter.

    Rationale: This prevents air and infection entering the vein. There are two ports to this type of catheter and ideally each cap should incorporate an on/off tap.

19. **Action:** From each port, withdraw any air and a little blood into a syringe containing a little heparinized saline.

    Rationale: This prevents an air embolism and ensures that the catheter is positioned intravascularly.

20. **Action:** Immediately flush through each port with heparinized saline.

    Rationale: To prevent clotting within the port.

21. **Action:** Place sutures through specific holes on the wing at the base of the catheter into the skin within the area.

    Rationale: To secure the catheter to the patient.

22. **Action:** Place a sterile dressing over the entry site and cover with a bandage.

    Rationale: This keeps the area clean and helps to hold the catheter in place. Make sure that the bandage is not too tight.

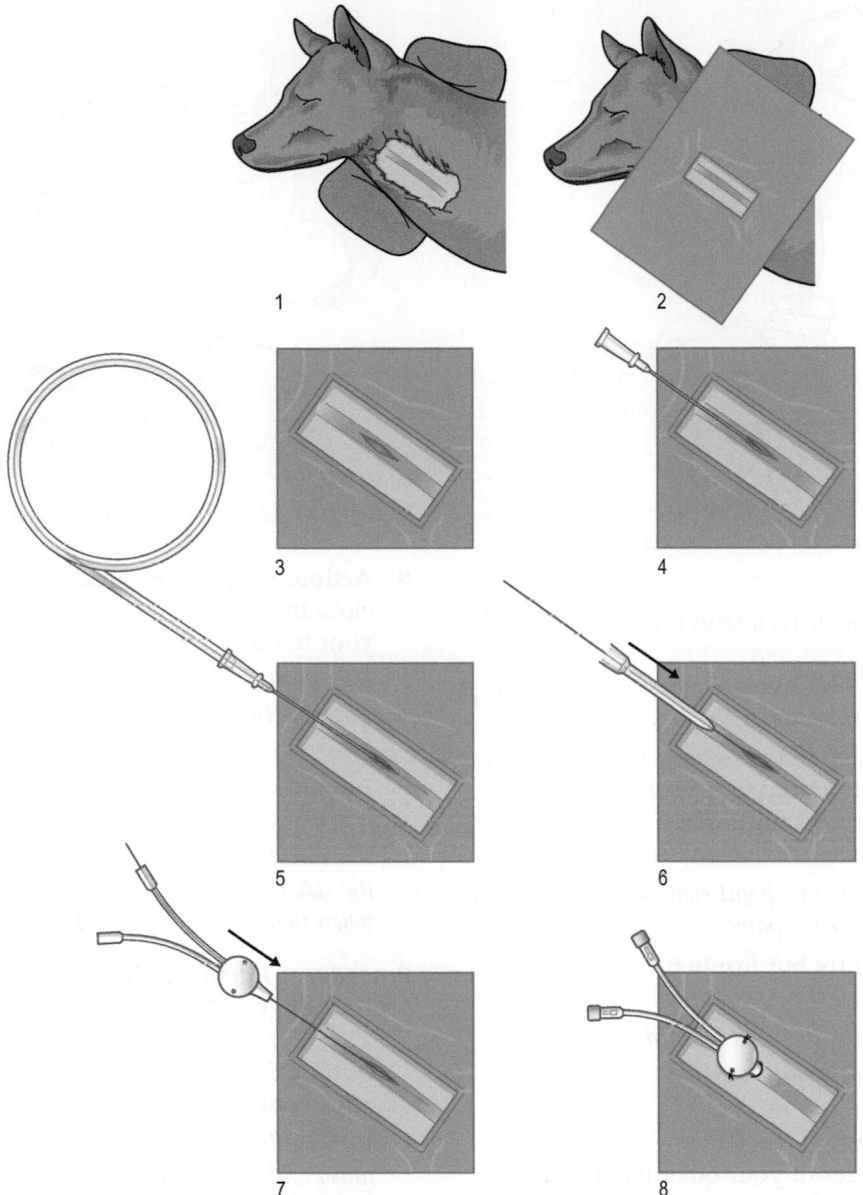

Figure 1.14 Steps involved in the modified Seldinger method of placing a catheter in the jugular vein. (Reproduced with permission from Nick Bexfield and Karla Lee: BSAVA Guide to Procedures in Small Animal Practice 2010, figs e-f, originally illustrated by Samantha J Elmhurst.)

CATS

Procedure: Administering a tablet

Assistance may be required, but it is perfectly possible to do this single-handedly providing that the cat is docile (Fig. 1.15).

1. **Action:** Place the cat in a sitting position on a stable examination table covered in a non-slip mat.

   Rationale: If the cat feels secure it will be less inclined to try and escape.

2. **Action:** If you have an assistant (often the client) ask him / her to hold the cat's forelimbs.

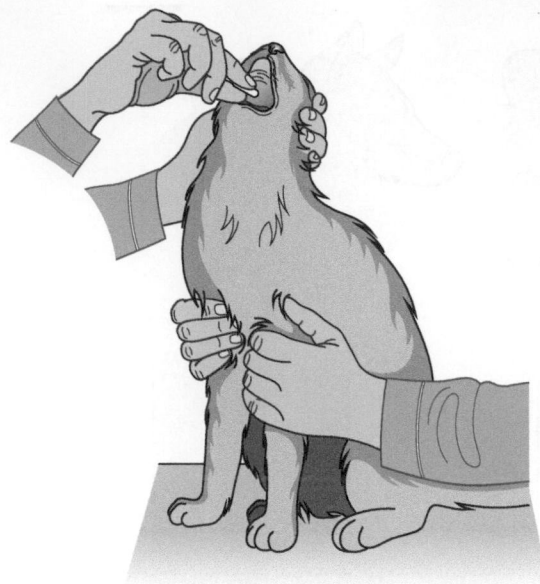

Figure 1.15 Administering a tablet to a cat.

Rationale: This prevents the cat from bringing its forelimbs up to scratch you.

3. **Action:** Grasp the cat's head by placing one hand over the head and your thumb and forefinger at the angle of the jaw, applying gentle pressure to the angle of the jaw.

   Rationale: At this point some unrestrained cats may raise their forepaws.

4. **Action:** Gently but firmly tilt the head backwards.

   Rationale: As the head is tilted the jaw will naturally relax and the mouth should be easier to open.

5. **Action:** Hold the tablet between the thumb and forefinger of your other hand.

6. **Action:** Use your second and third fingers to apply gentle downward pressure to the cat's lower jaw.

   Rationale: At the first attempt the jaws should open easily. At later attempts the cat may clench its jaws tightly making the procedure more difficult – an experience often reported by clients!

7. **Action:** As the jaw opens, place or drop the tablet on to the back of the tongue.

   Rationale: If the tablet is placed as far back as possible, the swallowing reflex will be induced.

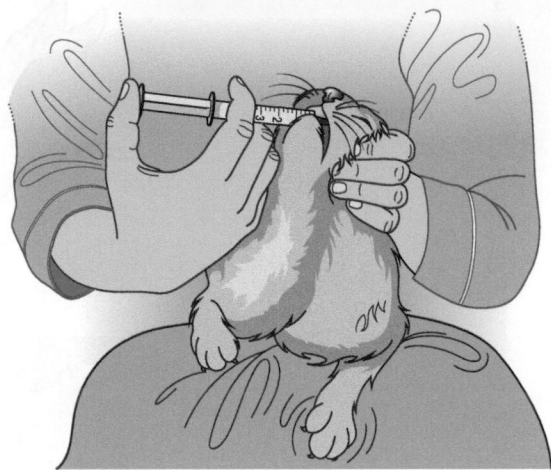

Figure 1.16 Administering liquid feed or medication.

8. **Action:** Keeping the head tilted vertically, close the mouth and hold it closed with your hand.

   Rationale: It is important to hold the mouth closed as this prevents the cat from spitting the tablet out.

9. **Action:** Gently stroke the throat until the cat is seen to swallow.

   Rationale: Some cats learn to hold the tablet in the side of their cheeks until the head is released when they then spit the tablet out!

Procedure: Administering liquid medication or oral fluids (Fig. 1.16)

1. **Action:** Sit on a chair with a towel or other absorbent material over your knees.

   Rationale: This procedure can be messy and the towel will absorb any spilt liquid.

2. **Action:** Take the cat on to your knee with its head pointing away from you.

   Rationale: In this position the cat will be comfortable and easy to restrain.

3. **Action:** Grasp the cat's head with one hand, with your thumb and forefinger at the angle of the jaw, and slightly tilt the head to one side.

   Rationale: If the cat raises its forepaws ask an assistant to hold them down or wrap them in the towel.

4. **Action:** Open the mouth slightly, creating a pocket at the angle of the jaw.

   Rationale: This pocket holds the liquid as it runs into the main part of the oral cavity.

5. **Action:** Using your other hand and a small syringe filled with the liquid, gently insert the end of the barrel into the mouth at the angle of the jaw.

   Rationale: Be as gentle as possible – rough handling can easily damage the mouth.

6. **Action:** Slowly depress the plunger so that the liquid trickles into the mouth.

   Rationale: If you depress the plunger too quickly the liquid may squirt out over you and the cat.

7. **Action:** Continue until the syringe is empty, refilling if necessary.

8. **Action:** When the procedure is complete, clean the cat's mouth, paws and any other parts which that are wet or covered in liquid.

   Rationale: Never leave the cat covered in liquid as it will become wet and cold and may attract flies.

Procedure: Applying ear medication

1. **Action:** Place the cat in a sitting position on a stable examination table covered in a non-slip mat.

   Rationale: If the cat feels secure it will be less inclined to try and escape.

2. **Action:** Ask your assistant to stand to one side of the cat and place his / her hands on either side of the cat bringing them forward to restrain the forelegs on the table.

   Rationale: Cats used to being handled prefer minimal restraint. This procedure does not usually cause too much discomfort and the cat is unlikely to struggle. However, if struggling does occur your assistant should hold the scruff with one hand and use the other to restrain the forelegs.

3. **Action:** Stand in front of the cat and take hold of the ear pinna on the side to be treated, with the finger and thumb of one hand.

   Rationale: In this position you can gain maximum access to the ear.

4. **Action:** Gently twist the head so that it faces upwards.

   Rationale: This brings the ear uppermost so that any medication runs down the ear canal by gravity. It also helps to restrain the head.

5. **Action:** Using the reverse position, apply medication to the other ear.

Procedure: Applying eye medication

1. **Action:** Place the cat in a sitting position on a stable examination table covered in a non-slip mat.

   Rationale: If the cat feels secure it will be less inclined to try and escape.

2. **Action:** Ask your assistant to place one hand on either side of the cat's rump.

   Rationale: This prevents the cat moving backwards and slipping off the table.

3. **Action:** Stand in front of the cat and take the cat's head in one hand, placing your thumb over the cranium and your fingers under the cat's chin. The affected eye should be on the far side of the head away from the palm of your hand.

   Rationale: In this position the head is held still, reducing the risk of damage to the eye. If the cat struggles the nozzle of the tube may penetrate the eye.

4. **Action:** Gently stretch the skin around the affected eye with the forefinger and thumb of this hand.

   Rationale: This will open the eyelids, allowing examination of the eye and the conjunctiva.

5. **Action:** Using your other hand, apply the medication around the edges of the conjunctiva.

   Rationale: If your hands are too rough you may cause damage to the delicate conjunctiva.

6. **Action:** Relax your thumb and forefinger so that the stretched tissues return to normal.

   Rationale: This enables the eyelids to close.

7. **Action:** Gently close the eyelids over the medication.

Rationale: This allows the drops or ointment to spread around the external tissues of the eye and the eyelids.

8. **Action:** It is important to maintain control of the forepaws for a short time to prevent the cat from clawing at the eye or rubbing its head on the table.

   Rationale: After a few minutes the ointment will have dissipated and the cat should feel no discomfort.

Procedure: Administering a subcutaneous injection. Site: Scruff of the neck

1. **Action:** Place the cat in sternal recumbency on a stable examination table covered in a non-slip mat.

   Rationale: If the cat feels secure it will be less inclined to escape.

2. **Action:** Grasp the scruff of the neck firmly with one hand.

   Rationale: This gives control of the head and the cat is unable to turn and bite. It also tents the skin ready for the injection.

3. **Action:** Make sure that your syringe is already filled and that a suitable-sized needle is attached.

   Rationale: To complete this procedure quickly and efficiently you must have your equipment prepared and ready to hand.

4. **Action:** Using your other hand, introduce the point of the needle, bevel-side uppermost, into the raised skin of the scruff.

   Rationale: Having the needle bevel-side uppermost makes it easier to push through the skin. Make sure that you do not push the needle right through the two layers of skin and squirt the contents out on to the cat or the client!

5. **Action:** Inject the contents into the subcuticular space and withdraw the needle.

   Rationale: If you wish, you may draw back on the syringe before injecting to check that you have not penetrated a small blood vessel but the blood supply to the area is relatively poor and the risk is low.

6. **Action:** Gently massage the site of the injection.

   Rationale: To disperse the drug. Absorption from this site takes about 30–45 minutes.

NB Most cats will not object to this procedure and it can usually be performed single-handedly, provided that you give the injection quickly. However, some cats may resent it and you may need the help of an assistant.

Procedure: Administering an intramuscular injection. Site: Quadriceps femoris muscle

1. **Action:** Place the cat on a stable examination table covered in a non-slip mat.

   Rationale: If the cat feels secure it will be less inclined to escape.

2. **Action:** Ask your assistant to stand to one side of the cat and follow step 3.

   Rationale: You should not perform this technique on your own as you could damage the muscle tissues if the cat moves.

3. **Action:** Restrain the head by grasping the scruff of the neck.

   Rationale: The head must be held tightly as this potentially painful procedure could cause the cat to bite.

4. **Action:** Make sure that a syringe is already filled and that a suitable-sized needle is attached.

   Rationale: To complete this procedure quickly and efficiently, you must have your equipment prepared and ready to hand.

5. **Action:** You, the veterinary surgeon, should take the nearest hindleg and locate the quadriceps group of muscles lying on the cranial aspect of the femur.

   Rationale: The quadriceps group is a large muscle mass that provides easy access for injection. The hamstring group and the gluteals may be used but there is a risk of bone and sciatic nerve damage.

6. **Action:** Fix the muscles between the thumb and forefingers of the hand closest to the

caudal end of the cat by encircling the top of the cat's thigh with that hand.

Rationale: This prevents the muscle mass moving as you insert the needle.

7. **Action:** Using the other hand introduce the needle, bevel-side uppermost, through the skin and the muscle mass in a direction running towards the femur and almost at right angles to the lateral aspect of the thigh.

    Rationale: At this angle the needle is unlikely to penetrate any major blood vessel or nerve.

8. **Action:** Draw back slightly on the plunger and look for blood in the hub of the syringe.

    Rationale: To ensure that you have not penetrated a blood vessel. Muscle tissue has a good blood supply and there is a risk of vascular penetration.

9. **Action:** If there is no blood in the syringe, inject the contents slowly.

    Rationale: Muscle tissue is very dense and rapid injections of any volume of fluid may be very painful. Avoid giving any more than 2 ml at a time.

10. **Action:** Withdraw the needle and massage the site gently.

Rationale: Gentle massage will help to disperse the drug into the blood stream. Absorption from the area usually takes about 20–30 minutes.

NB It is possible to use other muscle masses for intramuscular injections. The choice may be largely due to personal preference and the ability to restrain the cat appropriately.

Other muscles used include:

- Lumbar – approximately midway between the last rib and the wing of the ilium
- Hamstring group (semimembranosus / semitendinosus) – located on the caudal aspect of the hindlimb; insert the needle caudal to the femur and direct the tip caudally to avoid damaging the sciatic nerve, which runs along the line of and caudal to the femur
- Triceps – runs on the caudal aspect of the humerus; direct the needle caudally away from the humerus.

Procedure: Administering an intravenous injection. Site: Cephalic vein (Fig. 1.17)

(Assume that the skin has been clipped and cleaned with a swab soaked in spirit prior to the procedure.) The cephalic vein is the most common site for venepuncture and runs down the dorsal aspect of the lower forelimb.

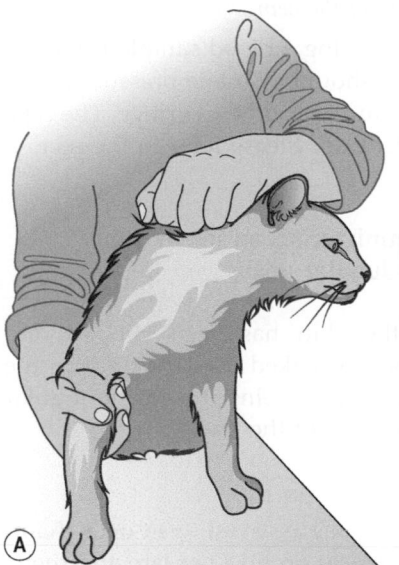
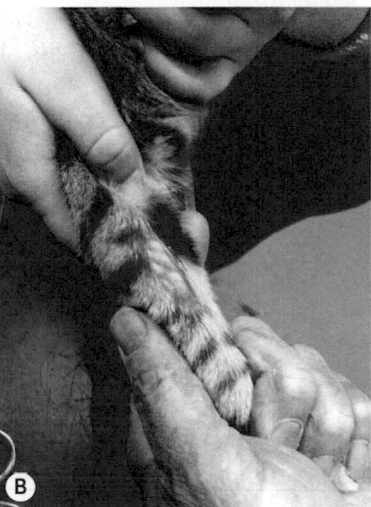
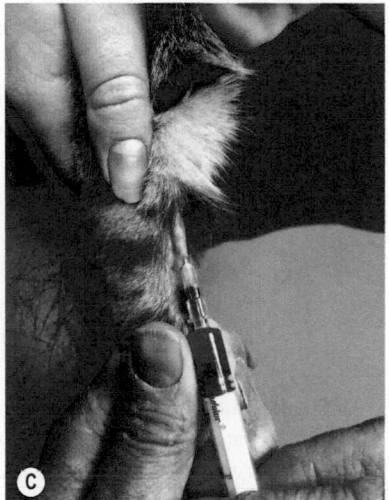

Figure 1.17 Restraining a cat for an intravenous injection using the cephalic vein.

1. **Action:** Place the cat in sternal recumbency or in a sitting position on a stable examination table covered in a non-slip mat.

   Rationale: *If the cat feels secure it will be less inclined to escape.*

2. **Action:** Ask your assistant to take a firm grasp of the cat's scruff with one hand and face it towards you and then follow steps 3–7.

   Rationale: *It is vital that the cat is held firmly as sudden movement may cause to injury to the patient, to the assistant or to you.*

3. **Action:** Your assistant should hold the cat's body close using his / her forearm and elbow of this same arm.

   Rationale: *Extra control can be achieved by changing the pressure exerted by the elbow.*

4. **Action:** Using the other hand, extend a foreleg towards the vet.

5. **Action:** Support the cat's elbow in the palm of your upturned hand and place your thumb across the crook of the elbow.

   Rationale: *Your hand can rest on the table, ensuring that the foreleg is supported and held firmly.*

6. **Action:** Apply pressure with your thumb and rotate your hand slightly outwards.

   Rationale: *This pressure acts as a tourniquet trapping blood as it flows up the forelimb and resulting in dilation of the vein – known as 'raising the vein'.*

7. **Action:** Maintain the pressure while the needle is inserted into the vein (Fig. 1.17).

   Rationale: *The cephalic vein should be clearly visible under the skin running down the dorsal aspect of the lower forelimb.*

8. **Action:** You, the veterinary surgeon, should make sure that your syringe is filled and that you have attached a suitable gauge and length of needle.

   Rationale: *The syringe should be of a size to hold the appropriate volume of drug, but not too large as this will make it difficult to control. Gauge of needle depends on the thickness of the drug and the species of animal – usually 23G is suitable for cats. The most common length is ⅝ inch (16 mm).*

9. **Action:** Insert the needle through the skin and into the cephalic vein, bevel-side uppermost.

   Rationale: *Inserting the needle bevel-side uppermost makes it easier to penetrate the wall of the blood vessel.*

10. **Action:** Draw back on the plunger of the syringe to check that you have penetrated the vein.

    Rationale: *If the vein has been correctly penetrated a small amount of blood will appear in the syringe. Perivascular injection may lead to tissue damage. Do NOT continue with the injection if you are not in the vein.*

11. **Action:** If you are certain that the needle is in the vein, ask your assistant to raise his / her thumb a little and slowly inject the contents of the syringe into the vein.

    Rationale: *Releasing the pressure allows the drug to flow into the vein.*

12. **Action:** When the procedure is complete, withdraw the needle slowly and apply gentle pressure to the entry point with a swab or small piece of cotton wool for about 30 seconds.

    Rationale: *This prevents haemorrhaging into the area around the vein.*

NB If you are collecting a blood sample from this site your assistant should maintain pressure on the vein while you draw back on the syringe. The type of restraint is identical. Please refer to the section on Dogs above.

Procedure: Administering an intravenous injection. Site: Jugular vein

(Assume that the skin has been clipped and cleaned with a swab soaked in spirit prior to the procedure.) The jugular veins run in the jugular furrows on either side of the trachea.

Method 1 (Fig. 1.18)

1. **Action:** Ask your assistant to sit on a chair and place the cat on his / her lap, and then follow steps 2 and 3.

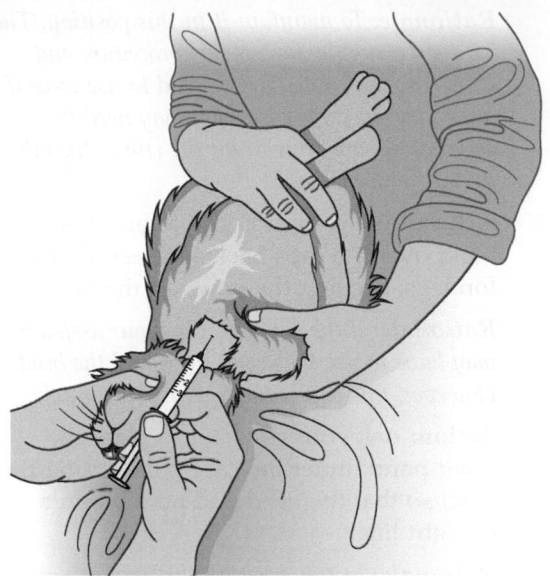

Figure 1.18 Restraint for an intravenous injection using the jugular vein (method 1).

Rationale: This ensures that the assistant is comfortable and enables the cat to be restrained more effectively.

2.   **Action:** Turn the cat over to lie in dorsal recumbency with its head directed towards the vet.

Rationale: In this position there is easy access to the ventral part of the neck. If the cat feels secure and comfortable it will be less likely to struggle.

3.   **Action:** Take all four legs in one hand.

Rationale: Control of the legs prevents scratching.

4.   **Action:** You, the veterinary surgeon, should extend the head with one hand, placing the thumb under the chin and cupping the cranium in the palm of the hand.

Rationale: Extending the head and neck stretches out the jugular as it runs beside the trachea and tenses the overlying skin, making it easier to penetrate the vein with the needle.

5.   **Action:** Ask your assistant to place his / her thumb of the hand not controlling the legs at the base of the jugular furrow, at the point where the trachea enters the thoracic cavity, and apply gentle pressure.

Rationale: The jugular vein on each side of the trachea runs in the jugular furrow and collects venous blood from the head, carrying it towards the heart. Applying pressure will prevent the flow of blood towards the heart causing the vein to dilate – known as 'raising the vein'.

6.   **Action:** Make sure that your syringe is filled and that you have attached a suitable gauge and length of needle.

Rationale: The syringe should be of a size to hold the appropriate volume of drug, but not too large as this will make it difficult to control. Gauge of needle depends on the thickness of the drug and the species of animal – usually 23G is suitable for cats. The most common length is ⅝ inch.

7.   **Action:** Your assistant should maintain the pressure on the vein while you insert the needle through the skin and into the underlying vein, bevel-side uppermost.

Rationale: The jugular vein should be clearly visible under the skin. Positioning the needle with the bevel-side uppermost makes it easier to insert through the skin and wall of the blood vessel.

8.   **Action:** Draw back on the plunger of the syringe to check that you have penetrated the vein.

Rationale: If the vein has been correctly penetrated a small amount of blood will appear in the syringe. Perivascular injection may lead to tissue damage. Do NOT continue with the injection if you are not in the vein.

9.   **Action:** If you are certain that the needle is in the vein, ask your assistant to release the pressure on the vein and slowly inject the drug.

Rationale: Releasing the pressure allows the drug to flow into the vein and around the circulation.

10. **Action:** When the procedure is complete, withdraw the needle slowly and apply gentle pressure to the entry point with a swab or small piece of cotton wool for about 30 seconds.

Rationale: This prevents haemorrhage into the area around the vein.

NB Jugular puncture can also be used for collecting a blood sample and may be a better site than the cephalic vein for collecting large volumes. If a blood sample is to be collected, maintain pressure on the vein until there is enough blood in the syringe.

Method 2 (Fig. 1.19)

1. **Action:** Place the cat in a sitting position on a stable examination table covered in a non-slip mat.

    Rationale: This ensures that the assistant is comfortable and enables the cat to be restrained more effectively.

2. **Action:** It may be necessary to ask another assistant to place a hand on either side of the cat's rump.

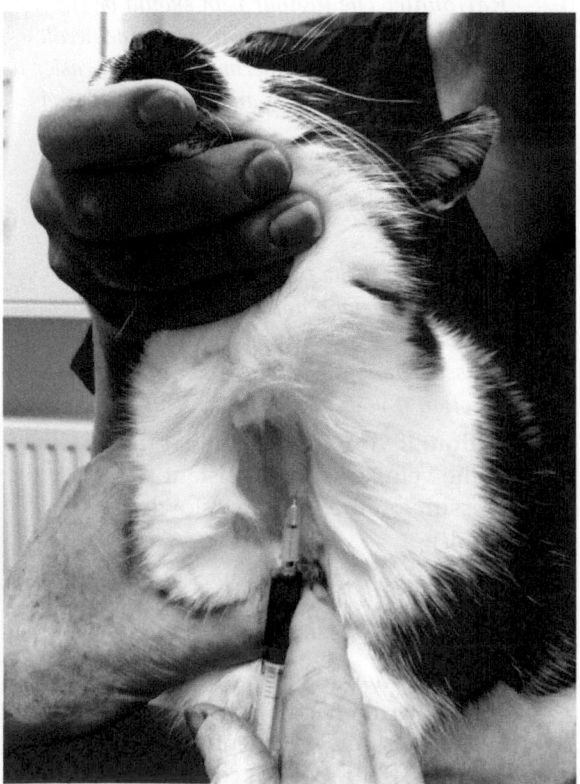

Figure 1.19 Raising the jugular vein of a cat by placing the thumb in the jugular furrow (method 2). The vein is clearly visible and is useful for collecting a blood sample.

Rationale: To maintain it in this position. The cat may struggle during this procedure and your assistant must be prepared to use force if necessary. In some cases you may need two assistants – one to restrain the rump, the other to deal with the head.

3. **Action:** Ask your assistant to bring one hand over the cat's back and restrain the forelegs, keeping the paws on the table.

    Rationale: If the cat struggles your assistant may have to use the scruff to extend the head. However, this leaves the legs free to scratch.

4. **Action:** Ask your assistant to place the other hand under the cat's chin raising the head so that the head and neck are in a straight line.

    Rationale: In this position the jugular vein and overlying skin are tensed making it easier to penetrate the vein with the needle.

5. **Action:** Make sure that your syringe is filled and that you have attached a suitable gauge and length of needle.

    Rationale: The syringe should be of a size to hold the appropriate volume of drug, but not too large as this will make it difficult to control. Gauge of needle depends on the thickness of the drug and the species of animal – usually 23G is suitable for cats. The most common length is ⅝ inch (16 mm).

6. **Action:** You, the veterinary surgeon, should apply pressure at the base of the jugular furrow with the fingers of one hand.

    Rationale: The jugular vein on each side of the trachea runs in the jugular furrow. It collects blood from the head and neck and returns it to the heart. Applying pressure to the base of the furrow causes the vein to distend.

7. **Action:** Using your other hand insert the needle, bevel-side uppermost, through the skin into the underlying vein, continuing to maintain the pressure on the vein.

    Rationale: The jugular vein should be clearly visible under the skin. Positioning the needle with the bevel-side uppermost makes it easier to insert through the skin and wall of the blood vessel.

8. **Action:** Draw back on the syringe.

   Rationale: *Perivascular injection may lead to tissue damage and a check must be made to ensure that the vein has been penetrated before attempting injection.*

9. **Action:** If blood appears at the hub of the needle, release the pressure on the vein and slowly inject the contents of the syringe into the vein.

   Rationale: *Releasing the pressure allows the drug to flow into the circulation.*

10. **Action:** When the procedure is complete, slowly withdraw the needle from the vein.

    Rationale: *This ensures that the vein is not damaged.*

11. **Action:** Apply gentle pressure, with a piece of cotton wool, to the injection site for about 30 seconds.

    Rationale: *This prevents haemorrhaging into the area around the vein.*

NB Jugular puncture can also be used for collecting a blood sample and may be a better site than the cephalic vein for collecting large volumes. If a blood sample is to be collected maintain pressure on the vein until there is enough blood in the syringe (Fig. 1.19).

Procedure: Administering an intravenous injection. Site: Lateral saphenous vein

(Assume that the skin has been clipped and sterilized ready for venepuncture.) The lateral saphenous vein runs over the lateral aspect of the hock.

1. **Action:** Place the cat in lateral recumbency on a stable examination table covered in a non-slip mat.

   Rationale: *The cat will feel secure and comfortable and will be less likely to try and escape.*

2. **Action:** Ask your assistant to grasp the scruff firmly and follow steps 3 and 4.

   Rationale: *The head must be restrained to prevent the cat from wriggling and biting.*

3. **Action:** Using the other hand, extend the cat's uppermost hindleg, at the same time stretching out the body.

   Rationale: *If the cat struggles or is aggressive, it may be necessary to exert extra control by wrapping the cat in a towel with the head out. The hindleg can be extended from the towel.*

4. **Action:** Place your hand around the lower leg at the level of the mid tibia / fibula and apply gentle pressure.

   Rationale: *The lateral saphenous vein collects blood from the hindpaw and runs superficially on the caudal aspect of the hock and distal tibia. Pressure applied around the distal tibia acts as a tourniquet, trapping venous blood as it returns to the heart and causing the vein to dilate – known as 'raising the vein'.*

5. **Action:** Make sure that your syringe is filled and that you have attached a suitable gauge and length of needle.

   Rationale: *The syringe should be of a size to hold the appropriate volume of drug, but not too large as this will make it difficult to control. Gauge of needle depends on the thickness of the drug and the species of animal – usually 23G is suitable for cats. The most common length is ⅝ inch (16 mm).*

6. **Action:** Your assistant should maintain the pressure on the vein while you, the veterinary surgeon, insert the needle, bevel-side uppermost, through the skin and into the underlying saphenous vein.

   Rationale: *The saphenous vein should be clearly visible lying just under the skin.*

7. **Action:** Draw back on the syringe.

   Rationale: *Perivascular injection may lead to tissue damage and a check must be made to ensure that the vein has been penetrated before attempting injection.*

8. **Action:** If blood appears at the hub of the needle, release the pressure on the vein and slowly inject the contents of the syringe into the vein.

   Rationale: *Releasing the pressure allows the drug to flow into the circulation.*

9. **Action:** When the procedure is complete, slowly withdraw the needle from the vein.

   Rationale: This ensures that the vein is not damaged.

10. **Action:** Apply gentle pressure with a piece of cotton wool, to the injection site for about 30 seconds.

    Rationale: This prevents haemorrhaging into the area around the vein.

NB The saphenous vein can also be used for collecting a blood sample; however, as the vein is quite small it is better to collect a large sample from another site such as the jugular vein. If a blood sample is to be collected, maintain pressure on the vein until there is enough blood in the syringe.

For the placement of intravenous catheters, please see the instructions for the dog and use the appropriate methods of cat restraint.

RABBITS

Most rabbits are easy to handle and rarely cause injury unless they are incorrectly or roughly handled. They are capable of using their teeth and their claws, and their back legs are extremely powerful and can inflict deep scratches.

Procedure: Administering fluids or liquid medication

1. **Action:** Place the rabbit in sternal recumbency on a stable examination table and wrap it in a towel as previously described.

   Rationale: By doing this, the legs are restrained but the head is exposed.

2. **Action:** You may need an assistant to hold the rabbit gently, but if the rabbit is docile you can do this single-handedly.

   Rationale: To prevent it leaping off the table.

3. **Action:** Take the head in one hand and tilt it slightly to one side.

   Rationale: In this position one corner of the mouth is uppermost.

4. **Action:** Using a syringe of an appropriate size filled with the liquid, place the nozzle into the uppermost corner of the mouth.

   Rationale: Do not use a large syringe as this can be difficult to control.

5. **Action:** Apply gentle pressure to the syringe and dispense the fluid into the mouth. Allow time for the rabbit to swallow.

   Rationale: Give fluid in boluses of 0.25–0.50 ml. If you give the fluid too quickly the rabbit may choke or the fluid may flow out of its mouth.

Procedure: Administering a subcutaneous injection. Site: Scruff of the neck

1. **Action:** Place the rabbit in sternal recumbency on a stable examination table covered in a non-slip mat.

   Rationale: If the rabbit feels secure it will be less likely to struggle and try to escape. You can use minimal restraint, but the animal must not be allowed to leap off the table and injure itself.

2. **Action:** Make sure that your syringe is filled and that you have attached a suitable gauge and length of needle.

   Rationale: The syringe should be of a size to hold the appropriate volume of drug, but not too large as this will make it difficult to control. Gauge of needle depends on the thickness of the drug and the species of animal – usually 21G or 23G is suitable for rabbits. The most common length is ⅝ inch (16 mm).

3. **Action:** Grasp the scruff of the neck with one hand.

   Rationale: The scruff of a rabbit is usually quite large and the site can be used to administer relatively large volumes.

4. **Action:** Using the other hand, introduce the point of the needle, bevel-side uppermost, into the raised skin of the scruff.

   Rationale: Having the bevel-side uppermost makes it easier to push through the skin. Make sure that you do not push the needle right through the two layers of skin and squirt the contents out onto the rabbit or the client!

5. **Action:** Inject the contents into the subcuticular space and withdraw the needle.

   Rationale: If you wish, you may draw back on the syringe before injecting to check that you have not penetrated a small blood vessel, but the blood supply to the area is relatively poor and the risk is low.

6. **Action:** Gently massage the site of the injection.

   Rationale: To disperse the drug. Absorption from this site takes about 30–45 minutes.

NB Most rabbits will not object to this procedure and it can usually be performed single-handedly, provided that you give the injection quickly.

Procedure: Administering an intramuscular injection. Site: Quadriceps femoris muscle

1. **Action:** Place the rabbit in sternal recumbency on a stable examination table covered in a non-slip mat.

   Rationale: If the rabbit feels secure it will be less likely to struggle and try to escape.

2. **Action:** Make sure that your syringe is filled and that you have attached a suitable gauge and length of needle.

   Rationale: The syringe should be of a size to hold the appropriate volume of drug, but not too large as this will make it difficult to control. Gauge of needle depends on the thickness of the drug and the species of animal – usually 23G is suitable for rabbits. No more than 0.5–1.00 ml can be given by this route. Large volumes will cause great pain and damage to the muscle tissue.

3. **Action:** Ask your assistant to restrain the rabbit by holding the scruff and then extend one of the hindlimbs.

   Rationale: In this position the rabbit is restrained and there is easy access to the muscle group.

4. **Action:** Hold the quadriceps muscle between the finger and thumb of one hand and introduce the needle, bevel-side uppermost, into the muscle with the other hand.

   Rationale: The quadriceps femoris muscle runs on the cranial aspect of the femur.

5. **Action:** Draw back slightly on the plunger and look for blood in the hub of the syringe.

   Rationale: To ensure that you have not penetrated a blood vessel. Muscle tissue has a good blood supply and there is a risk of vascular penetration.

6. **Action:** If there is no blood in the syringe, inject the contents slowly.

   Rationale: Muscle tissue is very dense and rapid injections of any volume of fluid may be very painful.

7. **Action:** Withdraw the needle and massage the site gently.

   Rationale: Gentle massage will help to disperse the drug into the blood stream. Absorption from the area usually takes about 20–30 minutes.

NB It is also possible to use the lumbar muscles, which run in a large mass on either side of the lumbar spine. Injection into this area can be done single-handedly if the rabbit is docile.

Procedure: Administering an intravenous injection. Site: Marginal ear vein (Fig. 1.20)

1. **Action:** Place the rabbit in sternal recumbency on a stable examination table covered in a non-slip mat.

   Rationale: If the rabbit feels secure it will be less likely to struggle and try to escape.

2. **Action:** Wrap the rabbit in a towel with the head uncovered as previously described.

   Rationale: This restrains the body while providing easy access to the ear.

3. **Action:** Clip the fur overlying the ear vein on one ear.

   Rationale: The marginal ear vein runs down the lateral side of each ear (Fig. 1.20).

4. **Action:** Clean the site, but avoid the use of spirit.

   Rationale: The vein must be cleaned to avoid the introduction of infection into the vein. Spirit may cause the vein to collapse, making injection and blood sampling more difficult.

5. **Action:** Apply local anaesthetic cream to the area and wait for 10 minutes.

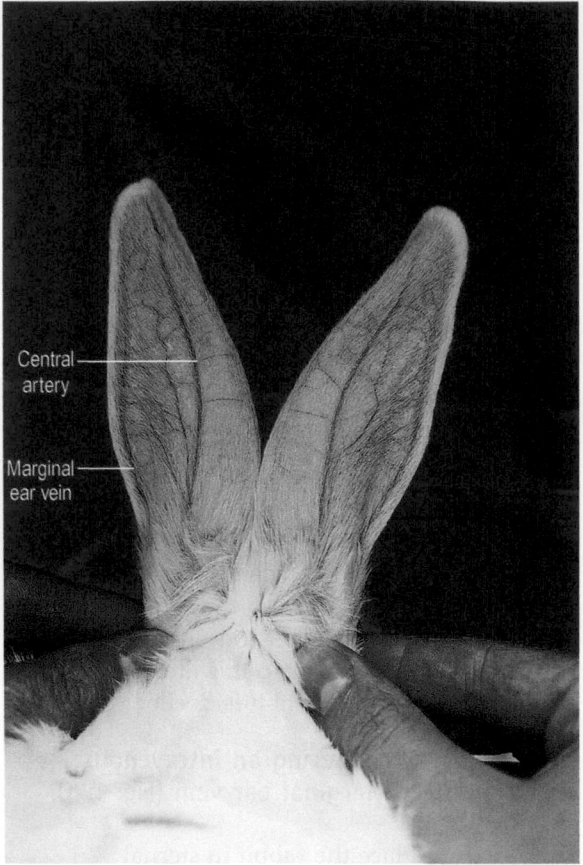

Figure 1.20 The blood vessels within the pinna of the rabbit: the central artery is clearly visible. The marginal ear veins can be used for venepuncture.

Rationale: This desensitizes the area so that the rabbit is less likely to shake its head when the needle is introduced.

6. **Action:** Place a ball of cotton wool soaked in hot water under the ear.

   Rationale: This causes the vein to dilate, making it easier to visualize.

7. **Action:** Ask your assistant to apply pressure to the base of the selected ear and maintain it.

   Rationale: This acts as a tourniquet preventing blood returning from the ear tissue to the heart. The vein will dilate and become more visible.

8. **Action:** Make sure that your syringe is filled and that you have attached a suitable gauge and length of needle.

   Rationale: The syringe should be of a size to hold the appropriate volume of drug, but not too large as this will make it difficult to control. Gauge of needle depends on the thickness of the drug and the species of animal – usually 23G is suitable for rabbits.

9. **Action:** Insert the needle bevel-side uppermost through the overlying skin and into the vein, directing it towards the ear tip.

   Rationale: Using the needle in this position makes it easier to penetrate the tissues.

10. **Action:** Draw back on the syringe.

    Rationale: Perivascular injection may lead to tissue damage and a check must be made to ensure that the vein has been penetrated before attempting injection.

11. **Action:** If blood appears at the hub of the needle, ask your assistant to release the pressure on the vein and slowly inject the contents of the syringe into the vein.

    Rationale: Releasing the pressure allows the drug to flow into the circulation.

12. **Action:** When the procedure is complete, slowly withdraw the needle from the vein.

    Rationale: This ensures that the vein is not damaged.

13. **Action:** Apply gentle pressure with a piece of cotton wool to the injection site for about 30 seconds.

    Rationale: This prevents haemorrhage into the area around the vein.

NB The marginal ear vein could be used to collect a blood sample; larger volumes can be collected from other veins. If repeated injections are to be given through this vein, use an intravenous or butterfly catheter attached firmly to the ear with superglue or sticky tape.

Other sites can be used for venepuncture in the rabbit:

Cephalic vein – restrain the rabbit in a similar way to the cat

Lateral saphenous vein – be careful with restraint as the hindlegs of a rabbit may be easily broken.

NB Use of the jugular vein is not recommended as rabbits do not like their heads being raised.

Procedure: Administering an intraperitoneal injection. Site: Mid abdomen (Fig. 1.21)

1. **Action:** Place the rabbit in sternal recumbency on a stable examination table covered in a non-slip mat.

   Rationale: If the rabbit feels secure it will be less likely to struggle and try to escape.

2. **Action:** Ask your assistant to grasp the scruff of the rabbit with one hand and the hindlegs with the other, and then follow step 3.

   Rationale: The rabbit must be held firmly to prevent it struggling during the procedure.

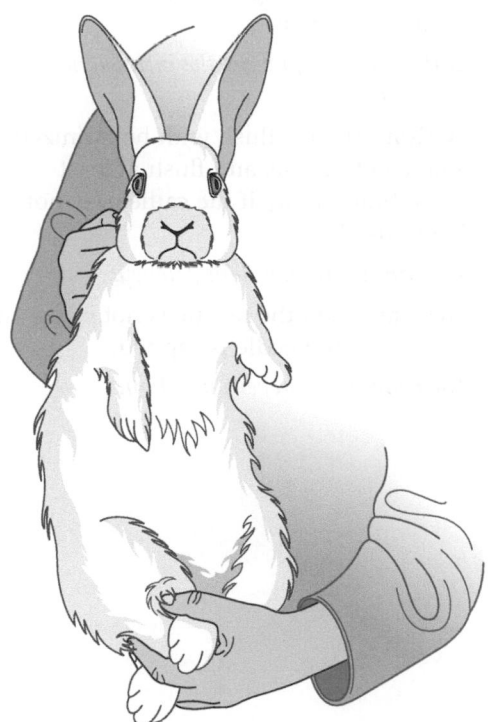

Figure 1.21 Restraining a rabbit for an intraperitoneal injection.

3. **Action:** Pick up the rabbit and hold it in dorsal recumbency with its spine against your chest.

   Rationale: This position exposes the ventral part of the abdomen for injection, but care must be taken with dyspnoeic patients.

4. **Action:** You, the veterinary surgeon, should make sure that your syringe is filled and that you have attached a suitable gauge and length of needle.

   Rationale: The syringe should be of a size to hold the appropriate volume of drug, but not too large as this will make it difficult to control. Gauge of needle depends on the thickness of the drug and the species of animal – usually 23G is suitable for rabbits. For this procedure you should use a short needle to avoid penetration of any of the viscera.

5. **Action:** You should introduce your needle bevel-side uppermost at a point midway between the xiphisternum and the pubis.

   Rationale: This position should avoid accidental penetration of the bladder or stomach. Rabbit skin is thin and a short needle easily penetrates the abdominal wall.

6. **Action:** Draw back on the syringe and examine the contents.

   Rationale: If blood, urine or gut contents appear, reposition the needle and try again. If nothing appears in the syringe, it is safe to proceed with the injection.

7. **Action:** If there is nothing in the syringe, gently inject the contents of the syringe.

   Rationale: Up to 50 ml of fluid can be given by this route.

8. **Action:** When the procedure is complete withdraw the needle.

NB This technique can be also used to collect samples of fluid from the peritoneal cavity and samples of urine from the bladder.

Procedure: Placing an intraosseus catheter

This technique is often used to provide fluid to a range of exotic species and is useful if the veins are damaged or are fragile. It is also used in the critical care of cats and dogs. The advantage is that absorption of fluids can be rapid and, if the needle is dislodged, haemorrhaging from the site is unlikely to occur. The disadvantages are infection, fat emboli and damage to the growth plates of the bone.

The patient should be heavily sedated or under a general anaesthetic as the procedure is very painful.

1. **Action:** Select a suitable site.

    Rationale: In the rabbit the proximal femur and the proximal tibia provide easy access and a medullary cavity from which fluid can be easily absorbed.

2. **Action:** Prepare the site aseptically.

    Rationale: To prevent the introduction of bacteria that would cause severe osteomyelitis.

3. **Action:** Infiltrate the area with local anaesthetic.

    Rationale: To desensitize the tissues.

4. **Action:** Select a spinal needle or 20–21G needle and insert into the bone using a screwing action.

    Rationale: The needle must be of an appropriate size to enter the medullary cavity. This can be assessed by radiography or previous experience.

5. **Action:** Flush the needle with heparinized saline.

    Rationale: This will ensure that the needle is patent as it may become blocked with tissue fragments.

6. **Action:** Fix the needle in place with tissue glue or by suturing.

    Rationale: It is important that the needle does not become dislodged.

7. **Action:** Apply antibiotic cream around the base of the needle.

    Rationale: To prevent infection.

8. **Action:** Attach a short length of tubing and a syringe or attach a fluid giving set to the needle.

    Rationale: This procedure may be used to give a bolus of fluid or a slow infusion. Absorption from this site is as rapid as the intravenous route.

9. **Action:** If the needle is to be left in situ, bandage the area.

    Rationale: To prevent the risk of infection, to reduce limb mobility and to prevent patient interference.

10. **Action:** If necessary use an Elizabethan collar.

    Rationale: To prevent patient interference. Intraosseus catheters are usually well tolerated.

11. **Action:** When giving further fluids or medication through the needle it is vital to maintain asepsis.

    Rationale: To prevent the introduction of infection.

12. **Action:** Always flush with heparinized saline before use, and flush at least three times a day if the catheter is not being used.

    Rationale: To maintain patency.

13. **Action:** When the needle is not in use make sure that the needle is capped.

    Rationale: To prevent infection.

CHAPTER 2

Basic consulting room techniques

The first time you find yourself alone in the consulting room with worried clients and their beloved animal can be terrifying. Knowing that you know how to do all the most common and most basic procedures that are likely to be presented will give you confidence. Appearing confident and competent in front of the client is the art of veterinary medicine as opposed to the science of veterinary medicine. If you are confident, the client will trust you and the animal will also respond positively.

Procedure: Basic clinical examination

When carrying out a clinical examination you must develop a logical, methodical, systematic approach and always stick to it. Always remember that 'common things are common' – the dog that walks into the surgery salivating is probably suffering from car sickness or dental problems not rabies!

Remember that your consultation should take about 10 minutes (depends on practice protocols) so time is of the essence – you have a lot to achieve in a short time!

1. **History** – This must be taken early on in the consultation process and should be as detailed as possible.

   a. When taking the history, remember to *listen* to the answers. Sometimes your brain is 'talking' to you, especially if you are nervous, and you do not hear what is actually being said to you.

   b. Avoid asking leading questions, that is, those that suggest something to the client; e.g. 'Is your cat drinking a lot?' suggests to the client that it is, even if it is not.

   c. Avoid asking closed questions, that is, those that can only be answered by Yes or No; e.g. 'Is your cat drinking a lot? It is better to ask an open question such as 'How much is your cat drinking?'

   d. Take notes – either directly on to the computer, or use a note pad for later transcription – it may be difficult to write a full history within the allotted time.

The history should include:

- **Client's details** – name, address and telephone number. Some practices may also take the email address. These details may have been taken by the receptionist and will appear on your computer screen in the consulting room. Find out the animal's name and use it! Get the sex of the animal right – if you consistently refer to him rather than to her, this is what the client will pick up on not on whether you have made the diagnosis of the century!

- **Patient details** – species, breed, age, vaccination status, any previous medical history, how long they have had him / her. Weigh the animal – this will be useful for calculating dose rates, but is also a useful measure of health. In any animal on a diet this is a useful measure of progress. All these details may already be on the computer screen in front of you, but checking the facts is a good way of getting into a conversation.

- **Presenting sign** – this is the symptom that has made the client get off the sofa and bring the dog to the surgery. It will be the most obvious sign to them (e.g. the dog is drinking a lot, diarrhoea, vomiting, scratching, etc.) although not necessarily the most significant diagnostically. Ask questions to develop your understanding

of this presenting sign (Box 2.1), then ask questions about other relevant symptoms as you begin to extract the facts and widen your knowledge of the patient, e.g. diet, how much, when was it last wormed or defleaed.

2. **Initial examination** – First stand back and observe. Delay your thorough clinical examination for a short time. As soon as you start to touch the animal you destroy some of the evidence; for example, the heart rate and respiratory rate may rise if the animal is nervous. Observe the animal's behaviour, including such things as the respiratory rate, as it stands on your table. Look at the animal's general demeanour. This may be done at the same time as you are taking the client's details – as you become more experienced you will find that you can multitask!

3. **Clinical examination** – This must be done in a logical order to avoid missing a piece of evidence (Fig 2.1). Develop your own system and follow it every time. For example, you could start by examining all structures on the head, then progress to the trunk, then the legs and finally the perineum; or you could examine the respiratory system, the digestive system, etc.; or you could examine the parts of the animal alphabetically. It does not matter how you do it, but you must develop your own system and stick to it. In this way you should not miss anything significant. Always make notes and record your findings, both normal and abnormal.

   It is a good idea to start with the basic assessment of temperature, pulse and respiration, check the mucous membranes and the palpable lymph nodes (Table 2.1). This provides essential clinical information and extra thinking time. (Note how clients always start to talk when you are listening to the chest!)

Box 2.1 Suggested questions to develop a presenting sign

Suppose the presenting sign is ... 'My dog is drinking a lot'

Ask the client:

- How long has this been going on?
- Has it got worse?
- How much is a lot?
- How often do you have to fill his bowl?
- How big is the bowl?
- Does he drink from puddles and ponds?
- Is he peeing excessively?
- Does he wet the floor at night?
- What does he eat? – a dog fed on a dry diet will naturally drink more than one on tinned food

Suggested format for a clinical examination – in a routine 10-minute consultation you will not be able to complete as much detail as is suggested below. Listen to the history and from this you will get an idea of which area to focus on; for example, if the owner says the dog has diarrhoea then look at the digestive system. However, keep an open mind and do not completely rule out the other systems.

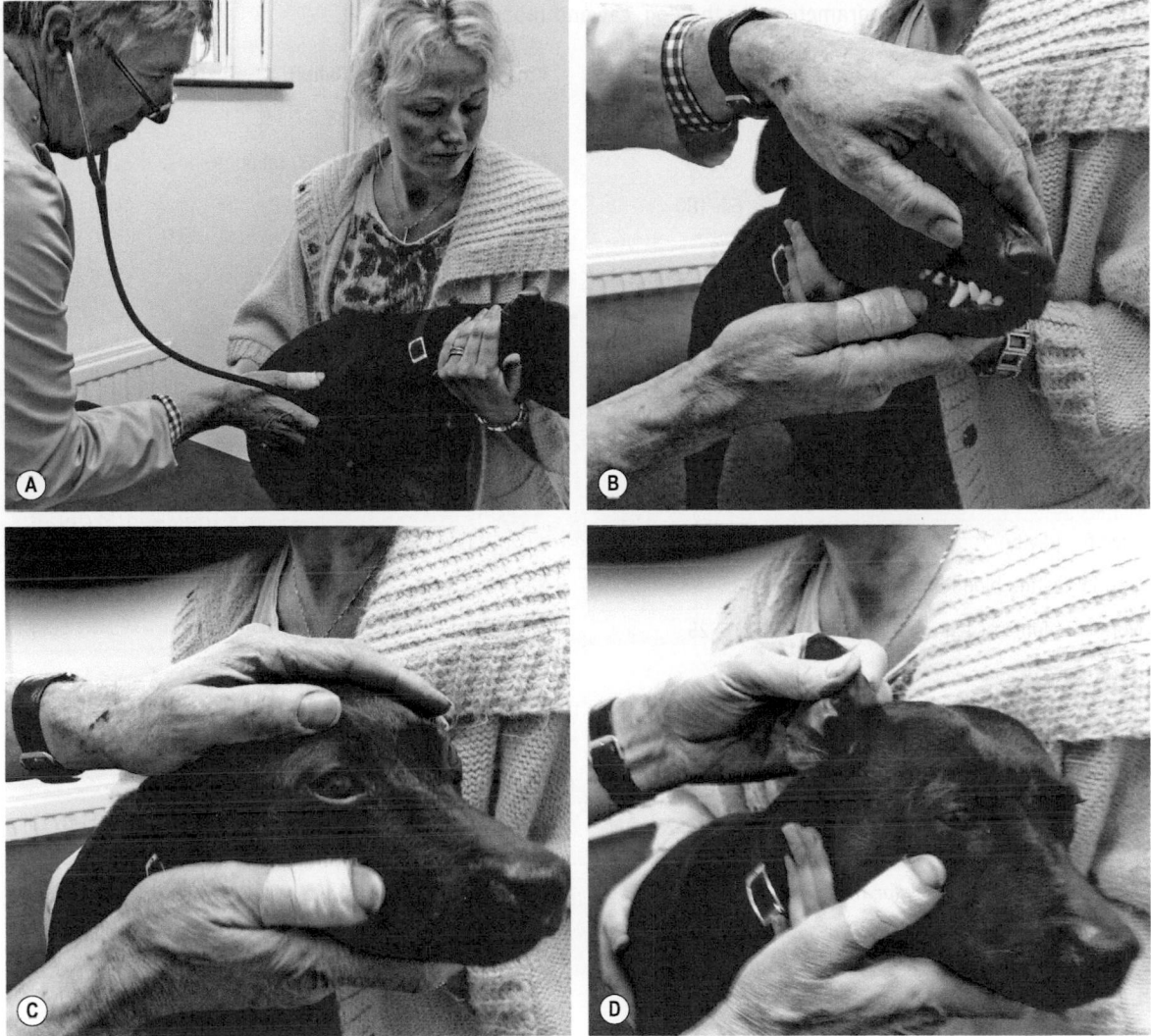

Figure 2.1 Carrying out a routine clinical examination: (A) auscultation of the heart; (B) examining the teeth and gums; (C) checking the eyes; (D) checking the ears.

Examine the following systems making notes about the indicated parameters.

• Palpable lymph nodes – these are indicators of local infection and inflammation:

1. **Action:** Submandibular and parotid.

    Rationale: Around the angle of the jaw and the base of the ear.

2. **Action:** Prescapular.

    Rationale: In front of the shoulder.

3. **Action:** Inguinal.

    Rationale: In the groin.

4. **Action:** Popliteal.

    Rationale: Caudal to the stifle joint within the gastrocnemius muscle.

• Cardiovascular system:

1. **Action:** Auscultate the heart using a stethoscope.

    Rationale: Listen to the rate and rhythm and make a note of any murmurs.

2. **Action:** Feel the pulse – use the femoral artery.

    Rationale: Count the rate for 15 seconds then multiply by 4. Notice the character.

3. **Action:** Check the colour of the mucous membranes.

Table 2.1 Normal clinical parameters for the dog, cat and rabbit*

Clinical parameter	Dog	Cat	Rabbit
Body temperature (°C)	38.3–38.7	38.0–38.5	38.5–39.5
Respiratory rate (b.p.m.)	10–30	20–30	35–60 (obligate nose breathers)
Pulse rate (beats/min)	60–180	110–180	130–325
Capillary refill time (seconds)	1–2	1–2	1–2
Mucous membranes	Salmon pink	Salmon pink	Salmon pink
Normal water intake (ml/kg/day)	50–60	50–60	120
Normal urine volume (ml/kg bodyweight/day)	20–25	20–25	20–350
Urine pH	5–7	5–7	7.6–8.8
Normal urine colour	Yellow and clear	Yellow and clear	Cream – yellow – red – all are normal
Specific gravity	1.016–1.060	1.020–1.040	1.003–1.036
Normal fasting blood glucose (mmol/l)	3.5–5.5	3.5–6.5	6–8.9
Normal volume of tears (ml/day)	15–25	15–25	–

*Taken from a range of sources.

Rationale: Take note of any change from the normal salmon-pink colour.

4. **Action:** Tent the skin.

   Rationale: To check for the level of hydration.

5. **Action:** Feel the extremities.

   Rationale: Note the temperature – are they cold or excessively hot?

6. **Action:** Look for signs of oedema.

   Rationale: Check the paws, legs, ventral abdomen and prepuce.

- Respiratory system:

1. **Action:** Note the respiratory rate.

   Rationale: Identify one area and watch it move over a period of 15 seconds then multiply by 4.

2. **Action:** Auscultate the chest using a stethoscope.

   Rationale: Listen to several areas to locate specific problems.

3. **Action:** Percussion of the chest.

   Rationale: To identify areas of consolidation.

4. **Action:** Check the colour of the mucous membranes.

   Rationale: To check for levels of oxygenation.

5. **Action:** Listen to the patient breathing.

   Rationale: Note whether any noise occurs during inspiration or expiration.

6. **Action:** Note any evidence of dyspnoea.

   Rationale: Inspiration or expiration?

7. **Action:** Elicit a cough.

   Rationale: By gently squeezing the larynx, note the type – dry and hacking or moist and productive.

8. **Action:** Nasal discharge.

   Rationale: Unilateral or bilateral?

9. **Action:** Check lymph nodes around pharyngeal area.

   Rationale: To check for areas of infection.

- Digestive system:

1. **Action:** Note any faeces on thermometer or around the anus.

   Rationale: Look at colour and smell. Note the presence of blood.

2. **Action:** Examine lips, inside of the mouth and teeth.

   Rationale: Check for colour, ulceration, injury and presence of gum or dental disease.

3.   **Action:** Check tongue and smell the breath.

     Rationale: Look for injury, ulceration, etc. A smell of pear drops indicates ketosis; foul smell may indicate gingivitis.

4.   **Action:** Check pharyngeal lymph nodes.

     Rationale: For signs of infection.

5.   **Action:** Check salivary glands.

     Rationale: For signs of mucocoele.

6.   **Action:** Palpate the abdomen.

     Rationale: Take note of any pain, very hard or soft areas, guarding.

7.   **Action:** Observe the patient's stance.

     Rationale: Arched back, praying stance, guarding.

8.   **Action:** Obtain a faecal sample.

     Rationale: Note colour, form and frequency. Faecal egg count will identify worm infestations.

9.   **Action:** Ask owner or obtain a sample of vomit.

     Rationale: Note colour, smell and contents. Note timing in relation to eating.

- Urinary system:

1.   **Action:** Palpate the bladder.

     Rationale: Note whether full or empty; presence of bladder stones.

2.   **Action:** Palpate the kidneys.

     Rationale: Size and consistency; painful or not.

3.   **Action:** Obtain a urine sample.

     Rationale: Carry out a full urinalysis.

- Reproductive system – female:

1.   **Action:** Check vulva.

     Rationale: For patency and injury.

2.   **Action:** Palpate vagina digitally.

     Rationale: To assess patency and potential damage.

3.   **Action:** Examine vagina with a speculum.

     Rationale: To assess mucous membranes for damage.

4.   **Action:** Check mammary glands.

     Rationale: Look for mammary tumours or evidence of false pregnancy.

5.   **Action:** Check inguinal lymph nodes.

     Rationale: For evidence of metastases or infection.

6.   **Action:** Timing and appearance of most recent season.

     Rationale: Only relevant in unspayed bitches or queens.

- Reproductive system – male:

1.   **Action:** Check scrotum and testes.

     Rationale: Only relevant in an uncastrated patient. There should be two testes, which should move freely within the scrotum.

2.   **Action:** Check the penis.

     Rationale: The penis should move easily within the prepuce, with no evidence of infection or trauma.

3.   **Action:** Check the prepuce.

     Rationale: For damage or infection.

4.   **Action:** Prostate gland.

     Rationale: In larger dogs this may just be palpated per rectum.

- Skin and coat:

1.   **Action:** Look at coat quality.

     Rationale: Provides a good indicator of general health.

2.   **Action:** Look for areas of alopecia.

     Rationale: Note the site and whether the areas are symmetrical.

3.   **Action:** Identify whether skin is pruritic.

     Rationale: May indicate parasite infestation.

4.   **Action:** Look for areas of scurf.

     Rationale: May indicate poor nutrition or parasite infestation.

5.   **Action:** Check for even pigmentation.

     Rationale: May indicate hormonal problems.

6.   **Action:** Variation in skin thickness.

     Rationale: May indicate trauma due to scratching or hormonal problems.

7.   **Action:** Check claws.

     Rationale: For length and damage.

- Ears:

1.   **Action:** Check both pinnae.

     Rationale: For damage or infection.

2.   **Action:** Examine external ear canal visually and with an auroscope.

     Rationale: For infection or parasite infestation. Also check for hairs, which may impede aeration. Check for smell.

3.   **Action:** Examine the tympanic membrane.

     Rationale: Using an auroscope. Look for damage due to infection or trauma.

- Eyes – always examine in a darkened room:

1.   **Action:** Note any evidence of photophobia, chemosis, blepharospasm and epiphora.

     Rationale: These clinical signs may indicate eye problems that require further investigation.

2.   **Action:** Check conjunctiva.

     Rationale: Look for inflammation and infection. Slight dullness could indicate 'dry eye'. Look for ulcers – use fluorescein stain.

3. **Action:** Check eyelids – remember to evert them as well.

    Rationale: Look for injury and foreign bodies.

4. **Action:** Check eyeballs.

    Rationale: Look for bruising, haemorrhage.

5. **Action:** Look at both eyes together and compare them.

    Rationale: Both eyes should look the same and function together.

6. **Action:** Check pupil size.

    Rationale: Should be the same.

7. **Action:** Check pupillary light response.

    Rationale: Pupil constricts in response to bright light.

8. **Action:** Check menace reflex.

    Rationale: Eyeball should pull back into orbit in response to a fast approaching object such as a hand.

9. **Action:** Check the lens.

    Rationale: Using an ophthalmoscope – look for evidence of cataracts.

10. **Action:** Check patency of the tear ducts.

    Rationale: Use fluorescein stain.

4. **Formulate a differential diagnosis** – This is based on the history and the clinical examination (Box 2.2). This will give you an idea as to how to proceed with the case.

5. **Treatment** – If you are certain of your diagnosis then you can proceed to the treatment. If you are unable to make a diagnosis then consider further tests which may include:

   a. Laboratory tests – e.g. haematology, blood biochemistry and electrolyte analysis, urinalysis

   b. Diagnostic imaging – e.g. radiology, ultrasonography, endoscopy, CT and MRI scans

   c. Hormonal tests – e.g. ACTH stimulation, dexamethasone suppression, water deprivation test

   d. Surgical exploration.

Finally remember that in some cases you may never reach a diagnosis and in other cases there is no treatment. Many patients recover well on symptomatic treatments such as

analgesics, antidiarrhoeal agents, antimicrobials, antiemetics, fluid therapy and dietary management.

6. **Euthanasia** – In some cases this may be best for the animal and it may be used:

   a. If the condition is going to progress to a painful end (e.g. neoplasia)

   b. To alleviate immediate and severe suffering from which there is unlikely to be recovery

   c. To prevent the spread of an infectious disease (e.g. FeLV), and often used in large animal / herd management

   d. If the cost of the treatment is above that which the client can afford or is willing to pay.

Box 2.2 Formulating a differential diagnosis based on an example of one clinical sign

'My dog is drinking a lot' – polydipsia – the dog is a 9 year old entire bitch who had a season 6 weeks ago. She is a bit lethargic and vomits occasionally. On examination you have found that she has a doughy abdomen and a creamy, smelly vulval discharge.

Prioritise the different clinical signs and formulate a differential diagnosis for each.

e.g. differential diagnosis for polydipsia includes:

- Diabetes mellitus – obtain urine and blood samples to confirm diagnosis. Look for presence of glucose in urine and blood.
- Chronic renal failure – obtain a urine and a blood sample to confirm diagnosis. Do full urinalysis and look at urea and serum creatinine levels.
- Diabetes insipidus – obtain a urine sample. Look at specific gravity and volume. Do a water deprivation test.
- Cushing's disease – obtain a urine and a blood sample. Do a ACTH stimulation test.
- Pyometra – obtain a blood sample and do a white cell count which may be raised although they may be lowered if the white cells are sequestered in the uterus. Use ultrasound on the abdomen.

Repeat for each clinical sign and the point(s) where they overlap will give an indication of the diagnosis.

On the basis of the laboratory findings, the history and your clinical examination this dog has a pyometra.

OTHER PROCEDURES

Procedure: Restraint and administration of all types of injection and blood sampling

See Chapter 1.

Procedure: Administration of tablets, liquids, ear and eye medication

See Chapter 1.

Procedure: Squeezing the anal sacs

Method 1

1. **Action:** Place the dog in a standing position on a stable examination table covered in a non-slip mat.
   Rationale: This position provides the best access to the anal sacs. If the dog feels secure on the table it will be less likely to try and escape.

2. **Action:** Ask the owner or an assistant to restrain the dog's head.
   Rationale: This will prevent the dog from turning around to bite you. It is always preferable for the owner to be bitten rather than you!

3. **Action:** Put on a pair of disposable rubber gloves.
   Rationale: These will protect you from contamination by faeces and by the anal sac discharge.

4. **Action:** Insert a well-lubricated index finger through the anal ring and have a small pad of cottonwool in the palm of your hand (Fig 2.2).
   Rationale: The anal sacs sit inside the anal ring.

5. **Action:** Angle the finger downwards to lie on the inside of the anal ring, while your thumb is on the outside. You should be able to feel the sac between the two.
   Rationale: The anal sacs lie in the 'twenty to four' position within the anal ring. Placing a finger on one side and the thumb on the other side enables you to feel the swollen gland between the two.

6. **Action:** Gently squeeze the anal sac, absorbing the discharge in the cottonwool pad.

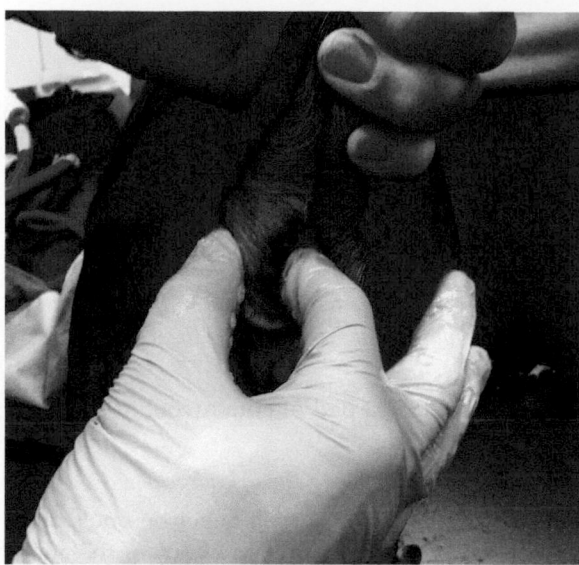

Figure 2.2 Squeezing the anal glands by inserting a gloved finger into the anal ring.

   Rationale: The discharge will be expelled from the sac and come out of through the anal ring. It will have an offensive smell and must be collected in the pad.

7. **Action:** Keeping your finger in the anal ring, angle your hand so that the finger and thumb can pick up the other anal sac.
   Rationale: There are two anal sacs.

8. **Action:** Gently squeeze this sac and collect the discharge.

9. **Action:** Remove your finger from the anal ring and dispose of the gloves and the cottonwool pad in the clinical waste bin.
   Rationale: It is not necessary to show the owner the discharge, but they may want to see it. It also helps to prove that something came out and you have done your job.

Method 2

1. **Action:** Place the dog in a standing position on a stable examination table covered in a non-slip mat.
   Rationale: This position provides the best access to the anal sacs. If the dog feels secure on the table it will be less likely to try and escape.

2. **Action:** Ask the owner or an assistant to restrain the dog's head.

   Rationale: *This will prevent the dog from turning around to bite you. It is always preferable for the owner to be bitten rather than you!*

3. **Action:** Put on a pair of disposable rubber gloves.

   Rationale: *These will protect you from contamination by faeces and by the anal sac discharge.*

4. **Action:** Place a pad of cottonwool in the palm of your hand.

   Rationale: *To absorb the discharge.*

5. **Action:** Place your index finger on one side of the anal ring over the area of one of the anal sacs and your thumb on the other side over the other anal sac.

   Rationale: *There are two anal sacs, lying in the 'twenty to four' position within the tissue of the anal ring.*

6. **Action:** Gently squeeze the anal ring.

   Rationale: *The anal sacs will be under pressure and should discharge their contents.*

7. **Action:** Remove your gloves and dispose of them and the cottonwool pad in the clinical waste bin.

   Rationale: *It is not necessary to show the owner the discharge but they may want to see it. It also helps to prove that something came out and you have done your job.*

NB This method is more difficult to do successfully, but many people prefer it.

Procedure: Clipping a dog's claws

1. **Action:** Place the dog in a sitting position on a stable examination table covered in a non-slip mat.

   Rationale: *If the dog feels secure on the table it will be less likely to try and escape.*

2. **Action:** Ask the owner or an assistant to restrain the dog by placing one arm under the dog's neck to restrain the head and using the other to steady the trunk.

   Rationale: *It is important that the dog does not wriggle as it may hurt itself or you.*

3. **Action:** If you think that it is necessary, put a muzzle on the dog. This may be a tape muzzle as shown in Figure 1.1 or a commercial muzzle of an appropriate size.

   Rationale: *Some dogs object to the procedure and may try to bite.*

4. **Action:** Pick up one of the forefeet.

   Rationale: *You can start with the hindfeet, but I prefer the forefeet.*

5. **Action:** With your left hand (or right hand if you are left handed) separate out one toe and gently extend the claw by pressing on the distal interphalangeal joint.

   Rationale: *This gives you the maximum chance of identifying the quick.*

6. **Action:** Identify the 'quick', which is easy in white nails, but quite difficult in dark nails (Fig. 2.3).

   Rationale: *The 'quick', which appears pale pink, comprises the blood supply to the growing nail tissue and its nerve supply. Cutting into it causes pain and bleeding.*

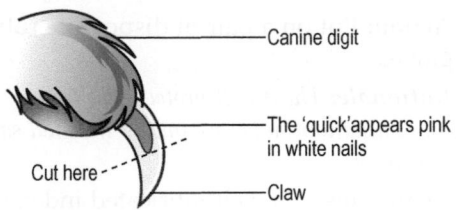

Canine digit

The 'quick' appears pink in white nails

Cut here

Claw

(A)

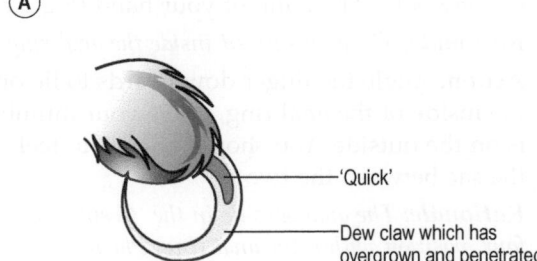

'Quick'

Dew claw which has overgrown and penetrated the associated pad

(B)

Figure 2.3 Diagram to show the position of the 'quick' within the claw: (A) a normal claw; (B) an overgrown dew claw.

7. **Action:** Place the clippers at the distal end of the 'quick' and cut quickly and firmly.

   Rationale: If you take too much time to do this the dog may move and this could result in you cutting into the quick.

8. **Action:** Repeat with all the other nails in the forefeet.

   Rationale: You may have difficulty with the two dew claws as they may have grown around and even have pierced the dew-claw pad (Fig. 2.3B). This makes it very difficult to slip some clippers over the end. You may have to nibble away at the end of the nail or even resort to doing it under a general anaesthetic or deep sedation.

9. **Action:** With the dog still restrained in a sitting position extend one of the hindfeet and repeat the procedure claw by claw.

   Rationale: Some dogs may prefer to stand when you do the hindfeet. There are usually no dew claws on the hindfeet, but make sure that you check.

NB Clipping the claws of any other species of animal or bird is more or less the same, but always check for the position of the 'quick'. Restraint for a bird is the same as for clipping the beak – see below.

Procedure: Clipping a bird's beak

This is most often done in small cage and aviary birds such as budgerigars, canaries, lovebirds cockatiels and finches.

1. **Action:** Make sure that all the doors and windows are closed and that extractor fans are switched off.

   Rationale: If the bird escapes from its cage or from your grasp it will not be able to get out of the room or be injured in the extractor fan.

2. **Action:** Remove all moveable objects from the cage such as perches, toys and feeding bowls.

   Rationale: This makes capture easier and quicker and therefore less stressful to the bird.

3. **Action:** Turn the lights off or if possible dim them.

   Rationale: Most common species of cage or aviary bird are diurnal. A dim light will simulate night and induce quiet behaviour.

4. **Action:** Tip the cage on its side.

   Rationale: This enables you to approach from the bottom of the cage and gives you more room for manoeuvre.

5. **Action:** Approach the bird slowly.

   Rationale: This avoids causing air movement, which will startle the bird.

6. **Action:** Quickly grab the bird around its neck or close your hand around its wings and body.

   Rationale: It is important to catch the bird quickly, firmly and gently to avoid causing distress. Closing your hands around the wings creates a 'net' that prevents the wings from flapping and possibly breaking.

7. **Action:** Using your left hand, hold the bird so that the head is sticking out between your thumb and index finger and the rest of your hand holds the wings close to the body (Fig. 2.4).

   Rationale: It is important to prevent the wings from flapping and thus being injured.

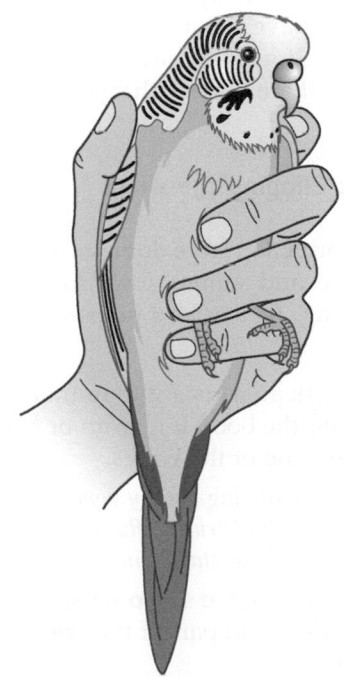

Figure 2.4 A budgerigar held in the hand. Note how the fingers form a net around the wings.

8. **Action:** Tilt the bird slightly so that you can clearly see and assess the beak.

    Rationale: Avoid tilting the bird horizontally as it is said to promote heart failure. Always be aware of the pressure you are applying to the chest with your fingers – it is easy to squeeze the chest because you are concentrating so hard on what you are doing. Some beaks may be excessively overgrown whereas others may be much less so.

9. **Action:** Identify the 'quick'.

    Rationale: The quick is the blood and nerve supply to the beak. It is often difficult to identify but, as it is usually fairly high up in the beak, in my experience it is rarely cut.

10. **Action:** Using sharp clippers, remove the bottom of the upper beak.

    Rationale: There is no need to trim the lower beak.

11. **Action:** Return the bird to its cage.

    Rationale: Always observe the bird for a few moments to make sure that it is all right.

NB If you are asked to cut the beak of a bigger bird such as a parrot, always wear clean strong gloves as these birds have vicious beaks. The use of gloves when handling smaller birds reduces your sense of touch and there is a risk that you will hold them too tightly.

Procedure: Clipping the wings

This is performed in large domestic fowl, e.g. hens, ducks, geese and guinea fowl, to prevent them from escaping. It may also be used in free-flying parrots.

1. **Action:** Ask an assistant to restrain the bird by placing the body under his or her arm and extending one of the wings.

    Rationale: Clipping is only done on one wing so that when the bird tries to fly, it is aerodynamically unstable and is forced to land.

2. **Action:** Using large sharp scissors cut through the main part of the primary feathers (Fig. 2.5).

    Rationale: Cutting through the main part of the feathers does not cause any pain. Avoid cutting

into the shaft at the point where it inserts into the skin as this will be painful and will cause bleeding. Wing clipping correctly done is no more painful than cutting hair.

3. **Action:** Leave the first one or two primary feathers uncut.

    Rationale: When the bird is at rest and its wings are folded you can hardly see that the rest of the primaries have been clipped – this is entirely cosmetic.

4. **Action:** Inform the owner that this procedure must be repeated annually.

    Rationale: Birds moult once a year so the clipped primaries will regrow allowing the bird to fly properly.

NB This procedure should not be confused with the technique of pinioning in which newly hatched birds have the bony tip of the wing removed. This is usually done in captive bird collections and is not recommended unless it is really necessary as it causes permanent disfigurement.

Procedure: Fluorescein test for the diagnosis of corneal ulcers or for assessing the patency of the tear duct

1. **Action:** The animal should be restrained by your assistant in a sitting or standing position on a stable examination table covered in a non-slip mat.

    Rationale: If the animal feels comfortable and secure it will be less likely to wriggle and try to escape.

2. **Action:** Remove a fluorescein strip from its wrapping and wet with a little sterile saline or distilled water.

    Rationale: Each strip is individually wrapped. Wetting the strip may not be necessary if there is ample tear production.

3. **Action:** Touch the test strip to the dorsal or ventral conjunctiva and if necessary irrigate the eye with a little more saline.

    Rationale: Irrigation will wash the excess fluorescein away.

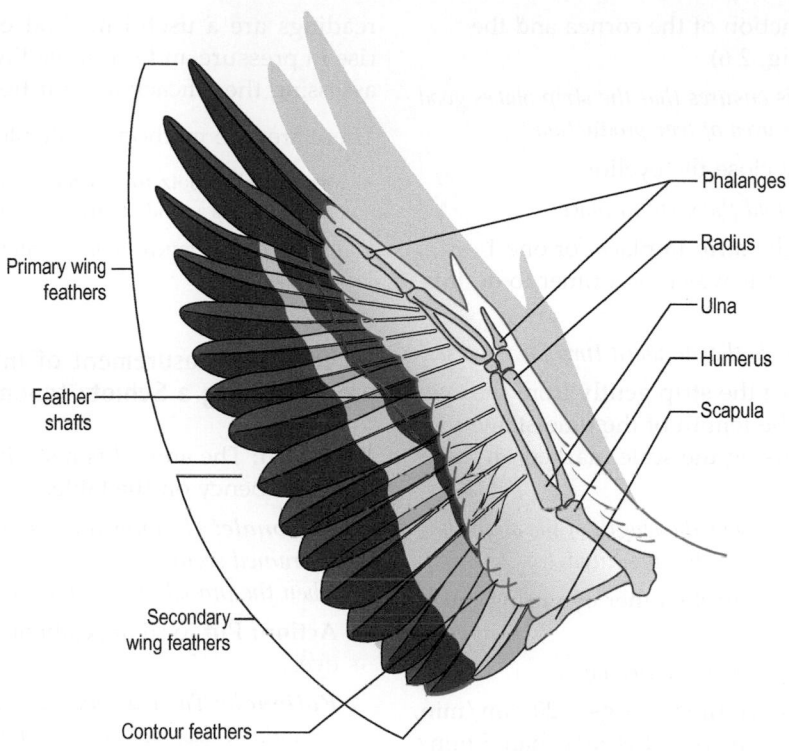

Figure 2.5 Where to clip the wings of a bird.

4. **Action:** Examine the eye using a blue light.

   Rationale: If there is a defect in the conjunctival epithelium, the fluorescein will stick to it indicating the presence of an ulcer.

5. **Action:** Examine the entrance to the nasal chambers at the point where the tear duct drains out. (Try to stop the animal licking its nose as it may remove all traces!)

   Rationale: If the tear duct is patent fluorescein will appear at the base of the duct having drained from the eye; if the duct is blocked fluorescein will spill over the edge of the eye and stain the cheek.

Procedure: Schirmer tear test to measure the amount of aqueous tear production

This simple test is a useful method of assessing tear production, aiding in the diagnosis of keratoconjunctivitis sicca (KCS) or 'dry eye'. This is a distressing problem in certain breeds such as the King Charles Spaniel and the test can also be used to monitor the effectiveness of treatment.

1. **Action:** The animal should be restrained by your assistant in sitting position or in sternal recumbency on a stable examination table covered in a non-slip mat.

   Rationale: You need to be able to reach the eye so if you are short the animal should be in sternal recumbency.

2. **Action:** Remove two Schirmer test strips from their sterile plastic envelope.

   Rationale: The strips are packaged to keep them sterile and dry.

3. **Action:** Fold the end of one strip at the notch close to the end. Try not to touch the strip with your fingers.

   Rationale: Touching the strip may cause lipids from the skin on your fingers to be absorbed and interfere with the absorption of aqueous tears.

4. **Action:** Gently roll out the lower eyelid and hook the short end of the strip so that it rests

against the junction of the cornea and the conjunctiva (Fig. 2.6).

Rationale: This ensures that the strip makes good contact with the area of tear production.

5. **Action:** Gently close the eyelids.

   Rationale: To hold the strip in place.

6. **Action:** Hold the strip in place for one 1 minute – use your watch or a timer to do this accurately.

   Rationale: This is the standard time for the test.

7. **Action:** Remove the strip gently from the eye and measure the length of the blue-stained area of paper using the scale marked on the strip.

   Rationale: The longer the length of the stain the greater the volume of tears produced.

8. **Action:** Repeat with the other eye using the second strip.

   Rationale: To compare the two eyes.

NB Average reference range: dogs = 20 mm/min, cats = 17 mm/min; in KCS it is less than 5 mm/min.

INTRAOCULAR PRESSURE

This rises if the eye starts to develop glaucoma. The increase in pressure can eventually destroy the internal structures causing severe pain, blindness and eventual collapse of the eye. Tonometry readings are a useful method of quantifying the rise in pressure and serial readings are a means of assessing the efficacy of your treatment.

There are two methods available:

- Mechanical Schiotz tonometer – less accurate and really only useful as a guide to the pressure
- Tono-Pen® – much more accurate and reliable but expensive.

Procedure: Measurement of intraocular pressure using a Schiotz tonometer

1. **Action:** The animal is restrained in lateral recumbency on the table.

   Rationale: The animal must be comfortable and restrained securely so that it does not hurt itself when the procedure is being carried out.

2. **Action:** Put local anaesthetic drops in both eyes.

   Rationale: These desensitize the cornea so that the animal does not blink or move when the cornea is touched.

3. **Action:** Calibrate the Schiotz tonometer by pressing it gently on to the metal test block. Different weights can be added to the plunger.

   Rationale: This sets the zero pressure level.

4. **Action:** Ask the assistant to hold the animal's head up so that the cornea is horizontal.

   Rationale: Readings depend on gravity so the instrument must be held as vertically as possible.

5. **Action:** Gently rest the instrument on the cornea and take a reading from the needle.

   Rationale: A soft eyeball will deflect the probe only a little thus producing a reading closer to the zero baseline. Conversely a harder eyeball will deflect the probe much more thus producing a higher reading.

6. **Action:** Take at least two readings from both eyes.

   Rationale: This allows comparison of the pressure in both eyes and by repetition checks the accuracy of the instrument. Each reading should be the same as the previous measurement.

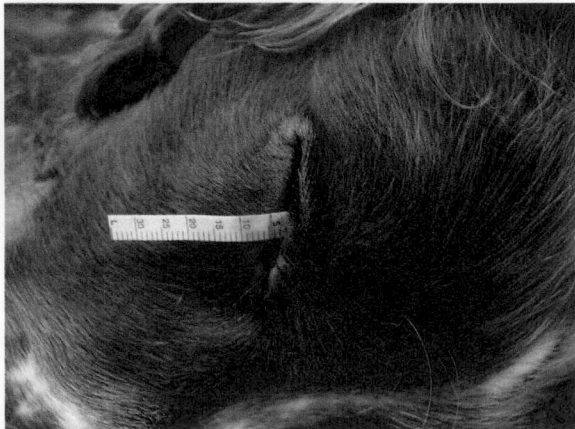

Figure 2.6 Use of Schirmer strips to measure tear production.

7. **Action:** Record the readings in the clinical records.

   Rationale: To allow comparison with later measurements and to monitor the efficacy of treatment.

Procedure: Measurement of intraocular pressure using a Tono–Pen®

1. **Action:** The animal is restrained in lateral recumbency on the table.

   Rationale: The animal must be comfortable and restrained securely so that it does not hurt itself when the procedure is being carried out.

2. **Action:** Put local anaesthetic drops in both eyes.

   Rationale: These desensitize the cornea so that the animal does not blink or move when the cornea is touched.

3. **Action:** Place a fresh latex sheath over the end of the Tono-Pen® using the cardboard applicator supplied by the manufacturer.

   Rationale: This protects the sensitive end of the instrument and prevents cross-infection.

4. **Action:** Calibrate the pen by pushing the button near to the tip with the Tono-Pen® held downwards. When it 'beeps' point the head vertically upwards. The machine should read 'good' on the display bar and readings can now be taken. If the display says 'bad' repeat the process until the correct response is obtained.

   Rationale: To calibrate and ensure the accuracy of the actual readings.

5. **Action:** Gently touch the latex tip onto the anaesthetized cornea. This should be done several times until a 'beep' is heard (Fig. 2.7).

   Rationale: The machine works by gentle corneal contact not by deforming the surface by pressure.

6. **Action:** Repeat the readings more than once and take them from both eyes.

   Rationale: This allows comparison of the pressure in both eyes and by repetition checks the accuracy. Each reading should be the same as the previous measurement.

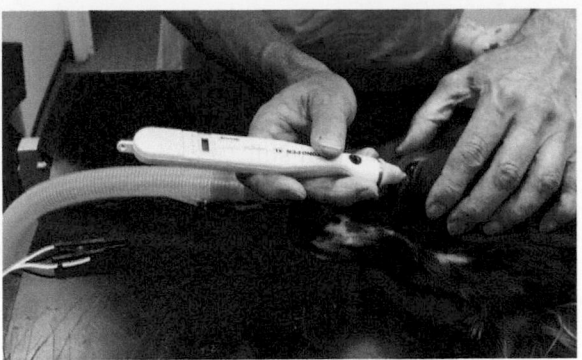

Figure 2.7 Use of a Tonopen® to measure intraocular pressure.

7. **Action:** Discard the latex sleeve in clinical waste.

   Rationale: To prevent cross-infection.

8. **Action:** Record the readings in the clinical records.

   Rationale: To allow comparison with later measurements and to monitor the efficacy of treatment.

Procedure: Collection of samples for ectoparasite identification

It is important to have an idea of which type of ectoparasite you think is the cause of the infestation.

Ectoparasites can be classified according to the depth of skin that they inhabit:

1. Surface dwellers e.g. *Cheyletiella, Otodectes, Neotrombicula* (harvest mites), lice and fleas; infestations usually cause pruritus
2. Burrowing mites:
   a. *Sarcoptes* – lives in the upper layers of the epidermis; infestations are pruritic
   b. *Demodex* – lives deep within the hair follicles; infestations are non-pruritic.

Coat brushings – used for *Cheyletiella, Neotrombicula*, fleas and lice

1. **Action:** Place the animal in a standing position on a stable examination table covered in a non-slip mat.

Rationale: If the animal feels secure on the table it will be less likely to try and escape. The position may be varied according to the site being sampled.

2. **Action:** Ask the owner to restrain the head of the animal to keep it still.

   Rationale: This is not a painful process so the animal should stand calmly.

3. **Action:** Comb through the coat thoroughly and collect the brushings in a Petri dish.

   Rationale: Make sure that you select an area that is obviously affected. When looking for fleas check under the chin, around the ears and base of the tail and in the axilla – fleas often select areas that are warm and dark.

4. **Action:** Examine under a low power or dissecting microscope (Fig. 2.8).

   Rationale: Fleas are less than 4.00 mm in length, which means they can be seen with the naked eye. You may also see flea faeces – this will turn reddish-brown if you add a drop of water to it. Cheyletiella is 0.4–0.8 mm in length so requires low magnification to be seen. You may find lice clinging to the hairs or louse eggs, known as 'nits', attached firmly to the hairs.

NB For *Otodectes* (ear mites) there is no need to brush the hair. These mites live within the external ear canal and can be identified by collecting a small sample of earwax, placing it on a glass slide and examining it under the microscope. Make sure that the sample is not too thick as this makes visualization of the mites quite difficult (Fig. 2.8C).

Sellotape® method

This is used for *Cheyletiella* and is also a useful means of collecting samples of the yeast *Malassezia pachydermatis*.

1. **Action:** Place the animal in a standing position on a stable examination table covered in a non-slip mat.

   Rationale: If the animal feels secure on the table it will be less likely to try and escape. The position may be varied according to the site being sampled.

2. **Action:** Ask the owner to restrain the head of the animal to keep it still.

   Rationale: This is not a painful process so the animal should stand calmly.

3. **Action:** Tear off a strip of Sellotape® about 2 inches (5 cm) long.

   Rationale: You need a long enough length of tape to cover a glass microscope slide.

4. **Action:** Part the coat and apply the tape sticky side down to an area that is obviously affected.

   Rationale: The sticky side should pick up skin flakes and debris, which may contain the parasites.

5. **Action:** Either place the Sellotape® sticky side down directly on to a clean glass slide or apply a drop of mineral oil to the slide before applying the Sellotape®.

   Rationale: The mineral oil increases the visibility of the parasites.

6. **Action:** If looking for *Malassezia*, the tape should be stained with the basophilic solution of Diff-Quik® (the 3rd one) before applying it to the slide.

   Rationale: Yeasts are too small and transparent to be easily seen without staining.

7. **Action:** Examine the slide under a microscope (Fig. 2.8).

   Rationale: You can easily see Cheyletiella *under low power, but you may need to increase the magnification to see* Malassezia.

Skin scraping

This is used for burrowing mites such as *Sarcoptes* and *Demodex*.

1. **Action:** Place the animal in a standing position on a stable examination table covered in a non-slip mat.

   Rationale: If the animal feels secure on the table it will be less likely to try and escape. The position may be varied according to the site being sampled.

2. **Action:** Ask the owner to restrain the head of the animal to keep it still.

   Rationale: This procedure may cause slight discomfort and the owner should be asked to hold the animal firmly.

3. **Action:** Select an appropriate area to be sampled.

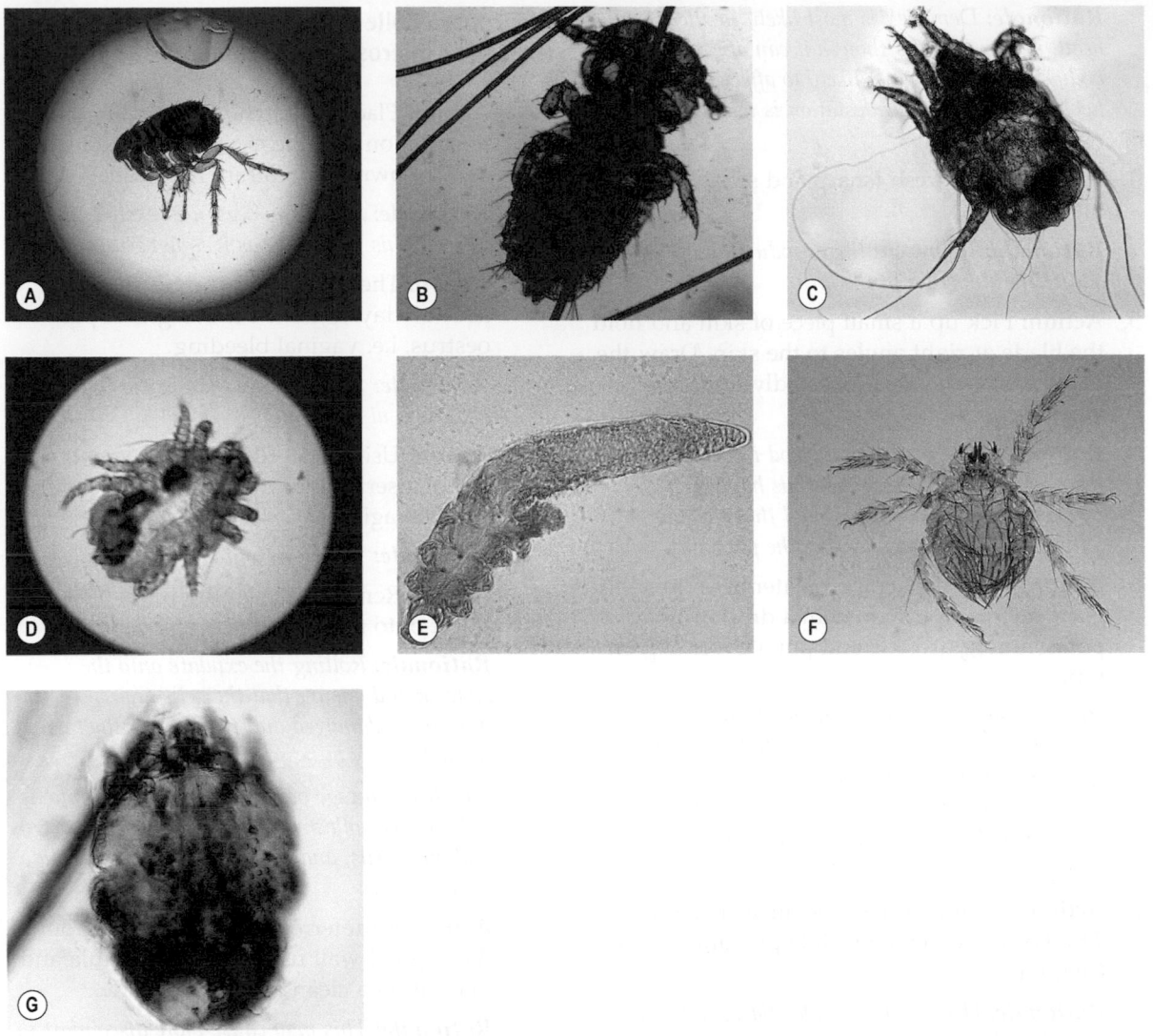

Figure 2.8 Ectoparasites that can be identified by skin scrapings or coat brushings: (A) Lateral view of an adult 'cat' flea, *Ctenocephalides felis*. Adult measures 1–2.5 mm in length. (B) *Trichodectes canis*, a biting louse of dogs. Adult is 1–2 mm in length. (C) The ear mite *Otodectes cynotis* can be recognized by the unjointed stalks or pedicels with suckers on the end that occur on the front two pairs of legs in all developmental stages. Adult mite is approx. 300 μm. (D) *Cheyletiella* spp. mites are large surface mites with long legs. They have a characteristic waist, large palps at the anterior end each carrying a heavy claw and 'combs' on the ends of their legs. (E) *Demodex* spp. mites are often described as cigar shaped. The legs are arranged in pairs at the front of the body. The mite measures approx. 0.2 mm. (F) The larvae of *Neotrombicula* or *Trombicula autumnalis* mites are hairy and have six legs. Measures approx. 200 μm. (G) *Sarcoptes* spp. mites are rotund with short legs. The back is covered in pegs and spines and the anus is terminal. The mite measures approx. 360 μm.

Rationale: Demodex *is most likely to affect the head, neck and feet although it can affect the whole body.* Sarcoptes *is most likely to affect the elbows, hocks and ears – the infestation is usually extremely pruritic.*

4. **Action:** Use a fresh (sharp and sterile) scalpel blade.

    Rationale: To prevent the introduction of additional infection to the area.

5. **Action:** Pick up a small piece of skin and hold the blade at right angles to the skin. Draw the blade across the area repeatedly until it bleeds.

    Rationale: The presence of blood indicates that the deeper layers of the epidermis have been reached. For Demodex *it is vital that the hair follicles are breached releasing the parasites.*

6. **Action:** Place the scraped material on to a glass microscope slide with a drop of 10% potassium hydroxide and put a cover slip on top.

    Rationale: Potassium hydroxide helps to break down any hair and skin cells in the debris and makes the parasites easier to see. Liquid paraffin is widely used but visibility of the parasites is less good and the slide can become very greasy.

7. **Action:** Examine under the microscope (Fig. 2.8). For more detail on slide preparation see Chapter 4.

    Rationale: Use ×4 objective for Sarcoptes; *use ×10 objective for* Demodex.

8. **Action:** On the patient, dress the area of the skin scraping with antiseptic powder.

    Rationale: To reduce the pain and prevent subsequent infection.

EXFOLIATIVE VAGINAL CYTOLOGY

This technique is based on the fact that the vaginal epithelium of the bitch changes in response to the hormones circulating during the oestrous cycle. Microscopic examination of cells shed from the epithelium will provide a guide to the stage of the cycle and will indicate when mating is likely to result in successful conception.

Procedure: Collecting and preparing a vaginal smear for microscopic examination

1. **Action:** Place the bitch in a standing position on a stable examination table and ask the owner to restrain her head.

    Rationale: A bitch in season is likely to tolerate this procedure as it is not painful.

2. **Action:** The first smear should be taken about 5 days after the first signs of pro-oestrus, i.e. vaginal bleeding.

    Rationale: Some bitches may be close to ovulation at this time.

3. **Action:** Using a sterile bacteriological swab, insert it into the vestibule and caudal vagina.

    Rationale: The swab will absorb the exudate.

4. **Action:** Remove it from the vestibule and roll it onto a clean microscope slide.

    Rationale: Rolling the exudate onto the slide should ensure that the cells are minimally damaged and remain as intact as possible.

    The disadvantage of this method is that mucus will also be collected, particularly in metoestrus and anoestrus, and this makes drying the slide rather slow.

5. **Action:** If preferred scrape material from the vaginal wall using a metal spatula and place it on a clean microscope slide.

    Rationale: This may cause more discomfort to the bitch.

    It is difficult to collect significant amounts of material by this method and the material is difficult to spread.

6. **Action:** If preferred, aspirate material from the caudal vagina using a catheter or a pipette and spread it on a clean microscope slide as you would a blood smear (see Ch. 5).

    Rationale: In metoestrus and anoestrus you may add a small amount of saline to collect a suspension of cells.

    This method produces a clear undistorted smear.

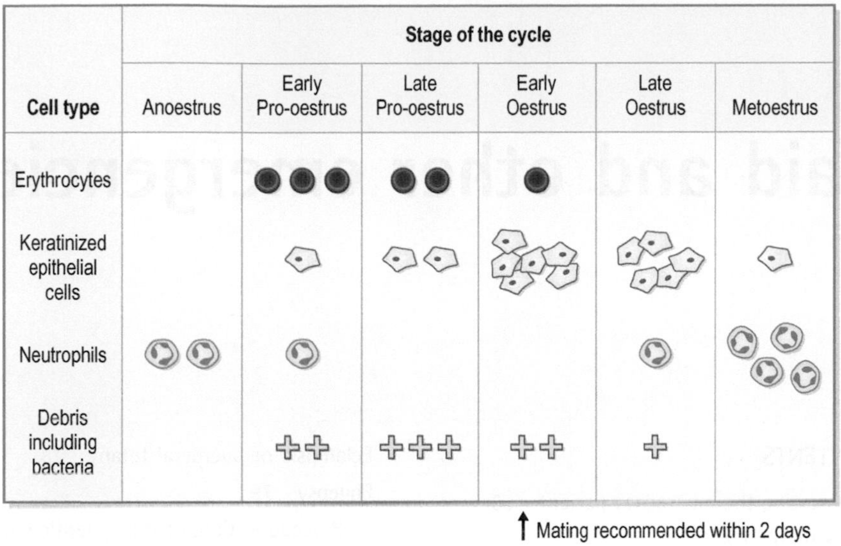

	Stage of the cycle					
Cell type	Anoestrus	Early Pro-oestrus	Late Pro-oestrus	Early Oestrus	Late Oestrus	Metoestrus
Erythrocytes		● ● ●	● ●	●		
Keratinized epithelial cells		⬠	⬠ ⬠	⬠⬠⬠	⬠⬠⬠	⬠
Neutrophils	◉ ◉	◉			◉	◉◉◉◉
Debris including bacteria		✛ ✛	✛ ✛ ✛	✛ ✛	✛	

↑ Mating recommended within 2 days

Figure 2.9 Changes in the vaginal epithelium of the bitch used in the technique of vaginal cytology to assess the stages of the oestrous cycle.

7. **Action:** Whichever method is used air dry the slide immediately.

    Rationale: To prevent distortion of the cells.

8. **Action:** Stain the slide using DiffQuik® by dipping into each of the three solutions six times, washing with water and allowing the slide to dry (see Ch. 5).

    Rationale: This stain gives rapid and consistent results although the solutions are expensive. You can also use Shorr's method, methylene blue and Leishman's stain (see Ch. 5).

9. **Action:** Examine under a microscope.

    Rationale: Interpretation is quick to do and you can provide an answer to the owner of the bitch while he/she waits.

10. **Action:** Repeat the procedure every 2–3 days.

    Rationale: If you repeat it every day the bitch may start to resent it and may then refuse to mate.

Interpretation of vaginal smears

Look for the presence of erythrocytes, neutrophils and keratinized epithelial cells sloughed from the vaginal lining. The relative proportions of these vary according to the stage of the oestrous cycle (Fig. 2. 9) and they can be used to identify:

- **Recommended time of mating** – this is not particularly important as the ova and sperm are long lived. Declining amounts of erythrocytes, keratinization of most of the epithelial cells and an absence of neutrophils will indicate that mating should occur within 2 days.

- **Artificial insemination** – may be carried out on the first day of returning neutrophils, which coincides with the last day of oestrus. The bitch may not allow normal mating at this time.

Vaginal smears can also be used to diagnose vaginitis, but not for pregnancy diagnosis.

CHAPTER 3
First aid and other emergencies

First aid is the first important action that is carried out when an animal suffers an accident. What is done to the animal will influence whether it lives or dies and will have an effect on its subsequent treatment and recovery.

Under the Veterinary Surgeons Act 1966, anyone may carry out first aid providing that it is:

- To save life.
- To prevent suffering.
- To prevent deterioration of the patient's condition.

What must happen afterwards is that the animal is handed over to a veterinary surgeon for further treatment. It is illegal for a layperson to keep the animal and continue treatment as this becomes an act of veterinary surgery requiring diagnosis, possible surgery and the prescribing of medication. Failure to do this may cause suffering, which will contravene the Animal Welfare Act 2006.

In many cases it will be a member of the public who administers first aid out in the 'field' (e.g. road traffic accident or a cut paw) but in some cases such as haemorrhage or anaesthetic arrest, which may occur within the practice, it will be the veterinary surgeon who is first on the scene. Obviously the chances of survival of the animal will be greatly increased by the degree of knowledge and experience of the person dealing with it; however, whoever this person is, the basic rules of first aid should be followed.

First of all, **keep calm and don't panic** – always ensure your own safety first. You will not be able to help the animal if you are injured. Levels of panic can be significantly reduced by knowledge and training and adhering to a well-rehearsed routine.

Now remember the acronym **ABC**:

- **Airway** – ensure that the animal has a clear airway allowing the passage of oxygen into the respiratory system and then into the circulatory system.
- **Breathing** – make sure that the animal is making some form of respiratory effort.
- **Circulation** – check that the heart is beating, i.e. there is a pulse, and look at the colour of the mucous membranes; a healthy pink colour will indicate oxygen is reaching the tissues.

When an animal is about to suffer cardiopulmonary arrest and requires resuscitation it is important to be able to recognize the clinical signs (Box 3.1) and to have a strict routine for cardiopulmonary cerebral resuscitation (CPCR). In an emergency everything seems to happen at once and successful treatment requires a trained 'crash' team who have defined roles and understand their responsibilities. The procedures that must be carried out by this team are:

- Intubation of the patient and attachment to an anaesthetic machine
- Provision of oxygen and manual compression of the reservoir bag if necessary
- External cardiac massage
- Placement of an intravenous catheter for the administration of fluids
- Attachment to an ECG machine to monitor progress and to assist in the provision of appropriate medication.

(In order to avoid repetition some procedures that may also be used as a first aid procedure or as continuing treatment are included in other chapters:

- Bandaging and stabilization of limbs – see Chapter 4
- Wound management – see Chapter 4
- Fluid therapy – see Chapter 7
- Anaesthetic emergencies – see Chapter 8.

Look inside the front cover for a life support algorithm.)

Procedure: Assessing the emergency patient

The steps in this assessment must, of necessity, be as rapid as possible and they will run into each other, making you feel that the steps must be carried out simultaneously. This may add to your feeling of panic but, in order not to forget anything, it is important to stick to a rigid protocol and remember the rules of **A**irway, **B**reathing, **C**irculation.

1. **Action:** Ensure that the environment is safe for you and the animal.

    Rationale: Do not attempt to rescue or treat an animal if there is any risk to you (e.g. electrocution, traffic, fire, radiation, falling masonry).

2. **Action:** Stand back from the animal and observe for a moment.

    Rationale: You must remain calm and in control. Touching the animal may destroy some evidence (see Ch. 2). Try to calm the owners or people around the animal as they may be panicking.

3. **Action:** Make sure that the animal is restrained appropriately. You may need to ask someone to help you. If the animal is

---

Box 3.1 Signs of cardiopulmonary arrest or impending death

- Loss of consciousness
- Absence of respiratory movements or agonal (gasping) breathing
- Either a very weak rapid pulse or lack of a pulse or heartbeat
- Fixed dilated pupils
- Lack of corneal or palpebral reflexes
- Cornea begins to dull
- Loss of control of the bowel and bladder

breathing normally you may have to apply a tape muzzle (see Ch. 1).

Rationale: The first reaction of an animal that is frightened and in pain is to bite and/or to run away. Never apply a tape muzzle to an animal that is having trouble breathing.

4. **Action:** Examine the airway to ensure that it is patent.

Rationale: The animal may be trying to breathe, but this will be difficult if the airway is blocked

5. **Action:** If necessary remove any blockage (e.g. blood clot, saliva, rubber ball).

Rationale: Both clotted blood and saliva can create as effective a blockage as a solid object such as a ball.

6. **Action:** Position the animal in such a way as to facilitate breathing (e.g. in lateral recumbency with the head extended, tongue pulled forward, loosen the collar). If the animal has been drowned, place the head lower than the rest of the body.

Rationale: In this position the airway should remain open. Never remove the collar as the animal may suddenly recover and run away and it will then be without its collar. Placing the head lower than the body enables water to drain out of the airway.

7. **Action:** Check that the animal is breathing. If necessary start artificial respiration (refer to later procedure).

Rationale: Lack of oxygen to the brain will kill the animal or cause irreparable brain damage within a matter of minutes.

8. **Action:** Check that the animal has a heartbeat. If necessary start cardiac massage (refer to later procedure).

Rationale: If the heart is not beating, oxygen will not be pumped around the body to supply the brain and other vital organs.

9. **Action:** Check the patient's capillary refill time, colour of mucous membrane, pulse and respiratory rate and body temperature. Record these parameters.

Rationale: These parameters will provide an indication of the animal's condition and provide a starting point on which to base your assessment as the animal's condition improves.

10. **Action:** Once the patient is stable and not going to die immediately, check for haemorrhage and take steps to control it (refer to later procedure).

Rationale: Haemorrhage must be dealt with quickly as severe blood loss will kill the animal within a few minutes or cause it to go into shock.

11. **Action:** Assess the animal for signs of shock and treat appropriately (refer to later procedure).

Rationale: In severe cases shock will set in rapidly and treatment must be instigated as soon as possible.

12. **Action:** Examine the animal for fractures and immobilize them (refer to Ch. 4).

Rationale: The presence of a fracture is not generally life threatening, but it will cause pain and the condition may be made worse by movement.

13. **Action:** Check the animal for all other wounds and provide a temporary dressing as appropriate.

Rationale: To prevent the entry of infection before you can clean, debride and provide proper wound dressings (refer to Ch. 4).

14. **Action:** Administer the appropriate medication (e.g. antibiotics and analgesics).

Rationale: Antibiotics will prevent sepsis and analgesia will help the animal to stabilize.

15. **Action:** Once you are satisfied that the animal is safe to move, take it to the surgery, or, if in the surgery, place it in a warm, quiet secure kennel and keep under observation.

Rationale: The first few minutes after an incident are vital, but once the animal is stable most wounds and immobilized fractures can be left for a short time while the animal begins to recover and poses less of an anaesthetic risk.

AIRWAY AND BREATHING

Procedure: Treatment of asphyxia

1. **Action:** Clear any obstruction from the mouth and the pharynx.

   Rationale: Obstructions may include clotted blood, saliva, vomit and solid material such as balls and wet leaves (if animal has drowned). A useful tip is to use the handle of a large spoon to lever out the obstruction without being bitten.

2. **Action:** Loosen the collar.

   Rationale: To facilitate breathing, but do not remove the collar as the animal may suddenly recover and run off. A dog running around without its collar is a stray.

3. **Action:** If water or a foreign body blocks the trachea then perform the Heimlich manoeuvre to remove the obstruction – hold the animal up by its hind legs or, if the animal is too big, hang it upside down over a table (Fig. 3.1). Administer a sharp punch to the abdominal wall, above the xiphisternum angled down towards the diaphragm.

   Rationale: This aim of this technique is to force foreign material from the trachea. The obstructing material may move down the trachea towards the pharynx in response to the pull of gravity.

4. **Action:** Repeat up to four times.

   Rationale: Repeating the procedure more than four times may cause damage.

5. **Action:** If attempts to remove the blockage fail then establish an emergency airway by pushing a wide gauge hypodermic needle through the ventral midline of the neck and into the trachea.

   Rationale: This will act as an airway until a proper tracheotomy can be performed.

TRACHEOTOMY VS TRACHEOSTOMY

A tracheotomy creates a temporary opening in the trachea in an animal with an upper airway obstruction allowing air to enter the trachea distal to the site of the blockage. If a tube is then placed in the stoma created by the tracheotomy this is then termed a tracheostomy. The procedures are usually performed as an emergency under local

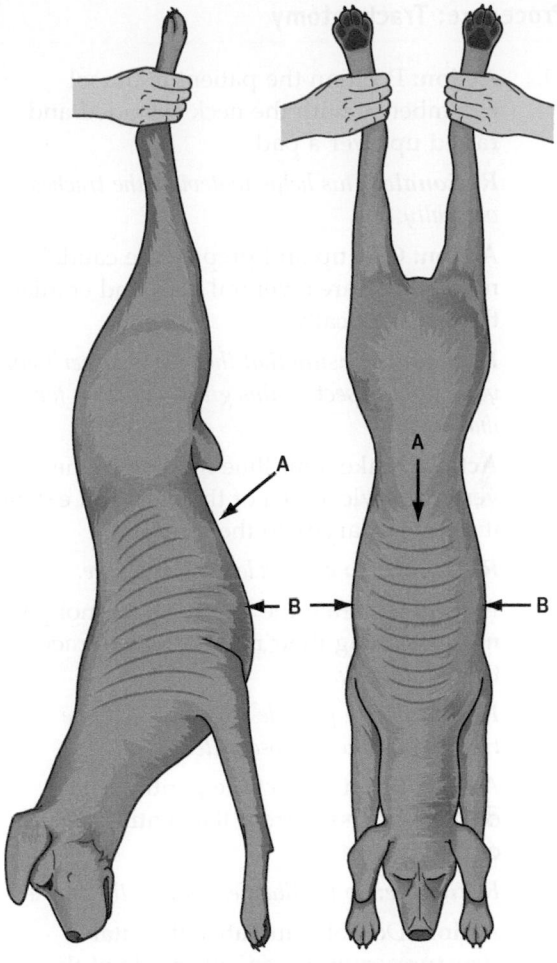

→ Direction and point of impact of blow

Figure 3.1 The Heimlich manoeuvre: A = standard version; B = modified version.

anaesthetic or sedation – dyspnoeic patients may present an anaesthetic risk. Aseptic preparation of the surgical site should be carried out (see Ch. 9), but if the animal is about to die it need not be done – provide antibiotic cover later on when the situation has improved.

The animal will present with increased inspiratory effort, dyspnoea, cyanosis, open mouth breathing and orthopnea. If the condition is acute, i.e. the animal is close to death, then a wide gauge hypodermic needle can be pushed through the ventral midline of the trachea as a temporary measure.

A tracheotomy may also be used to remove obstructions or to collect samples.

Procedure: Tracheotomy

1. **Action:** Position the patient in dorsal recumbency with the neck extended and raised up over a pad.

   Rationale: This helps to deviate the trachea ventrally.

2. **Action:** Clip up and prepare the caudal mandibular area, ventral neck and cranial thorax aseptically.

   Rationale: Ensure that the area is larger than you might expect as this gives you room for manoeuvre.

3. **Action:** Make a midline incision in the ventral cervical area of the neck and extend it from the larynx to the sternum.

   Rationale: To allow adequate exposure.

4. **Action:** Separate the overlying sternohyoid muscles along their midline and retract them laterally.

   Rationale: To provide a good view of the trachea and the proposed site.

5. **Action:** Blunt dissect the peritracheal connective tissue from the ventral surface of the trachea

   Rationale: To facilitate entry into the trachea.

6. **Action:** Do not traumatize the vital structures running on either side of the trachea (i.e. recurrent laryngeal nerve, carotid artery, jugular vein and thyroid vessels). Also look out for the oesophagus.

   Rationale: Keep in the midline and you should avoid these structures.

7. **Action:** Fix the trachea between your forefinger and thumb and make a horizontal or vertical midline incision through the wall of the trachea.

   Rationale: To create an opening into the trachea.

8. **Action:** Place sutures around the adjacent tracheal cartilages and use them to pull the edges of the incision apart.

   Rationale: To elevate the cartilages and separate the edges, allowing inspection of the tracheal lumen.

9. **Action:** Use suction to clear debris, blood and secretions from the lumen.

   Rationale: To remove any blockage.

10. **Action:** If possible find the source of the blockage and remove it.

    Rationale: This may not always be possible.

11. **Action:** If the airway is now clear the opening can be closed:

    - Oppose the edges of the trachea with simple interrupted sutures placing sutures through the annular ligaments (between the cartilage rings).
    - Lavage the area with sterile saline.
    - Oppose the sternohyoid muscles using a continuous suture.
    - Oppose subcutaneous tissue and skin edges as normal (see Ch. 10).

    Rationale: Make sure that the suture line is more or less airtight to prevent air under-running the tissues as the animal inspires. This will gradually improve as the wound heals.

Procedure: Temporary tracheostomy

1. **Action:** Prepare the patient as above and follows steps 1 to 7 (Fig. 3.2).

   Rationale: The procedure is very similar, except that a tracheostomy tube is placed so that the stoma created stays open for a longer period and the site is more prescribed.

2. **Action:** If placing a tracheostomy tube the tracheal incision should be horizontal and between the 3rd / 4th or 4th / 5th tracheal cartilages. Do not extend the length of the incision more than half of the circumference of the trachea (Fig. 3.2).

   Rationale: To allow room for the flange of the tube to be placed comfortably below the larynx. The tube is unlikely to be dislodged by movement of the neck.

   If the incision is too long there is a risk of bisecting the trachea completely.

3. **Action:** An alternative incision can be made vertically between the 3rd and 5th cartilages.

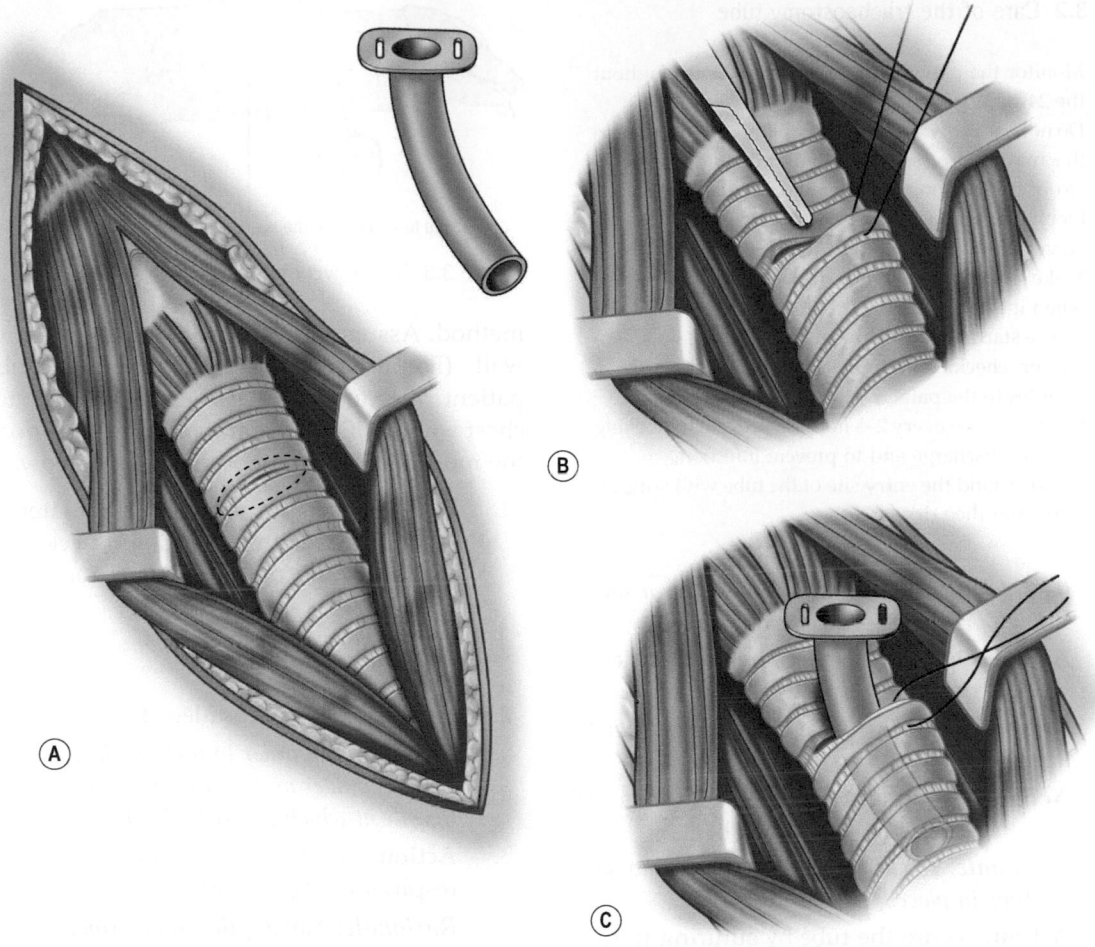

Figure 3.2 Tube tracheostomy: (A) Make a transverse incision through the annular ligament. Excise a small ellipse of cartilage from each tracheal cartilage adjacent to the tracheotomy incision to minimize tube irritation (dotted line). Facilitate tube placement by depressing the proximal cartilages with a hemostat (B) and elevating the distal cartilages with an encircling suture (C). Insert a tracheostomy tube that does not completely fill the lumen.

Rationale: It may be more difficult to place the tracheostomy tube using this approach.

4. **Action:** Using suction remove blood and other debris from the trachea.

   Rationale: To facilitate inspiration and clean up the surgical site.

5. **Action:** Select a tube that is non-reactive and that is no larger than half the size of the trachea. If the patient is to be placed on a respirator a cuffed tube must be used.

   Rationale: To prevent a reaction and to reduce resistance within the trachea. Use of a cuffed tube prevents breathing around the tube.

6. **Action:** Place a suture around the tracheal ring distal to the incision (Fig. 3.2).

   Rationale: This will be used to assist in opening the trachea prior to tube placement.

7. **Action:** Using a pair of closed artery forceps, depress the cartilage cranial to the opening.

   Rationale: To facilitate introduction of the tube.

8. **Action:** At the same time, using the suture around the distal cartilage, pull it up and insert the tube (Fig. 3.2).

   Rationale: This opens the incision making it easier to insert the tube. If there are difficulties

Box 3.2 Care of the tracheostomy tube

- Monitor the patient at regular intervals throughout the 24-hour period.
- Do not use fluffy bedding or cat litter in the kennel as this may become sucked into the tube and block it.
- Do not feed sloppy, dry or flaky food as this may block the tube.
- Never put a collar on the patient.
- Make sure that the patient does not occlude the tube when it is sleeping.
- Before starting or finishing any procedure, i.e. cleaning or checking, administer 100% oxygen for 5 minutes to the patient.
- Clean the tube every 2–3 hours to prevent it blocking up with discharge and to prevent infection.
- Clean around the entry site of the tube with surgical scrub and then dry.

the tracheal incision can be widened or a small ellipse of cartilage can be resected.

9. **Action:** Oppose the sternohyoid muscles with a continuous suture.

   Rationale: To close the dead space and to hold the tube in place.

10. **Action:** Close the subcutaneous tissues and the skin as normal (see Ch. 10).

    Rationale: To close the dead space and to hold the tube in place.

11. **Action:** Secure the tube by suturing it to the skin or by tying a gauze bandage around it and tying that around the patient's neck.

    Rationale: The patient must be checked regularly to make sure that the tube is still in place and the site is not becoming infected (Box 3.2).

NB Tracheostomy tubes used in emergency situations are not usually left in for more than a day or two. A permanent tracheostomy is achieved by the creation of a permanent stoma within the trachea and overlying skin, which may remain for life or until such time as the stoma is closed surgically.

Procedure: Artificial respiration

In some instances (e.g. out in the 'field') there may not be equipment available to intubate an animal so artificial respiration should be done by this

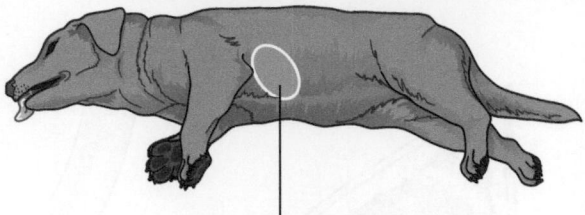

Area to which pressure is applied in artificial respiration

Figure 3.3 The recovery position.

method. Assume there is no damage to the chest wall. (For artificial respiration in an intubated patient refer to Ch. 8.) If there is damage to the chest wall, artificial respiration should be done by the mouth to nose method described below.

1. **Action:** Place the animal in right lateral recumbency with its head and neck extended, and pull the tongue forwards (Fig. 3.3).

   Rationale: This position allows maximum air intake.

2. **Action:** Pull the front legs forward.

   Rationale: In order to prevent the musculature of the shoulder and upper limb from obscuring the site at which pressure should be applied.

3. **Action:** Check that there are still no respiratory movements.

   Rationale: Moving the animal sometimes stimulates spontaneous respiration.

4. **Action:** Place the palm of your hand in the middle of the chest (Fig. 3.3).

   Rationale: Your hand will be directly over the majority of the lung field and will be used to force air into and out of the chest.

5. **Action:** Apply steady firm downward pressure and then release.

   Rationale: The elasticity of the rib cage makes the ribs spring back up, drawing air down the trachea.

6. **Action:** Apply the pressure at $\frac{1}{2}$–1-second intervals depending on the size of the animal.

   Rationale: The smaller the animal the faster is the respiration rate.

7. **Action:** Check the animal at regular intervals for signs of respiration.

Rationale: You may find it easier to ask an assistant to do this while you continue to administer artificial respiration.

8. **Action:** Continue until the animal begins to breathe on its own.

    Rationale: Continue artificial respiration for about 30 minutes; if the animal is still not breathing it may be pronounced dead.

9. **Action:** As soon as the animal starts to breathe provide oxygen.

    Rationale: If you are not in the surgery this can be difficult, but if in the surgery you should intubate and provide oxygen through a circuit. If intubation is impossible then provide oxygen by mask.

10. Check the animal every 5 minutes during its recovery and extend the time intervals as it regains consciousness.

    Rationale: Relapses can occur.

Procedure: Mouth to nose resuscitation

This is used to stimulate breathing when the chest wall is damaged.

1. **Action:** Place the animal in right lateral recumbency with its head and neck extended, and pull the tongue forwards.

    Rationale: This position allows maximum air intake.

2. **Action:** Grasp the nose firmly in the right hand so that the thumb and fingers curl around the nose and mouth, and hold the mouth closed (Fig. 3.4).

    Rationale: This creates an airtight seal.

3. **Action:** Place the left hand under the lower jaw (Fig. 3.4).

    Rationale: This supports the lower jaw.

4. **Action:** If possible use a facemask, a handkerchief or some form of cloth to blow through.

    Rationale: To prevent the potential transfer of pathogens.

5. **Action:** Place your mouth over the animal's nostrils forming a seal with your lips.

    Rationale: To maximize the effect of your expiratory effort.

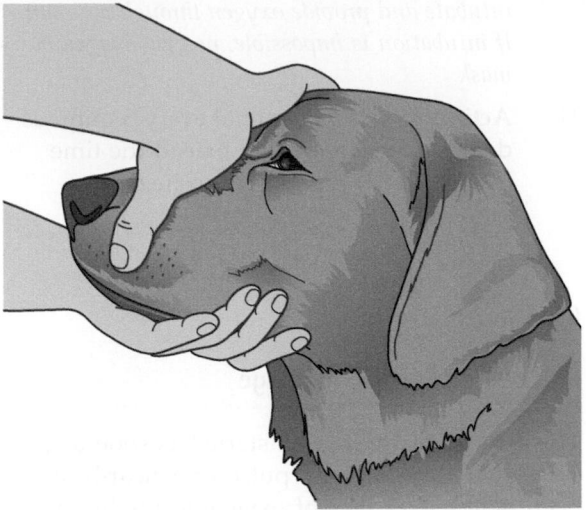

Figure 3.4 Mouth to nose resuscitation – holding the nose.

6. **Action:** Blow down the nose at 1-second intervals turning your head away after each expiration.

    Rationale: To avoid inhaling the animal's expired air and mucus. Your expired air contains carbon dioxide, which acts as a respiratory stimulant for the animal.

7. **Action:** Do not overinflate the lungs particularly if the animal is neonatal (i.e. resuscitation after a caesarean section). Use just enough force to raise the chest slightly.

    Rationale: Lung damage can occur as a result of sudden overinflation, especially in young animals.

8. **Action:** Periodically check for signs of respiration.

    Rationale: You may find it easier to ask an assistant to do this while you continue to administer mouth to nose respiration.

9. **Action:** Repeat the procedure until spontaneous respiration begins.

    Rationale: Continue for 20–30 minutes. If there is no response the animal may be pronounced dead.

10. **Action:** As soon as the animal starts to breathe provide oxygen.

    Rationale: If you are not in the surgery this can be difficult, but if in the surgery you should intubate and provide oxygen through a circuit. If intubation is impossible, provide oxygen by mask.

11. **Action:** Check the animal every 5 minutes during its recovery and extend the time intervals as it regains consciousness.

    Rationale: Relapses can occur.

CIRCULATION

Procedure: Cardiac massage

This procedure should be started as soon as possible after the lack of a pulse or a heartbeat has been detected as lack of oxygen to the brain and other tissues will very quickly result in permanent damage and / or death.

1. **Action:** Place the animal in right lateral recumbency.

   Rationale: In this position there is easier access to the heart for massage and for monitoring.

2. **Action:** Locate the position of the heart.

   Rationale: The heart lies between the 3rd rib and caudal border of the 6th rib.

3. **Action:** Using the heel of your hand, place it over the heart (Fig. 3.5a). Apply rhythmic pressure using enough force to depress the chest wall by 1–3 cm depending on the size of the animal.

   Rationale: This force will reach the heart wall and compress the muscle.

4. **Action:** Place your other hand under the animal's chest to support it (Fig. 3.5A).

   Rationale: You can also place a firm sandbag under the chest to provide something to push against.

5. **Action:** In feline patients or in very small dogs you can apply pressure by placing the thumb and forefinger around the sternum (Fig 3.5B).

   Rationale: As the animal is small your hand should fit around the sternum to reach the appropriate part of the chest wall.

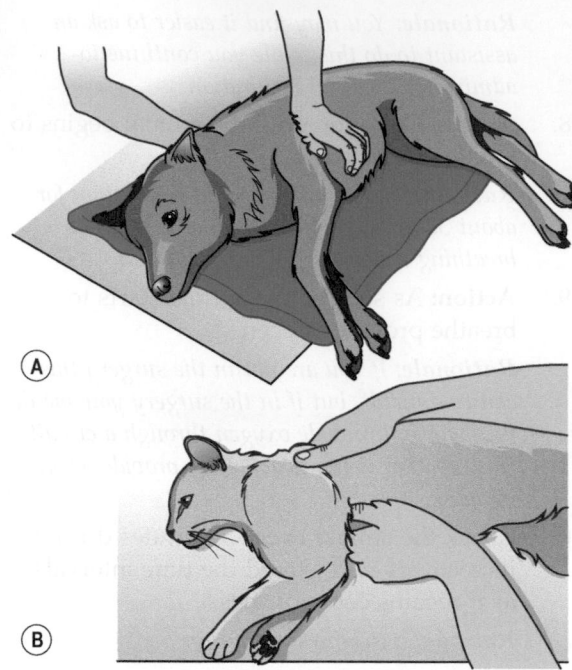

Figure 3.5 Technique used for cardiac massage in (A) a dog and (B) a cat.

6. **Action:** The ideal rate of chest compressions is 100 per minute giving equal time to compression and relaxation.

   Rationale: Singing 'Nellie the Elephant' will provide the appropriate beat to your compressions.

7. **Action:** Give a breath every 5th or 6th compression.

   Rationale: If the animal is intubated, squeeze the bag; if you are out in the 'field' breathe into the animal's nose as described above.

8. **Action:** Every 3–4 minutes check for signs of a returning heartbeat.

   Rationale: Look for improved mucous membrane colour, restoration of a pulse, decreased capillary refill time and reduction in pupil size.

9. **Action:** If cardiac function returns then stop chest compressions.

   Rationale: You may cause damage to the heart if chest compressions continue while the heart is beating.

10.   **Action:** If cardiac function does not return, assess the condition of the patient and then consider open-chest compressions.

   Rationale: *This cannot be carried out in the 'field'. If the animal is in the surgery this procedure can be considered but the prognosis is poor (see Ch. 8 – Anaesthetic emergencies).*

CONTROL OF HAEMORRHAGE

Any loss of blood can potentially be life threatening and should be taken seriously. Table 3.1 describes the types of haemorrhage and Table 3.2 describes the range of first aid treatments. Methods used to control haemorrhage are temporary and once haemorrhage has ceased the bandage should be removed and the wound cleaned and treated by suturing or by rebandaging (see Ch. 4 for bandaging techniques and Ch. 10 for suturing techniques).

Procedure: Control of haemorrhage

1.   **Action:** Place the animal on a stable table or on a surface that is at a comfortable height for you.

   Rationale: *If the animal feels secure it will be less likely to try and escape. If the procedure takes*

Table 3.1 Types of haemorrhage

Type	Clinical signs	Treatment
Arterial	Blood is bright red and pumps out in spurts. Bleeding point is usually easy to identify.	Very serious and a significant volume may be lost rapidly. Stop immediately using digital pressure until a more permanent method is put in place.
Venous	Blood is darker red and flows in a steady stream. Bleeding point is usually easy to identify.	Serious; stop as soon as possible by digital pressure or a pressure bandage.
Capillary	Multiple pinpoint haemorrhages. Blood oozes from the wound with little force. Commonly seen in surgical incisions.	Less serious, but capillary ooze for a long period may result in significant blood loss. Stop by means of a pressure bandage.
Mixed	Combination of the types described above. This is the most common type.	Depends on the extent of the haemorrhage.

Table 3.2 Range of first aid treatment for haemorrhage

Treatment	Method	Comment
Direct digital pressure	With a clean finger and thumb apply pressure to either side of the wound. Avoid pushing bone fragments or foreign bodies deeper into the wound.	Quick and easy, but only a temporary measure until a pressure bandage is applied.
Pressure bandage	Place sterile swab over the wound and apply pressure using a conforming bandage. If wound involves the neck or chest, make sure that breathing is not impeded.	Deep wounds may need packing with sterile gauze to spread the pressure. If wound includes a penetrating foreign body or bone fragments, place a ring pad over it before placing the bandage.
Pressure points	These are sites where pressure can be applied to a major artery by pushing it against a bone, thus stopping the blood supply to the area distal to it. Common sites are the brachial, femoral and coccygeal arteries.	Sites are not easy to locate. Venous bleeding still continues. Apply a pressure bandage or tourniquet as soon as possible.
Tourniquet	Ready-made or improvised strap is applied to a limb proximal to the injury and tightened. Pressure should be just enough to stop bleeding.	Never leave a tourniquet in place for longer than 15 minutes as tissue damage will occur. Relieve pressure for 1 minute then retighten.

some time you must feel comfortable and have easy access to the animal.

2. **Action:** Ask an assistant to restrain the animal so that you can reach the affected part of the body without the animal moving too much or biting you.

   Rationale: The animal may resent the wound being touched. Your assistant should be able to react quickly to prevent the animal moving or trying to escape.

3. **Action:** Wash your hands thoroughly with a surgical scrub.

   Rationale: It is important not to introduce infection into the wound, but as the wound is not sterile there is no need to scrub up.

4. **Action:** Assess what type of haemorrhage you are presented with (Table 3.1).

   Rationale: The extent of the haemorrhage depends on which blood vessels are severed and determines your treatment.

5. **Action:** As quickly as possible stop the bleeding using one of the first aid measures described in Table 3.2.

   Rationale: It is vital that the animal loses as little blood as possible. The method depends on where you are, for example, in the surgery or in the 'field'.

6. **Action:** Once the bleeding has stopped, or is showing signs of stopping, assess the animal's condition. Check for signs of shock and treat if necessary (see later procedure).

   Rationale: Blood loss may lead to hypovolaemic shock. Treatment must be instigated as soon as possible to prevent death.

7. **Action:** Monitor the animal closely. If blood soaks through the bandage, place another one over the top. Do not remove the original bandage.

   Rationale: If you remove the original bandage you may remove the blood clot and start the bleeding again.

8. **Action:** Once the animal's condition is stable, place it in a quiet warm kennel and check every 15 minutes.

   Rationale: Overexcitement may start the bleeding again.

9. **Action:** When the bleeding has stopped and the animal is stable, treatment to repair the wound can be carried out.

   Rationale: It may be necessary to anaesthetize the animal – this should not be done until you are certain that the animal is out of danger and anaesthesia no longer poses a risk.

SHOCK

To put it simply, shock occurs when the effective circulating blood volume is reduced so that the oxygen and nutrient requirements of the tissues are unable to be satisfied. In addition, the waste products resulting from normal metabolism are not removed so they build up to toxic levels within the tissues resulting in cell and eventually tissue death. If treatment is not instigated as rapidly as possible the patient will die.

All types of shock will reduce:

- The effective circulating blood volume
- The capacity of the blood to deliver oxygen to the cells
- The heart's ability to pump blood around the circulation
- The vascular system's ability to maintain vasomotor tone.

Shock can be classified according to its pathophysiology into:

1. **Hypovolaemic shock** – results from severe haemorrhage or severe vomiting and diarrhoea, which causes loss of fluid and electrolytes. The body responds by vasoconstriction to raise the blood pressure, but this is a short term solution and the animal will recover only if circulating volume is restored by fluid therapy (see Ch. 6).

2. **Traumatic shock** – results from tissue damage and the release of inflammatory mediators, which cause further cell damage. May be complicated by haemorrhage and sepsis and be followed by hypovolaemic shock. Initially heart rate and cardiac output increase. Vasodilation occurs and is followed by intense vasoconstriction.

3. **Cardiogenic shock** – results from failure of the pumping mechanism of the heart. Blood volume remains normal but cardiac output is reduced. Rising pressure in the atria leads to

congestion and oedema of the dependent organs (i.e. liver and lungs).

4. **Distributive shock** – results from the release of inflammatory mediators, which interfere with the normal regulatory mechanisms of blood pressure. Clinical signs are *different* from other types and include vasodilation, hypotension and unequal distribution of fluid.

It has two forms:

- **Septic shock** – resulting from infection. Starts with signs of sepsis, including pyrexia, and is followed by signs of shock.
- **Anaphylactic shock** – follows from an allergic reaction to an antigen to which the patient has become sensitized. Clinical signs such as urticaria, laryngeal oedema and bronchospasm accompany the signs of shock.

The general clinical signs of shock are listed in Box 3.3.

Procedure: Treatment of shock

1. **Action:** Assess the animal for clinical signs of shock (Box 3.3).

   Rationale: *This will determine the severity of the problem and the subsequent treatment.*

2. **Action:** Provide any first aid treatment as appropriate.

   Rationale: *Remember ABC and see previous procedures.*

Box 3.3 Clinical signs of shock

- Reduced mentation – reduced level of consciousness and altered behaviour
- Pale or dry mucous membranes
- Slowed capillary refill time
- Tachycardia
- Weak rapid pulse
- Tachypnoea
- Cold extremities – core temperature is normal unless septic shock is present
- Decreased skin turgor
- Reduced urine output
- Collapse, convulsions and death

3. **Action:** Provide intravenous replacement therapy to replace the circulating fluid volume.

   Rationale: *For choice of fluids see Chapter 6. Remember replacement fluid should resemble as closely as possible the fluid that is lost. In severe shock plasma expanders may be used.*

   For choice of administration route and method of restraint see Chapters 1 and 6.

4. **Action:** Provide oxygen to the animal. If the animal is unconscious intubate and attach to a closed anaesthetic circuit; if it is conscious use a mask or place in an oxygen tent.

   Rationale: *To correct the levels of hypoxia resulting from blood loss.*

5. **Action:** Provide warmth by indirect heat (e.g. warm environment) or by wrapping the animal in blankets or bubble wrap.

   Rationale: *Direct heat (e.g. heat lamps) will increase dilation of the surface capillaries taking blood away from the vital organs.*

6. **Action:** Administer the appropriate medication.

   Rationale: *Indications for drug therapy may include:*

   » Treating the developing acidosis – intravenous fluids and oxygen therapy
   » Treating anaphylaxis – intravenous adrenaline
   » Providing antibiosis – broad-spectrum antibiotics
   » Suppressing the inflammatory response – corticosteroids.

7. **Action:** When the animal is stable, place it in a quiet, warm, stress free kennel and monitor at regular intervals.

   Rationale: *Monitor the parameters (described in Ch. 6).*

OTHER EMERGENCIES

BURNS AND SCALDS

- A **burn** may be caused by dry heat, electrocution or corrosive chemicals.
- A **scald** is caused by moist heat such as boiling water, hot oil or hot tar.

Procedure: Treating burns and scalds

1. **Action:** Place the animal in a comfortable position on a stable examination table.

   Rationale: If the animal feels secure it will be less likely to try and escape.

2. **Action:** Ask an assistant to restrain the animal so that it is comfortable but cannot wriggle or escape.

   Rationale: The animal will be in pain and may try to bite you. It is likely to resent the wound being touched or examined.

3. **Action:** Wash your hands thoroughly using a surgical scrub.

   Rationale: To prevent the introduction of infection into the wound.

4. **Action:** As soon as possible after the damage is done to the animal, cool the area using cold water – a shower hose is ideal as it covers a large area with a minimum amount of pressure. Continue for at least 10 minutes. You may have to give this advice to the owner over the telephone.

   Rationale: Cooling the area stops the heat causing further damage to the cells and limits the size of the burn. Do not use ice as it puts pressure on the burned skin.

5. **Action:** Keep the animal warm by wrapping it in a blanket. Take care as the animal will be in pain.

   Rationale: The burned skin must be cooled, but the animal must be kept warm to avoid the onset of shock. Avoid the use of direct heat (e.g. heat pads or lamps).

6. **Action:** Gently clean the burned skin with sterile saline.

   Rationale: The area will be extremely painful and proper cleaning may be achieved only under a general anaesthetic. General anaesthesia is recommended only if the animal is in a stable condition.

7. **Action:** Dress the wound with wound gel and/or paraffin tulle.

   Rationale: The wound must be kept moist to promote healing. Paraffin tulle prevents the wound from drying out.

8. **Action:** Apply a light non-adhesive dressing on the top.

   Rationale: Heat must be able to escape and moisture must be retained – a light dressing will allow this.

9. **Action:** Wrap a plastic bag or cling film over the wound. Do not apply too much pressure.

   Rationale: This will retain moisture by preventing evaporation from the wound surface. Using too much pressure will be painful and may delay wound healing.

10. **Action:** Gently place a cold wet towel over the wound and replace at regular intervals.

    Rationale: This will keep the area cool.

11. **Action:** Observe the animal for signs of shock and give fluid therapy.

    Fluid replacement is essential to replace the fluid lost from the burned area.

12. **Action:** Give antibiotics and analgesia.

    Burns are extremely susceptible to infection and the pain will continue for some time after the initial treatment.

BITES AND STINGS

Dogs are more commonly affected by bites and stings than cats as they are more curious and will keep nuzzling at a bee or a wasp. Cats may investigate a bee, but will leave it alone very quickly. The most common areas to be affected are the nose, mouth and paws. Insect stings are an emergency only if they have affected the inside of the mouth, nose or throat as there is a risk that the consequent swelling will impede breathing; however, they are painful and will cause localized swelling so the owner is naturally concerned. Anaphylaxis is rare and will present as dyspnoea, urticaria, signs of shock and collapse.

Snake bites are rare in the UK and we have only one venomous species: the European adder (*Viperus berus*). Bites are seasonal, occurring in the spring and summer months. The reaction depends on the amount of venom injected and the individual's response. Dogs often pick up toads whose response to this harassment is to secrete a

Table 3.3 Treatment of bites and stings

Type of bite or sting	Clinical signs	Treatment	Complications
Wasp and hornet stings	Stings are usually around the mouth, nose and feet. The sting does **not** remain in the animal. Causes swelling, pain and salivation if the sting is in the mouth area.	Wash the area with a dilute solution of acetic acid (vinegar).	Watch out for anaphylaxis (rare) – dyspnoea, collapse and other signs of shock.
Bee stings	Stings are usually around the mouth, nose and feet. The sting does remain in the animal. Causes swelling, pain and salivation if the sting is in the mouth area.	The sting has a pumping sac attached to it – remove from the skin using tweezers to hold it at the point of entry. If you grasp it in the middle it will squeeze more liquid into the skin, worsening the effects. Wash the area with a solution containing 1 teaspoon of bicarbonate of soda in a pint of water.	Watch out for anaphylaxis (rare) – dyspnoea, collapse and other signs of shock.
Adder bite (*Viperus berus*)	Bites, usually around the head, neck and paws, are painful and oedematous. Look for a pair of fang marks. Sometimes cause bleeding, pyrexia and shock. Liver and kidney damage have been reported. *Always see an animal that has been bitten.*	Keep animal calm to reduce absorption of the poison. Wash the area thoroughly, but do not rub as this pushes the venom deeper into the tissues. Apply a cold compress to stimulate vasoconstriction in the area, which restricts absorption. Administer antivenom if available. If not use antibiotics and corticosteroids.	Patient's reaction depends on the amount of venom injected. Any snake's mouth is full of bacteria so always treat with antibiotics to prevent infection.
Toad (*Bufo bufo*) venom	Animal will salivate and froth at the mouth. Secretions from the toad's skin taste nasty. If the poison is ingested it may cause bradycardia and muscle paralysis, but this is rare.	If possible wash the animal's mouth out with water. Keep the animal warm and under observation.	Nervous symptoms sometimes develop.

bitter-tasting secretion from their skins, which causes the dog to salivate and froth at the mouth. Table 3.3 describes treatment protocols.

Remember:

- **B**ee stings are acid – use **B**icarbonate!
- **V**asp stings are alkaline – use **V**inegar!

POISONING

VETERINARY POISONS INFORMATION SERVICE (VPIS)

If you are presented with a poisoning case consult the VPIS for advice. It operates a poison specific advice service 24 hours per day, 365 days a year. A charge may be made for the service.

- VPIS, Mary Sheridan House, Guy's Hospital, 13 St Thomas Street, London SE1 9RY
- Tel no: 020 7188 0200
- Email: vpis@gstt.nhs.uk
- Web: www.vpis.co.uk

Poisoning is more common in dogs than cats as they are less discriminating in what they eat. Cats are more sensible, although many cases of feline poisoning are a result of their tendency to keep themselves clean. If anything gets on to the coat or paws (e.g. tar or creosote), a cat will clean it off and so ingest it. Cats will also eat grass that may have been sprayed with herbicide or pesticide and, if they are kept indoors, they may eat pot plants

Table 3.4 Questions to ask the owner of a poisoned animal

Question	Rationale
Do you know what the animal has eaten?	This makes everything much easier and vital time is saved, but often the clinical signs are the first indication that something is wrong. If possible the owner should bring in the packet or container to the surgery to aid identification of the poison.
If the poison was not eaten, by what route did it get into the body?	Not all poisons enter the body by ingestion, although this does account for the majority. They may enter through the lungs (e.g. smoke or gas) the eye, skin or as a bite or sting.
How long have the symptoms been going on?	If the animal is already showing signs this tells you that the poison has already been absorbed and emesis will not work.
How long ago did the animal eat the poison?	This will determine whether inducing emesis is likely to work.
Has the animal vomited?	This could indicate that the animal has got rid of the poison and it will influence your treatment, but it may be a symptom of the poison.
Did the animal eat anything unusual prior to the onset of symptoms?	If a sample is available the owner should bring it to the surgery.
Was the animal missing before the onset of symptoms? If so where?	If the owner knows where, e.g. trapped in a shed or garage, the premises should be searched for a possible source of poison.
Is there any substance on the animal's coat, paws or in the mouth?	This could provide direct evidence of the possible cause of the symptoms.
Have you noticed any human or animal medication that is missing?	This may help you to identify the poison. Ask the owner to bring in the packet.
Did the owner use any potentially harmful product in the house or garden prior to the onset of symptoms?	Animals may react to cleaning products or to garden chemicals. This may help you to identify the poison. Ask the owner to bring in the packet.

– such as spider plants (*Chlorophyton*) or cut flowers (e.g. lilies).

The first step towards treating a poisoned patient is to ask the right questions. These may be put to the owner over the telephone or when the animal is brought in, but in either case it is vital to get the information quickly as the longer a poison is in the stomach the sooner it will be absorbed into the system and cause clinical signs. Table 3.4 suggests questions that should be asked prior to treatment.

Procedure: General treatment of poisoning

Remember to keep calm and start some form of treatment as soon as you can. You may never know what the animal has eaten or breathed in, and your treatment will be based on the evidence of the clinical signs.

1. **Action:** Take a comprehensive history from the owner, either over the telephone or in the surgery (Table 3.4).

   Rationale: This will provide you with the facts on which to base your treatment.

2. **Action:** If the animal is still in contact with the poison it must be removed immediately – this is most likely to be done by the owner, who may be panicking.

   Rationale:

   a. *If the animal is suffering from inhalation of smoke or carbon monoxide it must be taken into the fresh air.*

b. *If the animal has coat/skin/paw contamination (e.g. tar), advise putting a T-shirt or towel around the animal and/or socks on the paws to prevent it licking the chemical while it is brought to the surgery. In the surgery, use an Elizabethan collar.*

3. **Action:** If possible identify the poison.

   Rationale: This will be deduced from the owner's information, the packet or label of the poison and the clinical signs. It will determine your treatment.

4. **Action:** Induce emesis.

   Rationale: This is done to prevent further absorption of the poison.

   » Emesis is ineffective if the poison has been ingested for more than 4 hours. If clinical signs are occurring it may be too late.

   » NEVER induce emesis if the poison is known to be irritant, corrosive, or if the animal is unconscious or fitting.

   » If emesis is an option, ask the owner to make the animal vomit while still at home. If he/she cannot do this, do not waste time but bring the animal into the surgery immediately. For suggested emetics see Table 3.5.

5. **Action:** If the animal has collapsed or is unconscious then administer oxygen.

   Rationale: Basic first aid procedure to maintain oxygen levels in the brain and other organs.

6. **Action:** Administer intravenous fluids, or if the animal is conscious give oral fluids.

   Rationale: Administration of fluids will dilute and flush out the poison and reduce damage to the tissues.

7. **Action:** Administer an antidote if there is one.

   Rationale: In ethylene glycol poisoning the antidote is intravenous ethanol – vodka is recommended. Very few poisons have an antidote.

8. **Action:** If the animal has swallowed an irritant or corrosive poison (e.g. white spirit, creosote, petrol), try to coat the lining of the stomach with a demulcent agent (Table 3.6).

   Rationale: Demulcents coat the stomach and help to bind the poison, reducing the chances of absorption.

9. **Action:** If the animal is unconscious, using a wide bore stomach tube, wash out the stomach with warm water or saline (gastric lavage) and repeat until the washings are clear. Then replace with absorbent granules e.g. BCK (Table 3.6).

   Rationale: Gastric lavage will wash out the poison and BCK granules will absorb any remains. This should be done only if the animal is unconscious or under a general anaesthetic.

Table 3.5 Emetic agents

Emetic	Method
Apomorphine	Dogs only; 20–40 μg/kg i.v. or 40–100 μg/kg s.c. or i.m. Emesis will occur within 10 min. Do not use in rabbits as they are unable to vomit.
Xylazine	Cats only; 1–3 mg/kg i.m. or lower dose i.v.
Washing soda crystals	Two crystals placed on the back of the tongue.
Mustard	2 teaspoons in a cup of warm water. Not very effective.

NB Do NOT use salt solution as an emetic as it may cause dehydration and electrolyte imbalance.

Table 3.6 Demulcent agents

Demulcent	Method
BCK granules	1–3 heaped teaspoons given orally. May have to be mixed with food or water and given by syringe or stomach tube.
Charcoal	1 g/kg orally. May have to be mixed with food or water and given by syringe or stomach tube.
Kaolin	1–2 ml/kg orally.
Raw beaten egg + 1 teaspoon of sugar + a little milk	Given orally. Egg and milk coagulate on the lining of the stomach.

10.   **Action:** If the skin is contaminated (a particular problem in cats) take steps to prevent ingestion and wash with an appropriate agent. Dry the animal and keep under observation.

Rationale: Different contaminants require different cleaning agents:

»   **Non-oily compounds** – e.g. disinfectants. Do not use detergents as they may increase skin absorption. Use copious amounts of water.

»   **Liquid oily compounds** – e.g. sump oil, creosote. Smear in Swarfega®, liquid paraffin or cooking oil and wash thoroughly until all smell has gone.

»   **Solid oily compounds** – e.g. tar. Cut away contaminated fur. Rub butter, vegetable oil or liquid paraffin into the area to soften the tar. Bandage for 15 minutes while warmth of the skin causes further softening. Wash thoroughly.

11.   **Action:** Identify any other clinical signs and treat appropriately.

Rationale: Different poisons will cause a range of different clinical signs that need treatment. (See list of most common poisons below.)

12.   **Action:** Once specific treatment has been completed make sure that the animal is warm by covering in blankets and placing in a warm kennel.

Rationale: Some poisons will lower the body temperature whereas others may raise it.

13.   **Action:** Monitor the animal's condition continually.

Rationale: The condition may change and it is vital to act quickly.

The most common poisons (VPIS 2011 – based on most frequent enquiries) are:

• **Chocolate** – particularly associated with dogs, although cats, rodents and rabbits are also susceptible. It contains theobromine, which is similar in its effects to caffeine and depends on the amount ingested and the type of chocolate; white chocolate is not really toxic; milk chocolate requires treatment for ingestion of over 9 g/kg body weight; dark chocolate requires treatment for 1 g/kg.

The *clinical signs* include diarrhoea, vomiting, dehydration progressing to hyperactivity, hyperthermia and hypertension, and often severe tachycardia. Muscular rigidity, tremors and convulsions may also be seen.

Treatment is largely supportive and includes fluid therapy, sedation and use of activated charcoal to speed up elimination. Regular monitoring is required over a period of time as theobromine undergoes enterohepatic recirculation.

• **Ethylene glycol** – this is found in antifreeze, screenwash and some deicers. It is toxic to all animals, particularly cats. It is sweet tasting so is palatable and just a few millilitres cause toxicity and death. Ethylene glycol is not the main poison but it is metabolized to glycolic acid, which causes acidosis. It is then further metabolized to oxalate, which causes renal damage and binds to calcium, forming calcium oxalate, resulting in hypocalcaemia. Calcium oxalate crystals will appear in the urine of affected animals.

The *clinical signs* of toxicity are those of acute renal failure and the treatment is aimed at blocking the formation of the toxic metabolites. The earlier treatment can be instigated the better is the prognosis.

The *specific antidote* is ethanol and its most obtainable form is as vodka. It should be given within the first 12 hours and no later than 24 hours after ingestion. It is detrimental if this is administered once the animal is in renal failure. Ethanol blocks the metabolism of ethylene glycol with no formation of the toxic metabolites.

• **Lily poisoning** (*Lilium* spp.) – cats are particularly susceptible. All parts of the lily are poisonous, even the flowers and the pollen, which may brush off on to the coat and be licked off. At present the toxic mechanism is unknown, but it is known that the poison causes renal failure.

Clinical signs begin within 2–6 hours of ingestion and vomiting is an early sign. Cats may show anorexia, depression and within 24–72 hours there will be signs of renal failure. These include a rise in urea, creatinine, potassium and phosphorus levels, haematuria, proteinuria and glycosuria. Other signs include polydipsia and polyuria, pancreatitis and convulsions. Chronic renal failure may occur in the long term.

Treatment should be started as soon as poisoning is suspected – treatment started 18 hours after ingestion has a poor prognosis. The aim should be to limit absorption by gastric decontamination and treat as for acute renal failure using aggressive fluid therapy and constant monitoring of kidney function.

• **Metaldehyde** – found in slug pellets, which are usually green or blue, and can cause significant signs within an hour of consumption. If the animal is suspected of having ingested pellets it should be treated as soon as possible, as rapid intervention can save the animal's life.

Clinical signs include hyperaesthesia and incoordination, muscle spasms and rigidity, opisthotonus and convulsions. *Treatment* is largely supportive and should include heavy sedation and control of the convulsions.

Be aware that not all slug pellets contain metaldehyde – some contain ferric phosphate and methiocarb. Ask the owner to bring in the packet to aid identification of the poison.

- **NSAIDS** – a range of non-steroidals are used in human medicine as anti-inflammatories and pain killers and it is not uncommon for them to be ingested by dogs. Ibuprofen is particularly poisonous.

  Clinical signs, which may develop quickly, include vomiting with the presence of blood, diarrhoea, weakness and depression, abdominal tenderness and gastric ulceration. Renal impairment may develop within 5 days and these animals are at greater risk.

  Treatment is aimed at getting rid of the toxin and protection of the gastrointestinal tract. Induction of emesis, fluid therapy and use of activated charcoal to protect the gastric mucosa are all recommended, as is the monitoring of renal function.

- **Permethrin** – found in some flea treatments available from supermarkets and pharmacies. Cats are very sensitive and poisoning often occurs when 'spot-on' treatments recommended for dogs are used on cats.

  Clinical signs can occur rapidly and may be seen as muscle twitching, tremors and convulsions, and fatalities are common. *Treatment* should be supportive including clipping the fur and washing the skin thoroughly with lukewarm water and detergent to prevent further absorption. Control the convulsions with diazepam, which is sometimes ineffective. Careful infusion of propofol may be effective in some cases.

- **Rodenticides** – two types are in common use:

  - **Anticoagulants** – often referred to as warfarin and its derivatives. These are designed to kill rats and mice by interfering with the clotting cascade, causing massive coagulopathy and haemorrhage. When eaten by dogs and cats the effects may be the same. However, small one-off doses may not cause any problems, but in excess or in repeated doses clinical signs may be seen but can be delayed for several days.

    Diagnosis and *treatment* include regular clotting tests in asymptomatic cases, oral vitamin K and in severe cases fresh plasma and blood transfusion.

  - **Alphachlorulose** – sometimes known as humane mouse killers because the victim falls asleep and dies of hypothermia. An animal eating the poison or possibly eating a dead mouse may become sleepy and suffer from hypothermia.

    Treatment should consist of keeping the animal warm and fluid therapy to prevent dehydration and flush out the toxin. Recovery should occur within 24 hours.

  It is important to determine which rodenticide has been ingested before beginning treatment.

- **Xylitol** – this is an artificial sweetener commonly used in chewing gum, sweets, human and veterinary medicines and as a sugar substitute in baking. When an animal eats its owner's medication it may be affected by xylitol as well as the core ingredient.

  Xylitol is extremely harmful to dogs and acts as a potent stimulator of insulin release causing hypoglycaemia. *Clinical signs* that may develop within an hour or be delayed for 24–48 hours include vomiting, ataxia, tachycardia, convulsions and coma. In severe cases dogs may develop metabolic acidosis, status epilepticus and cerebral anoxia. Liver failure has also been recorded.

  Treatment involves the management of hypoglycaemia and monitoring glucose levels and being aware of possible associated liver dysfunction.

DYSTOCIA – DIFFICULT BIRTH

Dystocia is rare in the queen but relatively common in the bitch, particularly those of brachycephalic breeds such as the bulldog.

Normal presentation of puppies and kittens is either anterior (head first) or posterior (feet first) with the head or hind legs fully extended and the dorsum uppermost (Fig. 3.6). Any other position may cause dystocia.

Procedure: Diagnosis of dystocia and subsequent obstetrical manipulation

1. **Action:** Make sure that you are familiar with the length of the gestation period and the timing of events associated with normal parturition in the dog and cat (Table 3.7).

   Rationale: This will enable you to make an accurate assessment of any problems when contacted by the owner.

2. **Action:** Take an accurate history from the owner and write it down.

   Rationale: Written notes can be referred to later on and they ensure that you do not forget any of the details. Take particular notice of the following:

   » Breed and age of bitch or queen
   » Date of mating – to estimate stage of pregnancy
   » Has the owner done anything to assist the bitch or queen – for example, administering herbal remedies such as raspberry leaf tea?

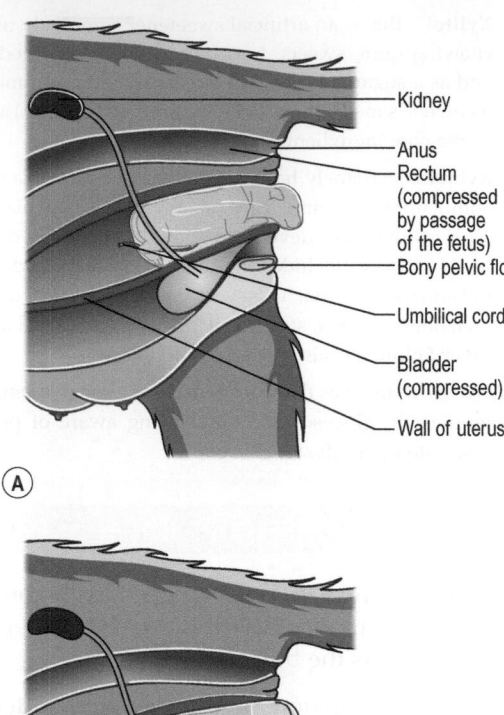

Kidney

Anus

Rectum
(compressed
by passage
of the fetus)

Bony pelvic floor

Umbilical cord

Bladder
(compressed)

Wall of uterus

(A)

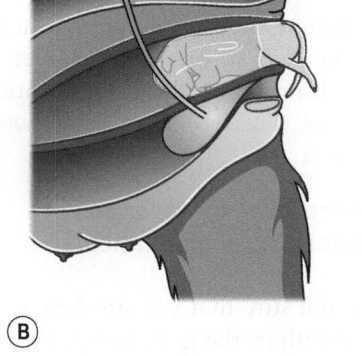

(B)

Figure 3.6 Normal birth in the bitch: (A) anterior presentation; (B) posterior presentation.

3. **Action:** Ask the owner to describe the course of events paying particular attention to the timing.

   Rationale: This will allow you to assess whether the birth is progressing normally or whether this is a case of dystocia. Table 3.7 describes the normal signs of parturition in the bitch and queen.

4. **Action:** If you are concerned you should ask the owner to bring the animal into the surgery. If some puppies or kittens have been delivered they should be placed in a warm, covered box and brought in with the dam.

Box 3.4 Possible causes for concern

- A bitch that has passed 70 days of gestation and is showing no sign of starting parturition.
- A queen that has passed 65 days of gestation and shows no sign of starting parturition. Be aware that Persians and Siamese often go up to 70 days' gestation.
- The dam is restless, strains forcefully but infrequently.
- Straining begins and then ceases.
- A black or greenish discharge has been produced but there are no signs of parturition.
- Parturition has not started within 48 hours of a drop in body temperature.
- Ineffectual straining for over an hour with no progress.
- Several fetuses have been produced, the last more than 2 hours ago, and the dam is restless.
- Several fetuses have been produced, the last more than 2 hours ago, and a large litter is expected. This may not be known by the owner, but can be deduced by the breed and examination of the abdomen.

Rationale: So that you can examine the animal and assess the problem. Box 3.4 lists possible causes for concern, but it is impossible to cover every eventuality. Any neonates must be kept warm when they are brought to the surgery so as to prevent hypothermia. If this happens in the early evening it is better to see the animal before you go to bed – you may be woken in the middle of the night!

5. **Action:** Place the dam on a stable table to make your examination.

   Rationale: The dam will feel more relaxed if she feels comfortable.

6. **Action:** Ask the owner to restrain the head of the dam while you examine her (see Ch. 1).

   Rationale: Some animals may resent palpation and try to jump off the table or to bite you.

7. **Action:** First check that the dam is pregnant by examination of the abdomen.

   Rationale: Some owners are so keen for their animal to be pregnant that they misinterpret the signs (e.g. weight gain and abdominal swelling could be due to obesity). This can be

Table 3.7 Normal stages of parturition in the bitch and queen*

Stage	Definition	Symptoms
Preparation	May last for several days and provides an indication that the parturition is imminent.	Nesting, restlessness, may seek out the company of the owner. Prepartum hypothermia, due to declining concentration of plasma progesterone, may occur and the body temperature may fall to below 37°C within 24–36 hours of birth. Relaxation and softening of the vulva.
Stage 1	Start of contractions until the cervix is fully dilated. May last for 24 hours in the bitch, but is difficult to assess as start of contractions is very gradual.	Onset of uterine contractions, which push against the dilating cervix. Allantoic fluid may drain from the vulva owing to the rupture of the allantochorion (first water bag). The dam may appear uncomfortable and restless. Vomiting, shivering and/or loss of appetite may occur.
Stage 2	Full dilation of the cervix until the delivery of the fetus. Puppies may be born every 20–30 minutes, whereas kittens may be born every 30–60 minutes.	Strong uterine contractions push the fetus through the dilated cervix and into the vagina. The fetus may be in anterior or posterior presentation and the amniotic sac surrounding the puppy or kitten may rupture. This is normal and allows the neonate to breathe when born. The dam may break the sac but if not, it must be broken rapidly.
Stage 3	Delivery of the placenta. Usually complete with 30–60 minutes.	Placenta is expelled from the vulva and may be eaten by the dam. Stages 2 and 3 may be mixed up in multiparous species.
Puerperium	Period during which the uterus involutes and returns to normal. It may last for several weeks.	A dark discharge known as the lochia may drain from the dam for up to a week after parturition. As long as this odourless and the dam is well there is no need to worry.

*After Aspinall 2008a, p 209, with permission of Elsevier Butterworth-Heinemann.

done by palpation, auscultation of the fetal heartbeats, ultrasonography and radiography.

8. **Action:** Clean the vulval area of the dam with antiseptic solution and, using a well-lubricated gloved finger, examine the vagina.

    Rationale: The area should be cleaned to prevent the introduction of infection. Gloves should be worn to prevent transmission of infection. Lubrication facilitates digital examination and prevents damage and drying of the vaginal mucosa.

9. **Action:** Check for the presence and presentation of a puppy in the birth canal (Fig. 3.6). Do not apply undue force as you may damage the bitch. Most live puppies make sucking movements when a finger is put in their mouths.

    Rationale: If a puppy is present you should be able to feel a nose and forepaws or the extended hindlegs. If you can feel the rump and tail the puppy may be in a breech position, which will cause a problem. Note: digital examination is

almost impossible in the queen as the vagina is too small.

10. **Action:** Take note of any bony or soft tissue abnormalities in the pelvic canal.

    Rationale: Problems such as a previous pelvic fracture, a vaginal polyp or a congenital malformation may make normal delivery impossible.

11. **Action:** If you can feel a puppy far down the birth canal and it appears to be normally presented give an injection of oxytocin. Put the bitch in a warm kennel and wait for 10–20 minutes.

    Rationale: Oxytocin should never be given if there is any sign of an obstruction or if the cervix is not thought to be relaxed as this can lead to uterine rupture. It produces powerful rhythmic contractions resulting in delivery within approximately 20 minutes (Box 3.5).

12. **Action:** If you can feel a puppy within the caudal birth canal you may be able to assist

Box 3.5 Dose rates of oxytocin and calcium salts

Oxytocin

- Dogs: 0.1–0.5 IU/kg i.m.
- Cats: 0.1–0.5 IU/kg i.m.
- Rabbits: 0.1–3.0 IU/kg s.c. or i.m.

Calcium salts

- Dogs: 50–150 mg/kg = 0.5–1.5 ml/kg of 10% solution of calcium borogluconate given i.v. over 20–30 min.
- Cats: 95–140 kg = 1–1.5 ml/kg of 10% solution of calcium gluconate given i.v. over 10 –20 min.
- Rabbits: 100 mg/kg i.m. or i.p.

NB If calcium (boro)gluconate is given too rapidly it may cause hypotension, cardiac arrhythmias and cardiac arrest.

delivery manually. This may be done using your fingers or whelping forceps. There is a risk of causing vaginal or fetal damage using whelping forceps; using a clean strong teaspoon, like a vectis, in conjunction with a forefinger to ease the head out may be preferable. Use water soluble lubricant to aid the passage of the puppy.

Rationale: Apply traction when the bitch is straining. Pressure on the roof of the vagina with your finger may elicit a contraction. Form a cradle using your thumb and forefinger or whelping forceps around the puppy's head or hips and pull gently; a sterile gauze swab may help you grip. Pull downwards towards the bitch's feet in a C-shaped arc. Avoid using undue force as it may cause damage to the head, neck or feet.

13. **Action:** When the puppy has been delivered it should be wrapped in a dry towel and rubbed vigorously to stimulate respiration.

    Rationale: The roughness of the towel will simulate the licking of the bitch and should result in the puppy taking its first gasping breath. If the puppy fails to breathe within a few minutes, use a respiratory stimulant such as an oral solution of doxapram applied sublingually.

14. **Action:** Once the puppy is breathing well, quickly check it over for any signs of damage or congenital abnormalities and place it with the bitch. It is vital to keep the puppy warm; if the bitch is busy delivering subsequent puppies, it may be better to place the puppy in a warm box covered in a towel (Box 3.6).

    Rationale: If there is evidence of a cleft palate or a harelip it may be better to euthanize the puppy at this stage. Hypothermia will kill a neonate more quickly than anything else so warmth is important. If the bitch is worried by the puppy being taken away, allow her to look after it.

15. **Action:** Give an injection of oxytocin intramuscularly.

    Rationale: To further strengthen uterine contractions. There is a risk of secondary uterine inertia if the bitch has been straining for some time.

16. **Action:** Place the bitch and her puppy in a warm kennel and cover the front with a blanket or towel. Keep under surreptitious observation every 10 minutes.

    Rationale: Many bitches will whelp only in private. All being well, the bitch should now deliver the rest of the litter but must be checked regularly to monitor her progress.

NB If a bitch still fails to deliver the puppies after the administration of oxytocin, a caesarean section should be considered. When dealing with a kittening queen, digital examination of the birth is difficult because of the size. Oxytocin can be used, but if there is no subsequent delivery a caesarean must be performed.

Table 3.8 describes the possible causes of dystocia.

CAESAREAN SECTION (HYSTEROTOMY)

This is a technique used to make a temporary opening into the uterus to remove as quickly as possible full term fetuses that are unable to be delivered as a result of some form of dystocia (Table 3.8). Caesarean section may also be performed as an elective procedure where dystocia is anticipated (e.g. in some brachycephalic breeds).

Box 3.6 Care of the neonate

Correct resuscitation and care of the neonate are vital for survival, no matter whether it has been delivered naturally or by caesarean section:

Clear the airway and establish respiration:
- Remove the amniotic sac from the head and the mouth.
- Clear any mucus from the mouth using a dry towel or lint-free swab to absorb the fluid.
- Rub vigorously with a towel and allow the animal to breathe. If it is not, gently compress the chest to massage the heart.
- Use suction with a small pipette to remove fluid.
- If necessary gently swing the body downwards, being careful to support the head and neck by placing two fingers along the cervical spine. This uses centrifugal force to remove fluid from the mouth and airways.
- Keep up resuscitation for at least 15 minutes – some animals take time to breathe and this may be due to the depressive effect of the anaesthetic protocol.

Cut the umbilical cord:
- Immediately after the neonate is delivered, place two pairs of artery forceps on the cord and cut between

them. Remaining length of cord should be about 3 cm – if it is too short it may result in a hernia; if too long the dam may bite it and eat into the abdominal wall.
- Excessive bleeding should be stopped by ligation.

Check that the dam is **producing milk** by gently squeezing a teat. If no milk is there give oxytocin to encourage 'let down'. Check that the neonates are **suckling** so that they receive their colostrum.

Maintain the litter at an **environmental temperature** of 25–30°C for the first few days and then reduce to around 22°C providing that there are no draughts. Hypothermia will kill.

On days 1, 2, 3 and then weekly, **weigh each neonate**. This enables you to check that they are feeding and to monitor their progress.

During the first few days examine each neonate and check for **congenital abnormalities,** e.g. cleft palate, hare lip, umbilical hernia, hydrocephalus, atresia ani, microophthalmia, polydactyly. If you think that the condition is life threatening or will affect the animal's quality of life then consider euthanasia.

Table 3.8 Possible causes of dystocia

Cause	Description	Treatment
Maternal dystocia – due to factors in the dam	Primary uterine inertia – contractions may fail to start or begin weakly and then cease. May be due to large litters, very small litters or seen in large, fat, unfit bitches. This is rare in cats.	Oxytocin, but monitor regularly as there is a risk of fetal death if placental separation has occurred. Do not leave too long before performing a caesarean section.
	Secondary uterine inertia – contractions start and then cease. May be due to exhaustion after delivery of a large litter or after obstructive dystocia.	Having made sure that this is not a case of obstructive dystocia, give i.v. oxytocin and calcium borogluconate (Box 3.5) to strengthen contractions. Monitor regularly and perform a caesarean section if delivery does not occur within 20 minutes.
	Obstruction of the birth canal – due to pelvic deformities, neoplasia or torsion of the uterus.	Obstruction may not be able to be rectified so caesarean section is required.
Fetal dystocia – due to factors caused by the fetus	Fetal oversize – may be a result of: • Breed conformation, e.g. large head size, brachycephalic breeds • Large fetus as a result of a small litter • Fetal monsters, e.g. conjoined twins.	Caesarean section will usually be necessary.
	Incorrect presentation – fetus is misaligned so that it cannot proceed through the birth canal.	It may be possible to reposition the puppy by gently pushing it back and repositioning, but this is possible only in large breeds. In most cases, caesarean section is necessary.

A midline incision is usually performed in both dogs and cats as this provides good access to the uterus and the dam can lie comfortably on both sides. There is a risk that the claws of the neonates might interfere with the wound while suckling, but this can be minimized by the use of subcuticular sutures.

Anaesthesia

Pregnancy may affect the requirements for anaesthesia and the dam may be debilitated by prolonged parturition, but whichever anaesthetic regimen is used it must:

- Ensure adequate oxygenation of the dam and fetus.
- Maintain blood volume and prevent hypotension.
- Minimize depression of the fetus and dam after surgery.

Various regimens are used and they must take into account the physiological status of the dam. To some extent the choice may be left to the personal preferences of the surgeon. Common methods are:

- Rapid intravenous induction agent (e.g. propofol or alfaxalone) followed by maintenance using a volatile agent (e.g. isofluorane). Propofol is rapidly metabolized by the bitch so recovery is quicker.
- Induction using a volatile agent delivered by mask. This may be used in small dogs and cats, but it may be stressful to the dam and result in a potentially damaging struggle.

Intravenous fluid therapy should also be considered especially if parturition has been going on for a long time, if a long operation is anticipated or if a hysterectomy is also to be performed.

Procedure: Caesarean section

1. **Action:** Before administering the anaesthetic, clip and do the preliminary preparation for a midline ventral abdominal incision.

   Rationale: This minimizes the time from induction to delivery, which is better for the well-being of the neonates.

2. **Action:** If possible, administer oxygen by mask to the dam.

   Rationale: This raises the blood oxygen levels to help the fetuses.

3. **Action:** Place an intravenous catheter in the cephalic vein (see Ch. 1).

   Rationale: To administer intravenous fluid therapy if necessary.

4. **Action:** Administer the chosen anaesthetic regimen as described above.

   Rationale: The aims of the regimen have been described previously.

5. **Action:** Move the dam into the operating theatre and place her on a sterile sheet of synthetic fleece. Position her in dorsal recumbency and slightly tilted to one side. Do the final aseptic preparation of the surgical site while the dam is being attached to the anaesthetic machine for maintenance of the anaesthetic using a volatile agent.

   Rationale: The surgical procedure must be as sterile as possible. Using a sheet of synthetic fleece keeps the body warm and helps to absorb parturient fluids, which would otherwise soak the fur. Slightly tilting the body to one side encourages venous return, which may be reduced by the weight of the uterus on the vena cava.

6. **Action:** Make a ventral midline incision from just cranial to the umbilicus to close to the pubis.

   Rationale: The incision must be long enough to allow exteriorization of the entire gravid uterus.

7. **Action:** Lift the external rectus sheath before making a stab incision through the linea alba.

   Rationale: To prevent accidental stabbing of the gravid uterus.

8. **Action:** Carefully lift the gravid uterine horns out of the incision.

   Rationale: Avoid pulling the horns through the incision as the uterine vessels are easily avulsed and the uterine wall may tear. Rough handling may cause a haematoma in the broad ligament.

9. **Action:** Isolate the uterus from the remainder of the peritoneal cavity using sterile towels or pads.

Rationale: To prevent contamination with amniotic fluids.

10. **Action:** For small litters, tent and then incise the uterine body; for larger litters, it may be necessary to make two incisions: one in the middle of each uterine horn. Make the incisions between adjacent placentae.

Rationale: To prevent laceration of the fetus and to prevent haemorrhage from the placentae.

11. **Action:** Extend the incision(s) using Metzenbaum scissors.

Rationale: The incision must be long enough to prevent tearing when the fetuses are brought out.

12. **Action:** Do not waste time trying to stop bleeding from the wound edges.

Rationale: This will stop quite naturally as the uterus involutes.

13. **Action:** Empty each horn by gently milking each conceptus from its cranial end towards the incision. Grasp it and gently pull it from the uterus.

Rationale: The wet coat of the fetus helps to prevent damage, but it should be treated gently and with respect.

14. **Action:** Rupture each amniotic sac, remove the puppy and clamp each umbilical cord with a pair of artery forceps as each fetus is presented (Fig. 3.7).

Rationale: The fetus should start to splutter and breathe as its head is freed from the amnion and the cord is clamped. Make sure that traction on the cord does not cause an umbilical hernia.

15. **Action:** Hand the neonate to your assistant who will rub it dry.

Rationale: It is important to carry out a resuscitation procedure immediately the neonate is delivered (Box 3.6).

16. **Action:** If the placenta has not separated, gently peel it away from the endometrium. Do not forcibly pull the placenta away as this may cause severe haemorrhage.

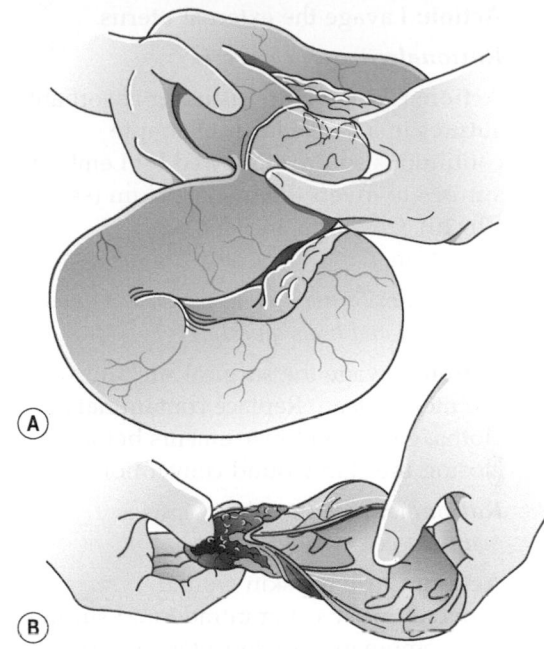

Figure 3.7 (A) A fetus is gently brought up to the incision site and removed with the placenta. (B) The amniotic sac is broken and removed from the fetus.

Rationale: At term the placenta is often expelled with the neonate. In elective caesareans carried out too early you may find it difficult to remove the placentae, in which case they should be left to pass out naturally per vaginum.

17. **Action:** Palpate the vagina and remove any fetuses from this position. The fetus may be dead and you should pack around the uterus with damp swabs while removing it. Remember to remove all swabs prior to closing the surgical site.

Rationale: To prevent contamination of the peritoneal cavity.

18. **Action:** Check the uterus before repairing your incision(s).

Rationale: To make sure that you have not left any fetuses in the uterus.

19. **Action:** Administer oxytocin if contractions are not visible (Box 3.5).

Rationale: To aid involution. Contractions often start when the fetuses are removed.

20. **Action:** Lavage the external uterus.

    Rationale: To remove debris.

21. **Action:** Close the uterus using absorbable sutures in a single layer of simple continuous sutures followed by Lembert sutures to invert the myometrium (see Ch. 10). Cover the incision with omentum.

    Rationale: To ensure that the wound seals effectively and heals quickly.

22. **Action:** Lavage the surgical site and wipe the uterus clean. Replace contaminated cloths, gloves and instruments before closing the skin wound conventionally.

    Rationale: To ensure that asepsis is maintained.

23. **Action:** Close the skin wound conventionally using intradermal sutures or a combination of subcutaneous and skin sutures (see Ch. 10).

    Rationale: These prevent the suckling neonates from interfering with the sutures.

24. **Action:** Give oxytocin if it has not already been given.

    Rationale: Oxytocin speeds up involution and the evacuation of the lochia. Blood-stained fluids may drain in diminishing quantities for several days. They may not always be noticed as the dam will clean herself, but it is important to ask the owner to observe quantity, colour and smell as this will provide evidence of the dam's recovery.

25. **Action:** Clean the wound and remove any debris from the ventral abdomen. Make sure that the dam is as dry as possible and put her in a warm kennel with her offspring to recover from the anaesthetic.

    Rationale: Both dam and offspring must be kept warm and dry. Wet fur will cause chilling and will not impress the owner. Use a hairdryer if necessary. If the dam shakes or struggles during recovery so that there is a risk of injuring the neonates, put them in a warm box and introduce them as soon as the dam is sufficiently recovered to take notice of them.

26. **Action:** Observe at regular intervals to make sure the dam has recovered and is taking notice of her offspring. When you are satisfied that they are suckling and that all is well, the dam can go home.

    Rationale: Taking a little time to ensure that everything is progressing as expected will save you time later and result in a healthy litter and client satisfaction.

Potential complications of caesarean section

1. Residual anaesthetic effect on the dam and the neonates. The dam may take time to recover and the neonates may be very sleepy until the effects wear off.

2. Risk of uterine rupture, haemorrhage and hypovolaemic shock.

3. Postoperative infection and wound breakdown.

4. Interference of the abdominal wound by the neonates.

5. Maternal rejection of the litter – may be more common in maiden dams. It may be helped by putting the litter with the dam as soon as possible after surgery. Try squeezing milk onto the neonates' heads so that they carry the smell of the dam. Keep the dam and her litter under observation until you are certain that all is well. If the dam does not accept her litter you must consider hand rearing or fostering.

ECLAMPSIA OR PUERPERAL TETANY

- This is mainly seen in the bitch and is physiologically related to milk fever in the cow.

- Caused by hypocalcaemia – milk contains high levels of calcium, which is taken from the blood and is unavailable for muscle and nerve function.

- Most often occurs at around 3 weeks post-whelping when production of milk reaches a peak and puppies are making high nutritional demands on the bitch prior to weaning. May occur earlier in lactation or in late pregnancy.

- Most common in small breeds (e.g. West Highland White terriers, Yorkshire terriers).

- May occur in large litters in which the puppies are doing particularly well.
- *Clinical signs* include shaking, muscle tremors, panting, whining, disorientation and salivation. If untreated the condition may progress to tonic or clonic muscular spasms.
- There is a risk that the bitch may die if untreated so these animals should be seen quickly.
- *Treatment* – give 5–20 ml of 10% calcium borogluconate intravenously. Administer this slowly (Box 3.5) and then give the same volume subcutaneously.
- Keep the bitch under observation until she has recovered. Recovery is usually rapid but there is a risk of relapse.
- Feed the puppies artificially for 24 hours.
- If the puppies are old enough consider weaning them. If not, consider removing half the litter and feeding them artificially and allow the remainder to suckle the bitch. Change the group around the next day and so on until they are old enough to wean.
- Oral calcium supplementation in at-risk breeds has not been found to work as it may depress the levels of parathyroid hormone and exacerbate the problem.

EPILEPSY

Epilepsy may be defined as an irritable focus within the brain that causes disorganized electrical activity resulting in convulsions or 'fits' or seizures. These convulsions are violent and uncoordinated contractions of the muscles due to abnormal cerebral stimulation; if they become continuous (i.e. one fit leads into another) this is described as **status epilepticus.**

There are many potential causes of epilepsy and these are listed in Box 3.7, but in the majority of cases the cause is never identified and treatment is symptomatic.

Clinical signs – these are divided into three phases:

1. **Pre-ictal phase** – warning signs. The animal is described as having an 'aura' in which it may appear to be apprehensive, seek out the

---

Box 3.7 Suggested causes of epilepsy

- Idiopathic – may be a familial or breed disposition
- Viral or bacterial infection, e.g. distemper or hepatitis
- Intracranial trauma leading to a rise in intracranial pressure
- Brain tumour
- Hydrocephalus – congenital
- Cerebral anoxia – most common cause is anaesthesia
- Portosystemic shunt – fits may develop soon after eating
- Hypocalcaemia – associated with eclampsia
- Hypoglycaemia – possible overdose of insulin in the treatment of diabetes mellitus, insulinoma
- Hypokalaemia
- Chronic liver disease – in the advanced stages
- Acute renal failure
- Chronic renal failure – in the advanced stages
- Poisons – such as lead, cyanide, metaldehyde

---

company of its owner and be generally restless.

2. **Ictal phase** – the actual fit. The animal falls onto its side, the limbs paddle and the jaws champ resulting in the formation of frothy saliva, described as 'foaming at the mouth'. The eyes will be open and staring and the animal is unaware of its surroundings. It may make a noise and may lose control of its bladder and anus. These convulsions may be:

   a. Tonic – sustained contractions with no periods of relaxation.

   b. Clonic – contractions that are interspersed with periods of relaxation.

3. **Post-ictal phase** – recovery. The animal will be exhausted by the fit and although it will be physically back to normal it will lie down and sleep for some time. The length of this episode will vary but the average time will be between 5 and 30 minutes.

Procedure: Care of the epileptic patient

In the majority of cases the fit will occur at home and advice to the owner will be given over the telephone. Little can be done during the fit and it is rare for an animal to die unless it is due to terminal liver or kidney disease or to some form of poisoning. When talking to the owner it is important to find out what might have caused the fit, how long it lasted and how often the fits occur.

1. **Action:** Make sure that the dog is left with just one person in the room.

   Rationale: A convulsing animal can be a source of interest/horror to people in the room. They should be discouraged from watching as their noise and presence will act as a stimulant, which may prolong the fit. One person should be present to ensure the safety of the animal.

2. **Action:** Advise the owner to avoid touching or talking to the animal.

   Rationale: Both sound and touch may stimulate the animal and as it is unaware of its surroundings it will not be comforted. There is a risk that the owner may be inadvertently bitten.

3. **Action:** The lights in the room should be dimmed, but leave a side light on. Draw the curtains if the sun is shining into the room.

   Rationale: Light will stimulate the animal, but there should be enough light to see what is happening.

4. **Action:** Make sure that the room is quiet; turn off the radio or television.

   Rationale: Noise will stimulate the animal. Radio and television produce high-pitched sound waves of which we are unaware, but which may be picked up by the animal brain.

5. **Action:** Move all furniture out of the way, paying attention to anything that might be dragged over by the animal's feet (e.g. stools or small tables).

   Rationale: To prevent damage to the animal.

6. **Action:** Ask the owner to observe the animal quietly and calmly, noting what happens and how the long the fit lasts.

   Rationale: These facts will help your subsequent diagnosis and treatment.

7. **Action:** Ask the owner to ring you when the fit is over or, if the fit does not stop, to ring you in 15–20 minutes.

Rationale: Most fits will stop within a few minutes and you need to know that it is over. If the fit does not stop you will need to consider status epilepticus.

8. **Action:** If the fit stops within the expected time you should warn the owner of what to expect and arrange to see the animal during the next surgery. Meanwhile the owner should allow the animal to sleep.

   Rationale: You can do little during the fit, but you should examine the animal and talk to the owner during the next surgery. At this stage you should be considering treatment versus quality of the animal's life.

9. **Action:** If the fit continues the animal may be in status epilepticus and it should be brought to the surgery for treatment as soon as possible.

   Rationale: When one fit runs into another there is a risk of cerebral oedema and consequent brain stem herniation and death. Treatment should be instigated as soon as possible and cannot be carried out at the owner's home.

Procedure: Treatment of the epileptic patient

NB Acepromazine and other phenothiazines are not recommended for epileptic patients as they lower the threshold to seizures.

1. **Action:** If the animal has had **one isolated fit** you should make a thorough examination, taking blood samples for tests and discussing with the owner the possible causes and consequences (Box 3.7).

   Rationale: If no obvious cause presents itself and the animal is otherwise well, treatment may not be needed. In many cases of idiopathic epilepsy the fit never recurs. Ask the owner to tell you if the animal has a repeat episode.

   If the results of the tests indicate an underlying cause then treat it as appropriate.

2. **Action:** If the animal has a history of **repeated fits** you should consider:
   - How often
   - How long each lasts
   - The animal's quality of life

and consider the appropriate treatment or euthanasia.

Rationale: Some types of medication make the animal depressed and sleepy and its quality of life may be poor. If the animal has a fit every day or every week, or the owners are unable to cope with or afford the treatment, euthanasia may be the more realistic outcome. If the animal is in the terminal stages of liver or renal failure, euthanasia is recommended.

3. **Action:** The initial drug of choice for the management of idiopathic epilepsy is oral phenobarbitone.

    Rationale: Not recommended in cases where there is an obvious cause. These should be treated appropriately.

4. **Action:** If the animal is in **status epilepticus** it should be admitted to the surgery as soon as possible and put into a warm, padded kennel.

    Rationale: Padding will prevent the animal damaging itself during the convulsions. Treatment focuses on stopping the seizure and preventing the recurrence, but do not forget normal survival factors (e.g. patency of the airway, oxygenation, maintaining normal body temperature, fluid and acid–base balance).

5. **Action:** Make a note of the animal's temperature, pulse rate and respiratory rate and the colour of its mucous membranes.

    Rationale: This will provide you with a baseline on which to assess recovery. Remember that touching the animal may stimulate repeated fits.

6. **Action:** Place an intravenous catheter. It is possible that the animal's movements may make this difficult.

    Rationale: This provides essential access for treatment and you should try hard to place it.

7. **Action:** Administer diazepam intravenously at a dose of 0.5–1.0 mg/kg.

    Rationale: Use the emulsion formulation (Diazemuls®) as the propylene glycol formulation of diazepam can cause thrombophlebitis. The antiseizure effect lasts for about 20 minutes in dogs. Note that Diazemuls® is denatured by saline so should be given separately from intravenous fluids.

8. **Action:** Expect a response within 2–3 minutes. If the fitting continues give a repeat dose of Diazemuls®.

    Rationale: Some animals take time to respond, but the longer the fits last the greater is the risk of brain swelling and subsequent brain stem herniation and acidosis.

9. **Action:** If there is no response the dose can be repeated 2–3 times over several minutes.

    Rationale: To stop the seizures. Diazepam maintains therapeutic blood levels for about 20 minutes.

10. **Action:** If the fit continues then give intravenous phenobarbitone at a dose of 2–4 mg/kg, or use other anaesthetic agents (e.g. propofol).

    Rationale: Onset of the anticonvulsant effect of phenobarbitone will be delayed for 15–20 minutes, but the dose can be repeated every 30 minutes until a cumulative dose of 20 mg/kg is reached.

11. **Action:** When control of the seizure is achieved give a maintenance dose of phenobarbitone at a rate of 2–4 mg/kg i.v. or i.m. every 6 hours for 24–48 hours.

    Rationale: To maintain level of control and prevent a relapse.

12. **Action:** If possible start oral anticonvulsants every 12 hours.

    Rationale: This should be started as soon as the animal is able to swallow.

13. **Action:** If the seizures continue beyond 20 minutes despite medication, give pentobarbitone to effect at a dose rate of 3–15 mg/kg i.v. Give slowly as diazepam and phenobarbitone potentiate its effects.

    Rationale: Respiratory depression may occur so the animal should be intubated and ventilated.

14. **Action:** In cases where status epilepticus lasts for longer than 30 minutes, it may take days or weeks to recover normal function or the animal may suffer permanent neurological deficit.

Rationale: For more specific treatment in long term cases consult a dedicated neurological textbook.

15. It is vital to consider the nursing care of the animal while being treated for status epilepticus:

- **Action:** Provide a well-padded bed and kennel.

  Rationale: To prevent the animal damaging itself and to prevent the development of bedsores.

- **Action:** Oxygen should be readily available and the animal should be intubated.

  Rationale: Risk of the champing jaws chewing the endotracheal tube.

- **Action:** Consider fluid therapy but be cautious, as if there is a risk of cerebral oedema and brain stem herniation then fluid therapy will make it worse.

  Rationale: Treat cerebral oedema with osmotic diuretics such as mannitol.

- **Action:** Monitor the body temperature.

  Rationale: Hyperthermia may develop during seizures; an animal lying still for some time may suffer from hypothermia.

- **Action:** Turn the patient at regular intervals.

  Rationale: To prevent hypostatic congestion in the dependent lung and the development of bedsores.

- **Action:** Monitor all clinical parameters and record on the hospital chart.

  Rationale: To assess progress and recovery.

GASTRIC DILATATION AND VOLVULUS

Gastric dilatation and volvulus (GDV) is a condition, mainly seen in dogs, in which fermenting food causes the stomach to expand with the accumulation of gas. The stomach becomes unstable and it may rotate (volvulus) at the distal oesophagus and cardia blocking the escape route for the

gases that continue to build up. Eventually the distended stomach presses on the surrounding organs and the hepatic portal vein and caudal vena cava and the animal goes into shock as a result of decreased venous return.

GDV is classically associated with:

- Deep-chested breeds of dog (e.g. Greyhounds, German shepherds, Dobermans, Wolf hounds) although it has been seen in other breeds.
- Feeding of large quantities of food – usually dried.
- Strenuous exercise after feeding.

The condition is rapidly fatal and is a true emergency. Suspected cases should be seen as soon as possible and have been known to die in the car on the way to the surgery. If treatment is not given, the animal becomes shocked and the blood supply to the stomach becomes compromised, leading to necrosis. Formation of toxins leads to endotoxaemia.

Clinical signs include:

- Dog is depressed and quiet – it may make moaning noises.
- Hypersalivation.
- Vomiting – this may help to relieve the situation because the fermenting food is voided.
- Abdomen may be visibly distended and this becomes more severe.
- Dog may look at its flank indicating the area of pain.
- As the condition worsens the mucous membranes become deep purple.
- Collapse and death.

Treatment is aimed at decompression of the stomach and prevention of shock by aggressive fluid therapy. Surgery to correct the gastric torsion and prevention of a recurrence must be done once the animal is stable.

Procedure: Treatment of gastric dilatation and volvulus

1. **Action:** Having taken an accurate history and made a rapid diagnosis over the telephone, ask the owner to come in to the surgery immediately.

Rationale: There is little point in visiting the animal at home as you need equipment and nursing support.

2. **Action:** If this occurs out of hours contact the nurse on call and / or another vet to come and help.

   Rationale: You need trained assistance and a panicking owner cannot be relied upon to help you.

3. **Action:** On arrival make a brief examination to confirm your diagnosis.

   Rationale: The presenting signs are usually very obvious and are unlikely to be confused with anything else.

4. **Action:** If you feel unsure, you should take a conscious right lateral radiograph to confirm the condition.

   Rationale: Sedation should be avoided as it may worsen the hypotension. Time is very important so do not delay unless you are really uncertain of your diagnosis. You may see a gas-filled pylorus dorsal and slightly cranial to the gas-filled gastric fundus.

5. **Action:** Place the dog in sternal recumbency and percuss the dog's right lateral abdomen where the distended stomach is likely to be touching the abdominal wall.

   Rationale: The gas in the stomach should produce a hollow tinkling sound. There is a slight risk that you may penetrate another organ, but if the stomach is really distended this is unlikely.

6. **Action:** Quickly clip an area on the right abdominal wall caudal to the last rib and ventral to the transverse vertebral process and prepare it aseptically.

   Rationale: Asepsis is important, but sometimes saving the dog is more important. You can give antibiotics when the animal recovers.

7. **Action:** Percuss the area and insert a 14G needle or a 16G or 18G over-the-needle intravenous catheter into the stomach.

Rationale: You should percuss to check that the spleen is not overlying the stomach risking its penetration. A wide gauge needle or catheter will allow the gas to evacuate as quickly as possible.

8. **Action:** If using a catheter, remove the stylet and allow the gas to escape.

   Rationale: There is no need to remove all the gas, but this technique will relieve the immediate pressure on the caudal vena cava and give you time to put the animal on fluids before you try to pass a stomach tube. Gastric decompression may make it easier to pass the stomach tube.

9. **Action:** Ask your assistant to restrain the dog while you place an intravenous catheter (see Ch. 1) ready for the administration of intravenous Hartmann's at a rate of 90 ml/kg over the first hour (see Ch. 7). Squeeze the bag while the fluid is going into the animal.

   Rationale: To prevent and/or treat hypovolaemic shock and prevent a metabolic acidosis. The fluids must be 'pushed' into the animal as rapidly as possible if it is to survive.

10. **Action:** If possible place two catheters, one in each leg.

    Rationale: To increase the speed at which fluid is given.

11. **Action:** While the fluid is being administered, place the dog in a sitting position in order to complete gastric decompression using a stomach tube.

    Rationale: Gastric decompression is best done in a sitting position but may also be achieved in right lateral recumbency.

12. **Action:** Using a wide bore stomach tube, place it on the outside of the dog and measure from the nose to the stomach (approx. 11th rib). Mark the position of the stomach on the tube with a biro.

    Rationale: When the tube is passed, this mark will be at the nose. The tube should not be pushed any further as it may rupture the compromised gastric wall.

13. **Action:** Using a 7.5 cm wide roll of adhesive bandage with a wide central plastic core, place it lengthways into the mouth.

    Rationale: This will create a 'tunnel' through which the stomach tube will be passed. The bandage on the roll makes it softer for the dog to hold on to with its teeth.

14. **Action:** Ask your assistant to hold the mouth shut to fix the bandage or apply tape around the mouth.

    Rationale: To hold the roll in place.

15. **Action:** Pass a lubricated stomach tube through the core of the bandage roll, gently through the pharynx and down the oesophagus into the dog's stomach. Stop when the biro mark is at the level of the dog's nose.

    Rationale: Slowing rotating the tube as it passes along may ease its passage.

16. **Action: If the tube successfully passes** into the stomach gas, fluid and ingesta will spontaneously escape by gravity and the use of suction.

    Rationale: Successful passage of the tube does not necessarily rule out volvulus and you should be aware of this.

17. **Action:** Once the stomach has been decompressed, lavage it with warm water or saline.

    Rationale: To remove any remaining debris.

18. **Action:** If you experience any difficulty in passing the tube into the stomach the distal oesophagus / cardiac sphincter may be twisted. Do not use excessive force. Slowly withdraw the tube from the stomach and repeat gastric decompression using a wide gauge needle or catheter into the stomach wall.

    Rationale: The entry into the stomach will be blocked and if you push too hard you may penetrate the oesophageal wall.

To remove more gas to enable the animal to stabilize.

19. **Action:** Once the immediate problems of gastric distension and shock have been dealt with and the animal stands a chance of survival, it should be given a short time to stabilize prior to surgery.

    Rationale: Surgery should be performed. Research shows that medical management alone results in a 75% recurrence rate within a year.

    Surgery is aimed at:

    » Restoring the stomach to its normal position.

    » Splenectomy – removal of the spleen, which may have been damaged in the volvulus or may prevent the stomach being restored to its normal position.

    » Gastropexy – attaching the stomach to the abdominal wall to prevent recurrence of volvulus. Research shows that this significantly increases the chances of survival post GDV.

20. **Action:** In the days after recovery watch out for a sudden relapse.

    Rationale: Of the dogs that die, 24% die within the first 7 days after surgery. This may be due to circulating toxins or to the development of cardiac arrhythmias.

21. **Action:** After surgery withhold food for 24–48 hours.

    Rationale: To allow healing to start without using the gastrointestinal tract.

22. **Action:** If vomiting continues treat with antiemetics (e.g. metaclopramide).

    Rationale: Vomiting sometimes continues post GDV.

23. **Action:** Once the dog has recovered you should advise the owner about its feeding routine:

    • Feed smaller meals twice or three times a day.

    • Soak dried food before feeding to reduce fermentation.

- Exercise the dog before feeding rather than afterwards.
- Raise the dog's bowl up when feeding to prevent aerophagia, which may predispose to gastric distension.
- Discourage drinking large volumes of water after exercise as this may cause gastric distension.

Rationale: *To reduce the chances of recurrence of GDV.*

CHAPTER 4
Bandaging techniques

A well-produced bandage that does the job it is intended to do, does not slip off and does not cut off the circulation is a technique that can be achieved by regular practice. Although in many practices it is the nurse who is left to bandage the limb after you, the veterinary surgeon, have carried out the clinical procedure, it is important that you know how to bandage competently. A neat bandage that stays on will impress your clients – after all, this may be the only bit that they can see.

Bandages have a number of functions and the main ones are shown in Table 4.1.

BANDAGING RULES

Before you start to bandage anything you should be aware of the following 'rules'. If necessary, practice your technique in private on a soft toy or on a partner!

1. **Action:** Wash your hands thoroughly before you start.

    Rationale: To prevent the introduction of infection. You may consider wearing gloves, but this may impede your dexterity.

2. **Action:** Collect all your equipment together and make sure that is it close at hand.

    Rationale: This saves time; when dealing with an animal you cannot expect it to sit quietly on the table while you search for different bandages. Plan ahead – you will appear much more competent and will feel better about the procedure.

3. **Action:** If applicable, remove any soiled bandages and dispose of them in the clinical waste bin.

    Rationale: To prevent the spread of infection the clinical waste will eventually be incinerated.

4. **Action:** When bandaging a lower limb, always include the foot.

    Rationale: To reduce the risk of swelling and cutting off the circulation to the toes. This can

Table 4.1 Reasons for bandaging

Function	Comment
Protection	From infection and dirt and from the environment. Also prevents self mutilation.
Support	Applies to fractures, strains, sprains, dislocations. Adequate support helps to reduce pain and swelling and promotes more rapid healing.
Pressure	To stop haemorrhage and reduce swelling.
Immobilization	Restricting the movement of joints or surrounding soft tissues will reduce pain and make the animal more comfortable.
Security	To hold an intravenous catheter in place, preventing infection and interference.

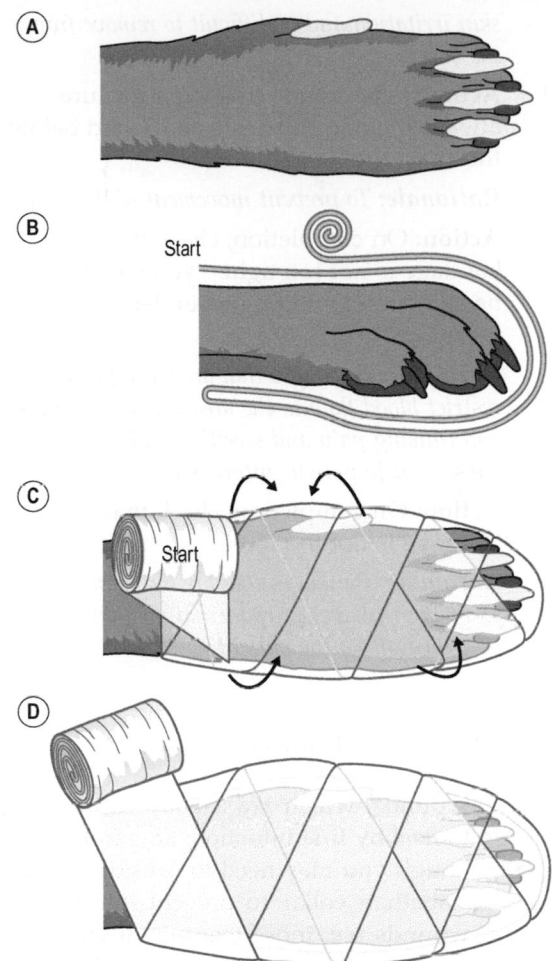

Figure 4.1 Limb bandage: (A) Pad the digits and pads with cottonwool. (B) Bandage over the toes. (C) Twist the bandage through 90°. (D) Continue winding the bandage up the limb.

result in sloughing off of the skin over the toes and in the worst case the complete loss of the toes.

5. **Action:** If the foot is included always place cottonwool pads between the toes (Fig. 4.1).

   Rationale: This absorbs sweat and prevents rubbing. (However, current thinking is moving away from this idea as the cottonwool may become soaked and cause rubbing rather than preventing it!)

6. **Action:** Keep the bandage rolled up and always have the roll on the top as you unwind (Fig. 4.1).

   Rationale: This helps you to control the bandage and to maintain tension.

7. **Action:** Always overlap the layers of a bandage by half of its width.

   Rationale: To prevent the development of gaps. This could let in infection or allow the patient to interfere with the area underneath. It may also cause swelling in the gaps.

8. **Action:** If bandaging tails or limbs always work from the distal to the proximal end of the area.

   Rationale: There is a risk of trapping blood or fluid if you interfere with the venous return to the heart. Results in painful swelling.

9. **Action:** Never use safety pins to secure the ends – use sticky zinc tape instead, although this is not recommended.

   Rationale: The patient may swallow a safety pin. Sticky tape such as zinc tape may cause skin irritation and is difficult to remove from the hair.

10. **Action:** When immobilizing a fracture, always include the joints above and below the area.

    Rationale: To prevent movement of the area.

11. **Action:** On completion, check that the bandage is not too tight – you should be able to get two fingers under the layers.

    Rationale: Bandages that are too tight will restrict blood flow to the area delaying healing, and causing pain and swelling and subsequently patient interference.

12. **Action:** On completion, check that the bandage is not too loose.

    Rationale: Bandages that are too loose will not serve their correct purpose and may fall off or be pulled off by the patient.

WOUND MANAGEMENT

Surgical wounds, which are usually sutured and allowed to heal by first intention, are rarely bandaged, although you may need to consider the use of an Elizabethan collar to prevent interference. Chronic wounds (i.e. those that may involve loss of tissue and are deep or infected) will be left to heal by second intention and may be protected by bandaging.

Before applying the bandage the wound must be decontaminated:

1. **Clip and clean the skin surrounding the wound** – all hair must be removed to keep the wound clean and to promote rapid healing.
   - Use disinfected, unchipped clipper blades to prevent dermatitis.
   - Prevent hairs going into the wound by applying water soluble gel or by temporarily closing it with towel clips or a continuous suture, or by covering it with a sterile swab.
   - Trim hair at the edges of the wound with scissors.

2. **Lavage** – wash the wound thoroughly with large volumes of sterile saline to remove any debris and to dilute any bacteria present. Do not be too vigorous as this will further damage the tissues.
   - Avoid the use of tap water as it is not sterile although it may be used initially.
   - Be aware that antiseptics will not stay in the wound for long enough to work.
   - Detergents in some surgical scrubs may irritate the wound.
   - Some lavage solutions may damage the host cells.

3. **Debridement** – this is the single most important step in promoting wound healing and is the removal of infected, necrotic or contaminated tissue from the wound that would otherwise delay healing. Tidy up the wound edges if surgical repair is to be attempted.

   There are three main ways of debriding a wound:
   - **Surgical** – under strict aseptic conditions, scrape away the necrotic or damaged tissue until the wound is clean.
   - **Dressings** – apply dressings such as dry or saline-soaked swabs to the wound and leave on for no more than 24 hours. These provide an optimal environment for healing to start and when removed they strip off the necrotic tissue.
   - **Enzymatic** – enzymes (available commercially) are applied to the wound and their action ceases when granulation tissue starts to form. Maggots (available in a sterile form) secrete enzymes that destroy necrotic tissue and allow granulation to begin.

ANATOMY OF A BANDAGE

Most bandages consist of the following layers:

1. **Wound dressings –** this layer is in direct contact with the wound and the aim is to promote healing and to prevent further harm. Dressings provide an environment

that is neither too wet nor too dry; the different types are summarized in Table 4.2.

2. **Primary layer** – this holds the dressing in place and absorbs any exudate. It also distributes the pressure evenly and provides padding to the wound. The most common materials are orthopaedic wool (e.g. Sofban®) and cottonwool sheets.

3. **Secondary layer** – the primary layer is stabilized using some form of conforming bandage that has a degree of stretch in it. It is important not to overstretch the material resulting in an overtight bandage, which will restrict blood supply to the area and could cause gangrene. Do not confuse firmness with tightness: the bandage must be firm but not too tight and you should be able to get two fingers under it.

4. **Tertiary layer** – this consists of an elastic cohesive bandage that protects the whole structure and prevents interference by the patient. This layer is very often coloured or may even have words printed on it, which is purely for the benefit of humans! At the top of the bandage the tertiary layer should not extend over the secondary layer as it may rub. Never use an adhesive tape to stick the bandage to the skin or fur as this will cause irritation and can be difficult to remove. If bandaging a lower limb always cover the foot. Increased protection from moisture and mud may be gained by covering the foot with a commercial canvas boot or by using an empty drip bag. Do not leave an impervious cover on the foot all the time as it restricts air and moisture flow and may lead to skin complications.

CARE AND MAINTENANCE OF BANDAGES

All bandages must be constantly monitored and the owners should be given written instructions at discharge. Poorly monitored bandages will delay healing and may result in sloughing of the skin.

1. Check the bandage every 4 hours for the first 24 hours.

2. Check twice daily for the duration of the bandage. This may be done by the owners, but the animal should be seen in the surgery every 4–5 days.

3. Make sure that the owners understand their responsibility to the patient and are aware of what to look for.

4. Exercise restriction is usually indicated, but this depends on the need for the bandage. In some cases exercise restriction may need to be enforced.

5. Monitor the bandage for the following: smell, wetness, swollen toes, cold toes, soiling, slippage and patient interference. Change the bandage if any of these have occurred.

6. If an open wound is present the bandage must be changed regularly – at least once a day. If no wound is present the bandage should be changed every 8–10 days.

7. Complications may include: maceration of the skin, swelling of the limb, wound contamination, dermatitis, necrosis of the skin and gangrene of the limb.

TYPES OF BANDAGE

Procedure: Limb bandage

This is used to support and protect wounds, reduce pain and swelling and prevent movement.

1. **Action:** Gather all your equipment together and arrange it within reach of the examination table.

   Rationale: This enables you to complete the bandage quickly and efficiently.

2. **Action:** Place the animal on a stable examination table covered in a non-slip mat.

   Rationale: If the animal feels secure it will be less likely to try and escape.

3. **Action:** Ask the owner or an assistant to restrain the animal appropriately so that you have access to the affected limb (see Ch. 1).

Table 4.2 Types of wound-dressing materials

Type	Material	Action
Adherent	Saline-soaked gauze swabs (wet to dry dressing)	*Passive.* Used to debride necrotic tissue. Stick to wound and are removed 24 hours later. Cheap, effective but painful to remove.
	Dry gauze swabs (dry to dry dressing)	*Passive.* Necrotic tissue sticks to the gauze and the swab is pulled off after 24 hours. Effective but painful.
Non-adherent – do not stick to the wound	Perforated polyurethane gauze and paraffin gauze, e.g. Melolin®	*Passive.* Used for wounds where there is little exudates, e.g. surgical wounds. Prevent the wound sticking to the bandaging layer.
Absorbent – absorb exudate from the wound preventing maceration of the tissues	Foam dressing, e.g. Allevyn®	*Passive.* Semipermeable membrane that allows fluid to move away from the wound keeping it moist, promoting epithelialization.
	Babies' nappies	*Passive.* Absorb fluid loss. Can be weighed before and after use to assess amount of fluid loss.
Complex	Alginate dressings, e.g. Kaltostat®, Algisite®	*Bioactive and interactive.* Sheets of protein from seaweed that release Na$^+$ and Ca^{2+} and form a gel when they come into contact with exudate. Gel keeps the wound moist. Controls low level bleeding, promotes inflammation and granulation. Disadvantage is that they can promote excessive granulation tissue.
	Hydrogel, e.g. Intrasite®, Biodres®	*Interactive.* Provide slow debridement, absorb exudate, reduce oedema and promote healing. Available as sheets or a gel. When gel is used put absorbent dressing over the top (e.g. foam) to prevent drying out.
	Hydrocolloids, e.g. Tagesorb®, Granuflex®	*Bioactive and interactive.* Sheets with an occlusive backing (waterproof), which prevents dehydration of the wound and encourages debridement. Later the structure becomes more gelatinous and fluid is able to escape from the wound site. May stick to the wound edges and prevent contraction and may promote excessive granulation. Not used for infected wounds as they must be changed regularly so are expensive.
Topical treatments	Aloe vera	Pure products will stimulate granulation.
	Silver sulfadiazine, e.g. Flamazine®	Topical broad-spectrum antibiotic with prolonged activity. Agent of choice to prevent sepsis in burns.
	Zinc bacitracin	Enhances epithelialization.
	Malic, benzoic and salicylic acid solution, e.g. Dermisol®	Debriding agent with a low pH. Toxic to granulation tissue so should not be left in the wound.
	Nanocrystalline silver	Good for infections that are resistant to commonly used antibiotics. Decreases use of antibiotics and reduces the risk of multi-drug resistance.
	Honey	Specific sterilized honey is becoming available. Originally used 2000 years ago. Has antibacterial activity and can be used in infected wounds showing evidence of antibiotic resistance, e.g. MRSA.

NB *Passive – no actio n on the wound; Interactive – responds to wound environment in some way; Bioactive – has a biological effect on the wound.*

Rationale: The animal may try to move during the procedure. Correct restraint will allow you to work quickly and efficiently.

4. **Action:** Apply cottonwool padding between the digits of the affected limb (Fig. 4.1).

   Rationale: This prevents rubbing and absorbs the sweat between the toes. (However, current practice is moving away from this idea and you will need to decide for yourself.)

5. **Action:** Apply an appropriate wound dressing to the affected area.

   Rationale: For example this may be used to cover a cut footpad or after the removal of a dew claw. This will promote healing.

6. **Action:** Apply the primary padding layer. Start on the cranial aspect of the limb, run the bandage down over the toes to the caudal aspect of the limb and then go back again (Fig. 4.1).

   Rationale: This holds the dressing in place, provides support and helps to absorb any exudate.

7. **Action:** Turn the bandage through 90° and, working from the distal to the proximal part of the limb, cover the toes in a figure-of-eight arrangement.

   Rationale: This makes the bandage firm and protective.

8. **Action:** Work up the limb until you are over the joint above the injury.

   Rationale: This helps to distribute the pressure of the bandage evenly.

9. **Action:** Apply a tertiary layer to the limb following the same pattern and working from distal to proximal.

   Rationale: This will hold everything together and protect the limb from daily wear and tear.

10. **Action:** Check the tension on the bandage.

    Rationale: If it is too loose the bandage will fall off very soon; it is too tight it may damage the underlying tissues.

Procedure: Tail bandage

This is used to protect the tail after traumatic injuries.

1. **Action:** Gather all your equipment together and arrange it within reach of the examination table.

   Rationale: This enables you to complete the bandage quickly and efficiently.

2. **Action:** Place the animal on a stable examination table covered in a non-slip mat.

   Rationale: If the animal feels secure it will be less likely to try and escape.

3. **Action:** Ask the owner or an assistant to restrain the animal in a standing position or sitting with the tail extended.

   Rationale: This depends on the size and nature of the patient.

4. **Action:** Apply an appropriate dressing to the wound on the tail.

   Rationale: This will promote healing.

5. **Action:** If the wound is on the end of the tail, cover the dressing with a large empty syringe case pierced with hole to provide ventilation.

   Rationale: This provides a quick and easy method of covering and holding the dressing in place. Good ventilation is important for wound healing.

6. **Action:** If the wound is higher up the tail, then apply a layer of conforming bandage over the dressing.

   Rationale: Even if the wound is on the proximal end of the tail, you should bandage the entire tail to prevent swelling towards the tip. In this area of the body there is no need to provide a layer of padding over the dressing.

7. **Action:** Cover either the syringe case or the conforming bandage with a layer of cohesive bandage, working from the caudal end to the proximal end of the tail.

   Rationale: This will protect the inner layers of the bandage and will prevent swelling of the tail tip.

8. **Action:** As you progress proximally towards the top of the conforming bandage, start to work the animal's tail hair into the cohesive bandage.

   Rationale: This will help the bandage to stay in place. Tail bandages will slip off easily and you may have to use sticky tape to hold it to the hair.

9. **Action:** Check that the bandage is secure and not too tight.

Rationale: Overtight bandages cause tissue damage and eventual necrosis.

Procedure: Ear bandage

This may be used following an ear canal ablation or after treatment for an aural haematoma or a cut pinna.

1. **Action:** Gather all your equipment together and arrange it within reach of the examination table.

Rationale: This enables you to complete the bandage quickly and efficiently.

2. **Action:** Place the animal on a stable examination table covered in a non-slip mat.

Rationale: If the animal feels secure it will be less likely to try and escape.

3. **Action:** Ask the owner or an assistant to restrain the animal in a sitting position or in sternal recumbency.

Rationale: This depends on the patient's comfort, but if you are short you will be able to reach over the head more easily if the animal is in sternal recumbency.

4. **Action:** Apply a dressing to the wound area.

Rationale: This is most likely to be on the pinna or over the external ear canal. The dressing will promote healing.

5. **Action:** Place a pad of cottonwool on the top of the head above the affected ear flap.

Rationale: This prevents the ear flap from rubbing on the top of the head. If both ears are affected then make the pad large enough to cover the entire top of the head.

6. **Action:** Fold the affected ear pinna up on to the pad and ask your assistant to hold it in place.

7. **Action:** Cover the ear pinna with another pad of cottonwool. Make sure that it is the same size as the ear pinna.

Rationale: The ear pinna is now lying between two pads of cottonwool, which prevent it rubbing on the top of the head.

8. **Action:** Apply a conforming bandage over the padding. Starting at the top of the head, run to the rostral side of the healthy ear, which will be hanging down, then down under the jaw and back up to the top of the head. Continue down again on the caudal side of the healthy ear flap under the jaw and back up again (Fig. 4.2). Continue in a figure-of-eight, going round and round, each time passing either side of the healthy ear until the affected ear and the cottonwool padding are neatly covered.

Rationale: The aim is to produce a figure-of-eight bandage anchored around the healthy ear which hangs down. If the animal has pricked-up ears the technique is exactly the same, but the healthy ear may not hold the bandage in place quite as effectively.

9. **Action:** Check that the bandage is not too tight around the larynx and trachea.

Rationale: This could impede the animal's breathing. You should be able to get two fingers between the bandage and the ventral part of the neck.

10. **Action:** Repeat the figure-of-eight technique using a cohesive bandage.

Rationale: This secures and protects the other layers.

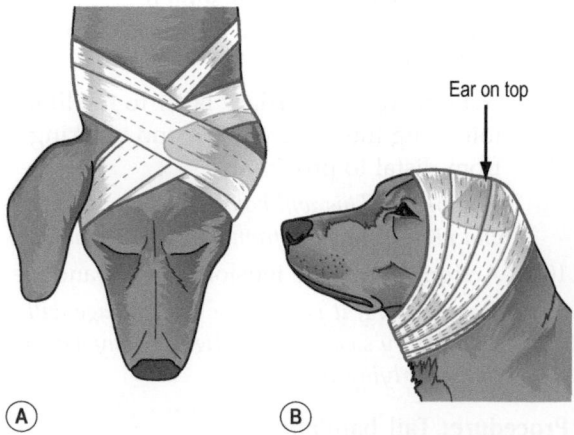

Figure 4.2 The figure-of-eight design for an ear bandage: (A) Wind the bandage around the head in a figure-of-eight. (B) Mark the position of the ear with an arrow.

11. **Action:** Tuck any bits of cottonwool or conforming bandage under the cohesive bandage.

    Rationale: This makes the bandage look neat and tidy and is purely to impress the owners.

12. **Action:** On the outside of the cohesive bandage, draw the outline of the affected ear using a felt pen.

    Rationale: If you use scissors to remove the bandage, these marks will tell you where the ear is so that you can avoid cutting into it.

Procedure: Chest bandage

This is used to secure and cover a chest drain, or as a first aid measure in cases of thoracic injury or flail chests.

1. **Action:** Gather all your equipment together and arrange it within reach of the examination table.

    Rationale: This enables you to complete the bandage quickly and efficiently.

2. **Action:** Place the animal on a stable examination table covered in a non-slip mat.

    Rationale: If the animal feels secure it will be less likely to try and escape.

3. **Action:** Ask the owner or an assistant to restrain the animal in a standing position (Fig. 4.3).

    Rationale: You must be able to wrap the bandage around the chest so you need complete access to the area.

4. **Action:** Apply a sterile wound dressing to any wounds.

    Rationale: To maintain sterility and to promote healing.

5. **Action:** If dealing with a chest drain, it may be necessary to place sterile dressings around the point of insertion.

    Rationale: To maintain sterility and to hold it in place.

6. **Action:** You can use either a synthetic padding bandage (e.g. Sofban®) or a conforming bandage. Start the bandage

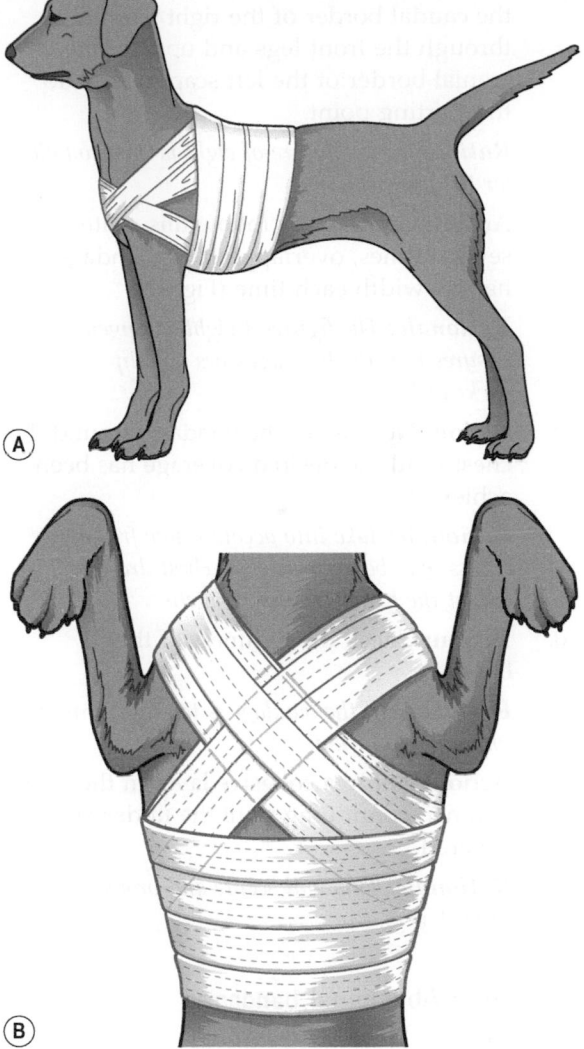

Figure 4.3 Figure-of-eight design for a chest bandage: (A) Lateral view. (B) Ventral view.

between the shoulder blades. Run over the cranial border of the right scapula, bringing the bandage down through the front legs and then run up towards the caudal border of the left scapula back to the starting point (Fig. 4.3).

Rationale: A padding layer will make the bandage comfortable, but in most cases you need only a conforming bandage as your base layer. Following this route creates half of a figure-of-eight.

7. **Action:** Continue to run the bandage over the caudal border of the right scapula, through the front legs and up over the cranial border of the left scapula back to the starting point.

   Rationale: The figure-of-eight is now complete for the first time.

8. **Action:** Continue to follow this route several times, overlapping the bandage by half its width each time (Fig 4.3).

   Rationale: The figure-of-eight arrangement ensures that the bandage does not slip backwards.

9. **Action:** Now wind the bandage around the chest until the desired coverage has been achieved.

   Rationale: Take into account how frequently access may be needed to the chest drain and adjust the bandage appropriately.

10. **Action:** Check the tightness of the bandage.

    Rationale: If the bandage is too tight it will impede respiration.

11. **Action:** Apply a cohesive layer in the same manner, continuing until the under layer is covered.

    Rationale: This will secure and protect the inner layers.

Procedure: Abdominal bandage

This is used to protect wounds following trauma or after surgery to support the ventral midline. May also be used as a pressure bandage.

1. **Action:** Gather all your equipment together and arrange it within reach of the examination table.

   Rationale: This enables you to complete the bandage quickly and efficiently.

2. **Action:** Place the animal on a stable examination table covered in a non-slip mat.

   Rationale: If the animal feels secure it will be less likely to try and escape.

3. **Action:** Ask the owner or an assistant to restrain the animal in a standing position

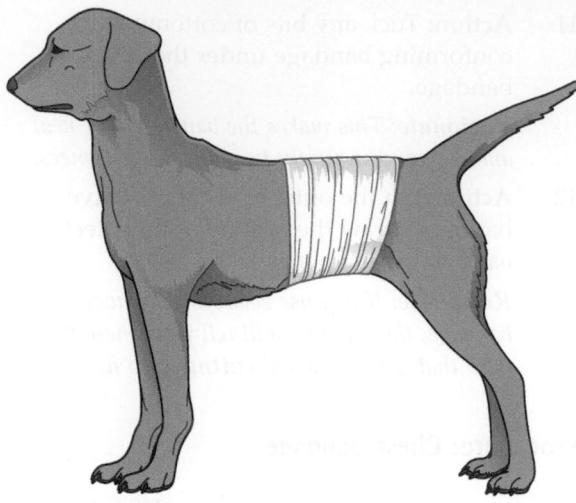

Figure 4.4 Abdominal bandage.

(Fig. 4.4) or in lateral recumbency if the animal is still anaesthetized post surgery.

Rationale: You must be able to wrap the bandage around the abdomen so you need complete access to the area.

4. **Action:** Apply a sterile wound dressing to any wounds.

   Rationale: To maintain sterility and to promote healing.

5. **Action:** Use a padding bandage such as Sofban® or cottonwool around the abdomen (Fig 4.4).

   Rationale: This will prevent rubbing as the hair over the abdomen is usually thinner than in other areas of the body. In male dogs, do not cover the prepuce as the animal will be uncomfortable and the bandage will become urine soaked.

6. **Action:** Apply a layer of conforming bandage over the padding layer until the desired coverage has been achieved.

   Rationale: This will hold the padding layer together. You may have to extend the bandage cranially to partially cover the thorax – this should prevent the bandage slipping towards the dog's 'waist'. Make sure that respiration is not impaired.

7. **Action:** Apply a layer of cohesive bandage.

   Rationale: This will protect the bandage but may not always be necessary.

8. **Action:** Check the tension.

   Rationale: If the bandage is too tight the animal will be uncomfortable.

Procedure: Robert Jones bandage

This is used to immobilize a limb fracture, control swelling and oedema and provide support to a limb postoperatively.

1. **Action:** Gather all your equipment together and arrange it within reach of the examination table.

   Rationale: This enables you to complete the bandage quickly and efficiently.

2. **Action:** Place the animal on a stable examination table covered in a non-slip mat.

   Rationale: If the animal feels secure it will be less likely to try and escape.

3. **Action:** Ask the owner or an assistant to restrain the animal in lateral recumbency with the relevant leg extended.

   Rationale: At first the limb may be painful so restraint is important. As the supporting layers start to work the pain should diminish a little.

4. **Action:** Cut two strips of 2.5 cm wide zinc oxide tape approximately 20 cm long and attach them to the dorsal and palmar (or plantar if it is a hindleg) sides of the lower limb (Fig. 4.5).

   Rationale: These form the stirrups which hold the bandage together later on in the procedure.

5. **Action:** Allow 10 cm to extend beyond the toes and stick the two lengths of tape lightly together.

   Rationale: This prevents them sticking to the other layers.

6. **Action:** Wrap cottonwool around the entire limb. Use at least three layers and try to make sure the bandage is of even thickness throughout. Pay attention to any bony prominences such as the elbow or hock and include all the joints as far up as the hip or the shoulder within the bandage.

   Rationale: This layer provides support for the limb and this is increased by the number of layers of cottonwool.

7. **Action:** Make sure that at least two toes protrude from the end of the bandage.

   Rationale: These are used to check that the blood supply to the distal limb is not impeded by the pressure of the bandage.

8. **Action:** Using conforming bandage of an appropriate width for the animal, compress the cottonwool layer. Starting distally and working towards the proximal part of the limb, continue winding the bandage until the cottonwool is under tension. Try to maintain the natural angles of the limb.

   Rationale: The bandage should now be approximately three times the thickness of the animal's leg and when 'flicked' with your finger should sound like a ripe melon.

   Maintaining the angles of the limb prevents the bandaged limb from becoming longer than the unaffected one, and, because it will be more comfortable, the animal is more likely to walk on it.

9. **Action:** Separate the two zinc oxide tapes from each other. Twist each tape through 180° and stick it to the conforming layer.

   Rationale: These stirrups will prevent the bandage from slipping down the limb.

10. **Action:** Apply an even layer of cohesive bandage over the conforming bandage (Fig. 4.5).

    Rationale: This will protect the bandage.

11. **Action:** Check the toes at regular intervals.

    Rationale: To assess temperature and sensation. Leaving the toes exposed may also encourage the animal to walk on the leg.

Procedure: Velpeau sling

This is used to support and immobilize the shoulder after luxation or surgery. It may also be used for conservative treatment for minimally displaced scapular fractures.

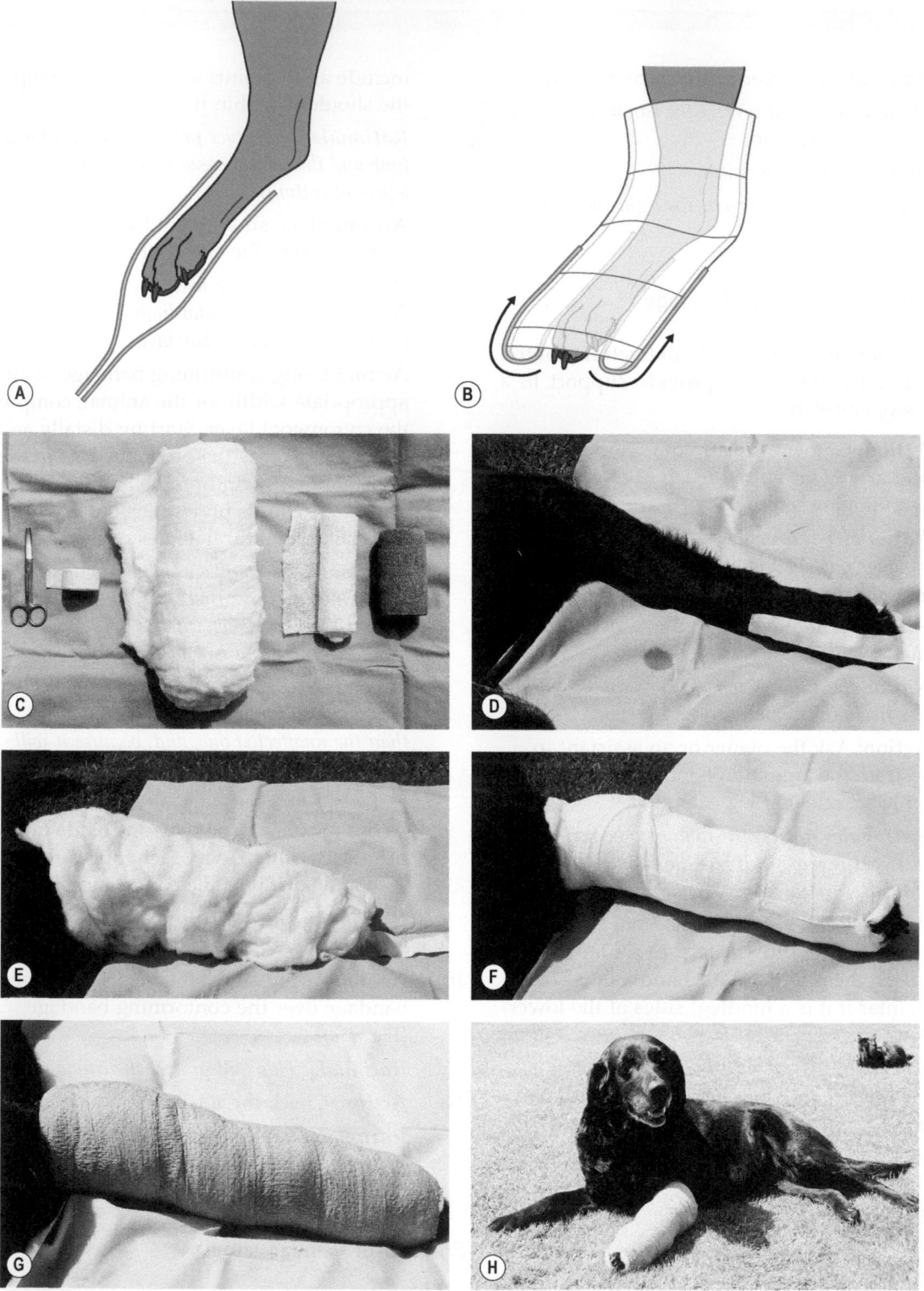

Figure 4.5 The Robert Jones bandage: (A) Stick the stirrups gently together. (B) Stick the stirrups to the conforming bandage. (C) Materials required for Robert Jones bandage. (D) Zinc oxide tapes are applied to the limb to act as 'stirrups'. (E) Cotton wool is wrapped around the entire length of the limb. (F) Conforming bandage is wrapped over the cotton wool and the stirrups are twisted and stuck to the outside. (G) Cohesive bandage is applied as a protective layer. (H) Patient with a correctly applied Robert Jones bandage.

1. **Action:** Gather all your equipment together and arrange it within reach of the examination table.

   Rationale: This enables you to complete the bandage quickly and efficiently.

2. **Action:** Place the animal on a stable examination table covered in a non-slip mat.

   Rationale: If the animal feels secure it will be less likely to try and escape.

3. **Action:** The animal may still be anaesthetized, but if it is conscious it should be restrained in lateral recumbency.

   Rationale: You need full access to the affected elbow.

4. **Action:** Apply a layer of cottonwool padding to the carpal and metacarpal areas of the affected limb.

   Rationale: These joints are going to be flexed and require padding for the comfort of the animal.

5. **Action:** Apply several turns of conforming bandage to the limb just above the carpus (Fig. 4.6A).

   Rationale: This secures the end of the bandage and provides a means of pulling the limb up into flexion.

6. **Action:** Flex the elbow and shoulder and at the same time run the conforming bandage up over the shoulder, down under the chest medial to the other limb and back to the carpus (Fig. 4.6B).

   Rationale: This will hold the elbow and shoulder in flexion against the body.

7. **Action:** Flex the carpus and include this within the bandage. Continue up over the shoulder and under the chest as before.

   Rationale: The entire limb is now held in flexion against the body.

8. **Action:** Continue winding the bandage until the whole limb is held securely.

   Rationale: The animal should not be able to move the limb but check that respiration is not impeded.

9. **Action:** Apply a layer of cohesive bandage over the conforming bandage (Fig. 4.6C).

   Rationale: To protect the other layers.

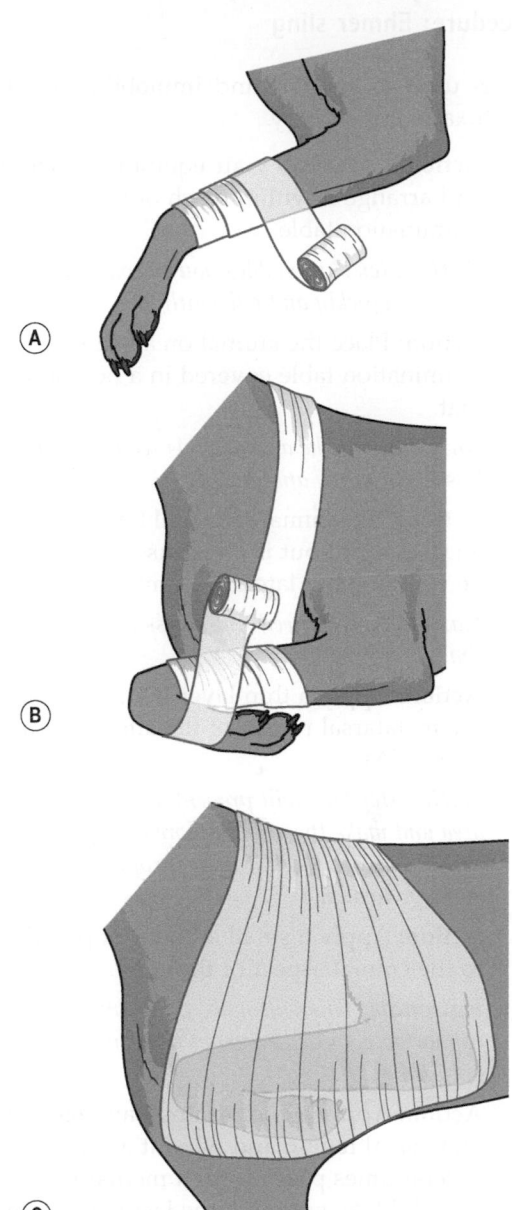

Figure 4.6 The Velpeau sling: (A) Wind the conforming bandage around the carpal. (B) Flex the carpus. (C) Apply a layer of cohesive bandage over the top.

Procedure: Ehmer sling

This is used to support and immobilize the hip after luxation or surgery.

1. **Action:** Gather all your equipment together and arrange it within reach of the examination table.

   Rationale: This enables you to complete the bandage quickly and efficiently.

2. **Action:** Place the animal on a stable examination table covered in a non-slip mat.

   Rationale: If the animal feels secure it will be less likely to try and escape.

3. **Action:** The animal may still be anaesthetized but if it is conscious it should be restrained in lateral recumbency.

   Rationale: You need full access to the affected limb.

4. **Action:** Apply a thin layer of padding to the metatarsal region of the affected limb (Fig. 4.7A).

   Rationale: This will prevent swelling of the area and make the animal more comfortable. If the layer is too thick it may encourage the bandage to slip.

5. **Action:** Apply a small amount of padding to the cranial aspect of the stifle.

   Rationale: This will make the animal more comfortable, but this part of the bandage is optional.

6. **Action:** Apply a conforming bandage to the metatarsal region and wind it around several times passing from medial to lateral. Make sure that the last turn finishes on the lateral side

   Rationale: This secures the start of the bandage.

7. **Action:** Flex the whole limb turning the foot inwards.

   Rationale: This will turn the hock outwards and the stifle inwards, which ensures that the femoral head is pushed into the acetabulum.

8. **Action:** Bring the bandage up to the medial aspect of the stifle, then down over the

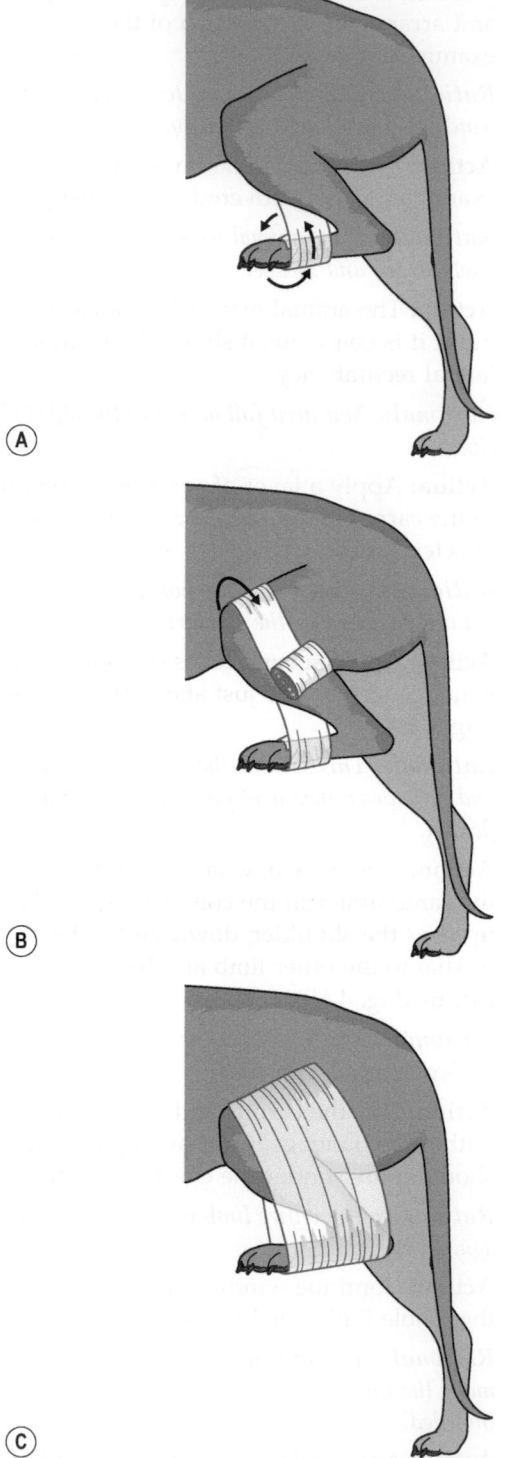

(A)

(B)

(C)

Figure 4.7 The Ehmer sling: (A) Wind the bandage around the metatarsal. (B) Bring the bandage over the lateral thigh. (C) Apply a layer of conforming bandage.

padding to the lateral aspect of the thigh (Fig. 4.7B).

Rationale: The limb will be held in flexion and the bandage has described a figure of eight.

9. **Action:** Take the bandage down to the medial aspect of the metatarsals and around to the lateral aspect.

Rationale: You are now back to your starting point.

10. **Action:** Continue to follow this route several times until the whole limb is held securely in place.

Rationale: The limb should not be able to be moved at all.

11. **Action:** Apply a cohesive bandage over the conforming layer (Fig. 4.7C).

Rationale: This provides protection for the deeper layers. Conforming bandages tend to slip and the use of a cohesive layer will prevent this.

NB When applying an Ehmer sling to a short-legged dog or one that has large amounts of loose skin, the bandage can encircle the abdomen to prevent it slipping.

Procedure: Ring pad

This is used to protect an area that is rubbing e.g. bedsores and keeps the overlying bandage clear of the area. It may be placed around a protruding foreign body to prevent further penetration by the object. The pad is made on your own fingers and is then applied to the patient (Fig. 4.8). Commercially made pads are available.

1. **Action:** Assuming that you are right handed, wrap several layers of conforming bandage around your left hand at the junction of your fingers to your palm (Fig. 4.8).

Rationale: This will form the basis of your ring pad.

2. **Action:** Do NOT cut the bandage. Carefully remove the ring of bandage from your hand and start to wind the remaining bandage around the ring.

Rationale: This holds the base of the bandage together and pads it out to form a ring.

3. **Action:** Continue to wind around the ring until the desired shape and size is created.

Rationale: This creates a firm ring-doughnut-shaped structure that can be placed over a penetrating foreign body or a bedsore.

NB If you are left handed, use your right hand!

CASTS AND SPLINTS

The use of casts and splints to repair fractures, which may be referred to as external coaptation, is less often used nowadays as modern internal and external fixation techniques are more effective and allow the animal to resume normal activity more quickly. However, the use of casts and splints is cheaper and is useful in the following instances:

- In young animals with relatively stable fractures (e.g. greenstick fractures)
- Simple closed fractures that are distal to the elbow or stifle and are non-articular – these allow sufficient immobilization to prevent twisting
- Fractures with a minimum of 50% contact
- Fractures in which healing should take place within a minimum of 4–6 weeks – these are more likely in younger animals.

The main use of casts and splints is as an adjunct to internal fixation to provide support and protection, which aids analgesia and reduces swelling. Their sole use is contraindicated where there is soft tissue swelling or in working animals.

CASTS

Procedure: Applying a cast

Materials: traditional casting material was plaster of Paris, but this is irritant, messy, radiopaque and takes time to reach weight-bearing strength. Modern materials are based on polyurethane resins, which are activated by immersion in hot water. They reach weight-bearing strength within 40 minutes and are radiolucent, enabling follow-up radiography to be carried out without removing the cast. The disadvantage is cost and some are irritant to the skin – make sure that you use an

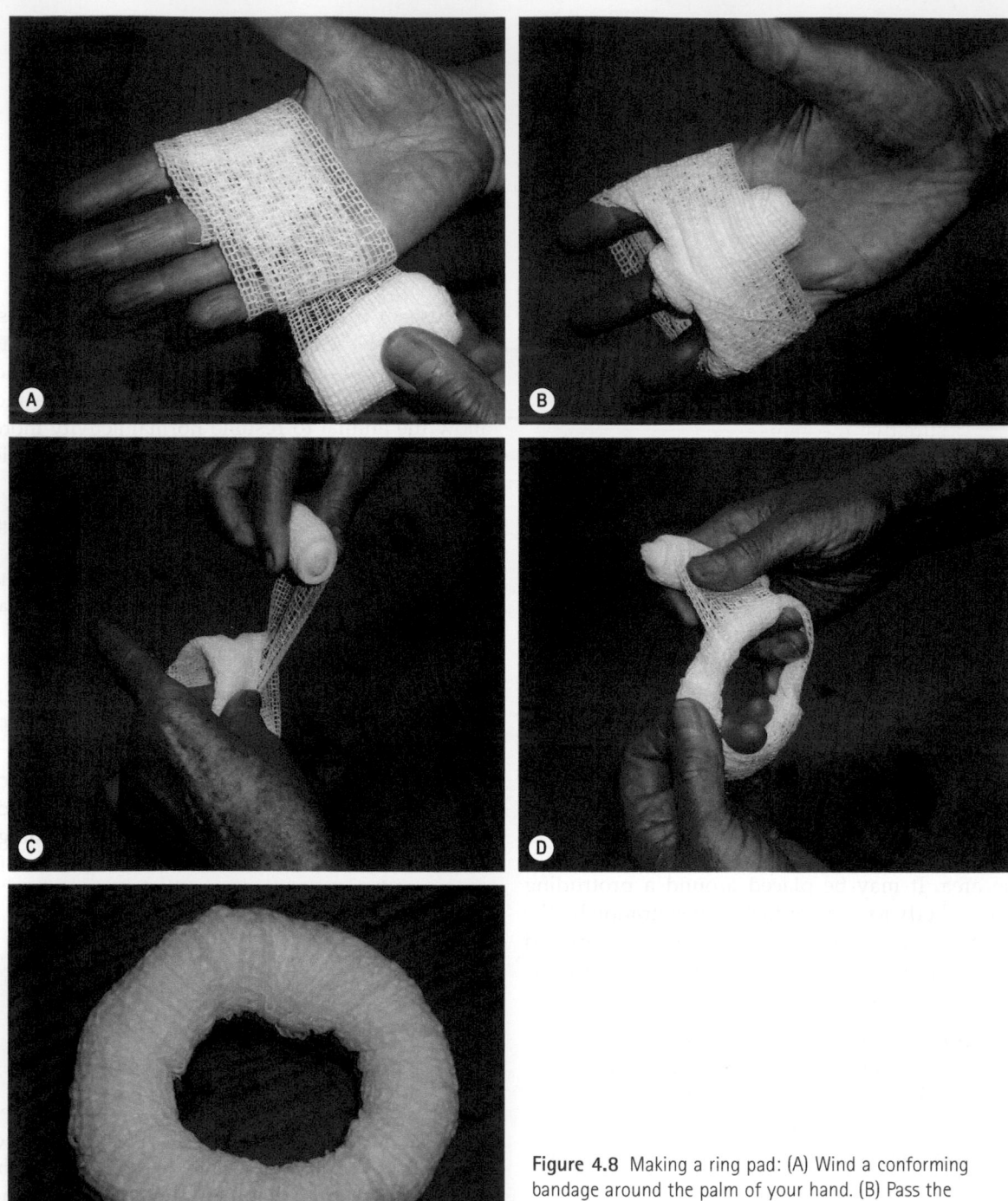

Figure 4.8 Making a ring pad: (A) Wind a conforming bandage around the palm of your hand. (B) Pass the bandage under the loop. (C) Carefully move the bandage from your hand. (D) Continue to wind the bandage around the ring until the desired shape and size is created. (E) The finished ring pad.

underlying layer of bandage and wear gloves when applying the material.

1. **Action:** Gather all your equipment together and arrange it within easy reach.

    Rationale: This enables you to complete the cast quickly and efficiently.

2. **Action:** The patient should be anaesthetized or heavily sedated.

    Rationale: This provides adequate muscle relaxation to reduce the fracture and ensure the limb is in the correct position. It also provides a degree of analgesia.

3. **Action:** Clip the fur from the limb, making sure that the joints distal and proximal to the fracture are included.

    Rationale: The fur will interfere with the application of the cast. The joints above and below the fracture must be immobilized within the cast to prevent twisting of the limb.

4. **Action:** Ensure that the whole limb is clean and dry.

    Rationale: Any moisture will absorb into the gauze layer and predispose to rubbing and/or maceration of the skin.

5. **Action:** Reduce the fracture.

    Rationale: This must be done prior to application of the cast as once it has hardened you cannot move the ends of the bone.

6. **Action:** Place the animal in lateral recumbency with the affected limb uppermost and held, by an assistant, in a weight-bearing position.

    Rationale: This is the shape that the cast will set and it is important that it is comfy for the patient. If the leg is too long or too short it will affect the patient's mobility.

7. **Action:** Cover the leg with tubular gauze appropriate to the animal's size. Ensure that the joints above and below the fracture are covered.

    Rationale: The gauze layer will prevent the cast material causing skin irritation. Enclosing the joints prevents subsequent twisting of the limb, which would mean that the fracture heals in an abnormal position.

8. **Action:** Apply a degree of tension to the gauze.

    Rationale: To eliminate creases from the bandage, which may rub on the animal's skin inside the cast.

9. **Action:** Allow 2 cm of extra gauze at either end.

    Rationale: This will be folded back later to ensure a smooth and comfortable end.

10. **Action:** Apply a layer of synthetic padding in a spiral fashion running from the distal limb to the proximal limb. Overlap by 50% at each turn. Extend by approximately 2 cm at either end.

    Rationale: This makes the cast more comfortable. Ensure that there is more padding over the joints and bony prominences, but make sure it is even. If there are any depressed areas on the limb, these can be filled in with padding to achieve a smoother outline to the final cast.

11. **Action:** Apply a layer of conforming bandage over the padding.

    Rationale: This will compact the padding layer.

12. **Action:** Make sure that you follow the manufacturer's instructions for handling and wetting the casting material.

    Rationale: Different types of casting material vary as to how they are used.

13. **Action:** Put on a pair of disposable gloves.

    Rationale: Some casting materials are irritant to the skin.

14. **Action:** Apply the casting material over the layers of bandage. Overlap each turn by 50%. Use 2–4 layers according to the instructions. Leave 1–2 cm of exposed padding at the proximal end of the cast.

    Rationale: The exposed padding will act as a soft protective border to the cast and prevent rubbing.

15. **Action:** Increase the tension of the cast material proximal to the stifle or elbow.

    Rationale: This makes a snug fit over the main muscle masses of the limb and prevents the cast loosening or slipping.

16. **Action:** Avoid making indentations in the cast with your fingers.

    Rationale: This may press on the limb underneath and cause areas of rubbing.

17. **Action:** Allow time to dry.

    Rationale: The material should be dry within 10 minutes, but must be supported until it is. Depending on the type of material the cast should be weight bearing within 40 minutes.

18. **Action:** While drying is occurring, roll back the gauze and any of the padding layer to cover the ends of the cast and secure with adhesive tape. The pads and nails of the longest digits should remain exposed.

    Rationale: This creates a neat and tidy cast and prevents rubbing at the top and bottom. The digits, pads and nails can be used to monitor the health of the underlying tissues.

MAINTENANCE OF THE CAST

Owners should be given written instructions about the signs to look out for and their responsibilities towards their animal and the cast.

1. Check the cast every 4 hours in the first 24 hours.
2. The cast should be checked in the surgery at least once a week unless the owner is concerned. Casts on young animals may need more frequent monitoring.
3. The cast must not be allowed to become wet.
4. Exercise should be restricted.
5. The cast may be kept clean by placing a plastic bag, such as an old drip bag, over the foot while the animal is outside. This must be removed when the animal is inside.
6. If the animal is interfering with the cast consider the use of an Elizabethan collar. Try to find out the reason for the interference – the animal may be experiencing some discomfort and you may be able to alleviate it.
7. Monitor the cast for the following: swelling, coldness and discoloration of the toes or the proximal limb, skin damage to the toes or proximal limb, foul odour, loosening of the cast, change in angulation of the cast, chewing or any damage to the cast, change in weight bearing, signs of general ill health.
8. If any of these are seen, the cast must be removed and replaced as soon as possible.
9. Complications may include: skin maceration, swelling, moist dermatitis, pressure necrosis and sores and wound contamination. If the cast loosens or changes shape this will affect the healing process which may result in deterioration in the apposition of the bone ends and ultimately a non-union, malunion or delayed union. The associated joints may also become lax or stiff. Complications are more likely to be found in growing and obese animals and in chondrodystrophic breeds.

Procedure: Removal of a cast

1. **Action:** The animal may be conscious or lightly sedated depending on its demeanour.

   Rationale: This is not a painful procedure, but some animals may object to it.

2. **Action:** Always take a radiograph of the fractured limb before making the decision to finally remove the cast.

   Rationale: This will show the extent of the callus formation indicating how well the fracture has healed. Manual restraint of the patient for radiology should be kept to a minimum – a sedated patient may stay still for a short while.

3. **Action:** Ask an assistant to restrain the patient on a non-slip examination table in an appropriate position.

   Rationale: If the animal feels comfortable and secure it will be less likely to try and escape.

4. **Action:** If possible use an oscillating circular saw to cut through the cast.

   Rationale: Plaster scissors can be used, but they take time to cut through and require a degree of strength.

5. **Action:** Make an incision along the length of the cast on the medial and lateral sides being careful not to injure the underlying tissues.

   Rationale: By making two cuts you can then more easily lift off the top part of the cast.

6. **Action:** Using cast spreaders, prise apart the two halves.

   Rationale: The two parts of the cast may be stuck to the underlying bandage.

7. **Action:** Remove the underlying bandage with scissors or by gently unwinding it.

   Rationale: To reveal the healed limb.

8. **Action:** Treat any damaged or sore areas of skin appropriately.

   Rationale: If the cast has been applied and maintained correctly there should be little damage to the skin underneath.

9. **Action:** Institute a regimen of gently increasing controlled exercise and physiotherapy.

   Rationale: The aim is to stimulate callus remodelling without damaging the fracture repair. Gentle physiotherapy such as passive joint mobilization and active therapeutic exercise may be used.

SPLINTS

A splint is a piece of rigid material applied to one aspect of the limb. Splints are not usually considered to be rigid enough for the primary repair of fractures but may be used in a first-aid situation to provide temporary support and a means of reducing pain before a definitive repair is instituted. They may also be used to repair fractures in exotic and wildlife species where it may be necessary to be inventive. A fractured phalanx may be repaired by binding it to the next intact digit, which acts as a splint and provides stability.

Procedure: Applying a splint

Materials: there are many types of commercially available splints, although it is possible to make your own in an emergency.

1. **Action:** Gather all your equipment together and arrange it within easy reach.

   Rationale: This enables you to complete the splint and bandage quickly and efficiently.

2. **Action:** The patient should be anaesthetized or heavily sedated.

   Rationale: This provides adequate muscle relaxation to reduce the fracture and ensure the limb is in the correct position. It also provides a degree of analgesia.

3. **Action:** Apply two layers of synthetic padding to the affected limb working from the distal to the proximal part of the limb. Do not use too thick a layer of padding.

   Rationale: This provides comfort and protects the limb from the splint itself; however, to be effective the splint must be in relative proximity to the limb to provide sufficient immobility. Some commercial splints are ready-padded so the amount of synthetic padding can be reduced.

4. **Action:** Cover both the joint above and the joint below the fracture.

   Rationale: Both joints must be involved within the splinted area to prevent rotation of the bone ends.

5. **Action:** Make sure any bony prominences are well padded.

   Rationale: To ensure that these areas do not become rubbed and sore.

6. **Action:** Apply the splint to the limb, making sure that it is long enough to immobilize the joints above and below the fracture.

   Rationale: To prevent rotation of the fractured ends of the bone.

7. **Action:** Hold the splint in place at two or three sites with micropore tape.

   This keeps the splint in place while you apply the next layer of bandage.

8. **Action:** Apply a layer of cohesive bandage over the splint.

   This holds the splint firmly in place and protects the whole bandage.

CHAPTER 5

Laboratory techniques

CHAPTER CONTENTS

Laboratory tests are used as an aid to diagnosis following taking a history and making a clinical examination. This evidence leads to a differential diagnosis and laboratory tests will then help to eliminate some possibilities and confirm others.

Some results will come back as normal; these are used to rule out some of the possible diagnoses and you can then pay more attention to the abnormal findings. Never discount an abnormal or unexpected result. It is easy to have a fixed idea of the diagnosis in your mind and to fit all the evidence to support it; however, if you think a result contradicts your diagnosis, repeat the test – it may have been an error due to inaccuracy, but it may be that the result is indicating something other than your original theory.

Many laboratory tests are carried out within the practice, although some will be sent away to a commercial laboratory; the proportion varies between practices, but most practices have a small 'in-house' lab. Some larger practices have designated lab technicians who do all the work, but it is important for the veterinary surgeon to know how to carry out the basic techniques, as there will be times, such as weekends or at night, when the support staff are not available.

As with all aspects of veterinary practice, the laboratory is subject to health and safety legislation. It is not the brief of this chapter to go into any detail except to say that precautions must be taken to ensure the safety of yourself and everyone around you. Make sure that you take steps to prevent yourself becoming infected by the samples; for example, wear protective clothing and eye protection, always wash your hands, avoid mouth pipetting and do not eat in the lab. Make sure that the lab itself is kept clean and tidy and that used equipment is cleaned immediately or disposed of in the correct manner (e.g. sharps bins or clinical waste bags).

Laboratory tests must be carried out correctly and accurately. Remember that the quality of your result reflects the quality of your sample – correct methods of collection, preservation and storage play a significant part. There are some rules that should be observed for all tests:

- Collect samples before you begin treatment unless doing follow-up tests to assess progress.
- Collect the appropriate samples and preserve them correctly.
- Perform the test as soon as possible after collection.
- Know how to perform the test correctly and accurately.
- If dispatching to a commercial laboratory, separate plasma or serum, enclose all the relevant details of the case, use the correct types of packaging and post as soon as possible by a traceable route.

LABORATORY EQUIPMENT

A routine practice laboratory will have the following pieces of equipment.

THE MICROSCOPE

The type of microscope found in a practice laboratory is the light microscope, which will have an inbuilt light source, although older ones may use a mirror and an external light source. Microscopes are expensive precision instruments and should be handled with care. They may be monocular or binocular, but both types are equally effective.

General rules for the care of microscopes are shown in Box 5.1.

Box 5.1 General rules for the care of light microscopes

- After use always switch off the machine and replace the cover to prevent contamination by dust and chemicals.
- Make sure that the microscope has regular electrical safety checks.
- Do not put the microscope close to the window or to sources of heat or moisture.
- Always site the microscope on a stable surface.
- Clean the microscope after use with the correct tissues and chemicals – incorrect materials may cause damage.
- When carrying the microscope, pick it up by the limb and always support it under the base.
- Keep spare bulbs in stock and do not touch the bulb when replacing it.
- Make sure that the machine is regularly serviced.

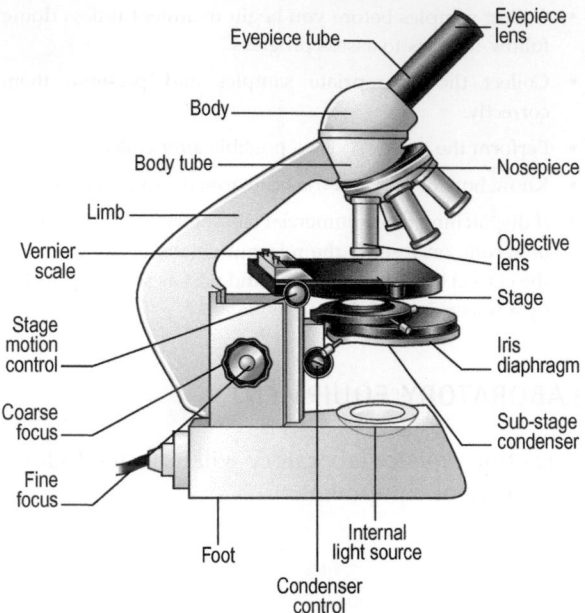

Figure 5.1 A light microscope.

Procedure: Care and use of the microscope (Fig. 5.1)

1. **Action:** Place the microscope on an even, stable surface.

   Rationale: The slightest vibration will be magnified when looking down the eyepiece making viewing an object very difficult.

2. **Action:** Before use, clean the eyepieces (Fig. 5.1), objective lens and the condenser with special lens tissue.

   Rationale: Lens tissue is lint free so that bits are not left on the surfaces. Other types of tissue or cloth may cause scratches. Cleaning should be done after you finish using the microscope, but you may need to do it again.

3. **Action:** Clean the oil immersion lens with the proper cleaning fluid.

   Rationale: This lens should be cleaned after every use with isopropanol. Oil left on the lens may damage the lens and cause it to consolidate.

4. **Action:** Turn the light control to a minimum and turn on the instrument.

Rationale: This prevents the sudden power surge breaking the microscope bulb.

5. **Action:** Adjust the eyepieces.

   Rationale: If using a binocular microscope arrange the eyepieces so that both fields converge as one. If you normally wear glasses remove them – you can alter the focus of the microscope to suit your eyes. Make sure that you are comfortable.

6. **Action:** Rotate the nosepiece in a clockwise direction so that the ×10 objective lens clicks into the viewing position.

   Rationale: Always start viewing a slide through the lowest magnification.

7. **Action:** Rack up the sub-stage condenser until its top surface is as high as possible.

   Rationale: This condenses the light source onto the specimen to make it bright and sharper.

8. **Action:** Looking from the side of the microscope, adjust the iris diaphragm control lever so that it is in its middle position.

   Rationale: This regulates the amount of light passing through the condenser. As the lens magnification is increased the aperture of the iris diaphragm should be increased.

9. **Action:** Place the slide on the stage over the hole in the centre.

   Rationale: The stage is made of black vulcanite with a hole in the centre through which light from the condenser illuminates the slide. There may be clips on the stage to hold the slide firmly in place.

10. **Action:** Position the area to be viewed over the light source by using the control knobs on the mechanical stage.

    Rationale: This allows the slide to be examined smoothly and accurately without touching the slide with your fingers.

11. **Action:** Focus using the coarse adjustment knob and then with the fine adjustment knob.

    Rationale: Always focus up from the slide to prevent the objective lens descending on to the slide and cracking it. Avoid using the fine focus to excess – if you have to do this it means you are not near enough to focus with the coarse focus.

12. **Action:** To increase magnification, turn the nosepiece clockwise until the next objective lens clicks into place.

    Rationale: There will usually be three objective lenses screwed into the nosepiece and one oil immersion lens. These provide different levels of magnification:

    » Blood and bacterial smears should be examined under ×10, ×50, then ×100 with oil immersion.
    » Urine sediments and faeces should be examined under ×10, then ×50.
    » Parasite slides should be examined with the naked eye followed by ×5, ×10, and if necessary ×50.

13. **Action:** After you have finished, remove the slide from the stage.

    Rationale: Slides should be stored in an appropriate box or, if not needed, should be disposed of in the sharps bin.

14. **Action:** After use, wipe the objective lenses with lens tissue and turn the nosepiece so that the lowest-powered lens is in position. Reduce the light and switch off and cover the microscope with its cover.

    Rationale: The microscope is now clean and ready to use the next time.

Procedure: Use of the oil immersion lens

When used correctly, this technique increases the magnification to the maximum achievable with a light microscope. This is required for the examination of bacteria and blood smears.

1. **Action:** Set up the microscope as described above and place the slide on the stage.

   Rationale: You are now ready to use oil immersion.

2. **Action:** Rotate the nosepiece so that neither the ×50 or ×100 lens is in position.

   Rationale: You need to have clear access to the slide when you place the drop of oil.

3. **Action:** Place a drop of oil on the slide (Fig. 5.2).

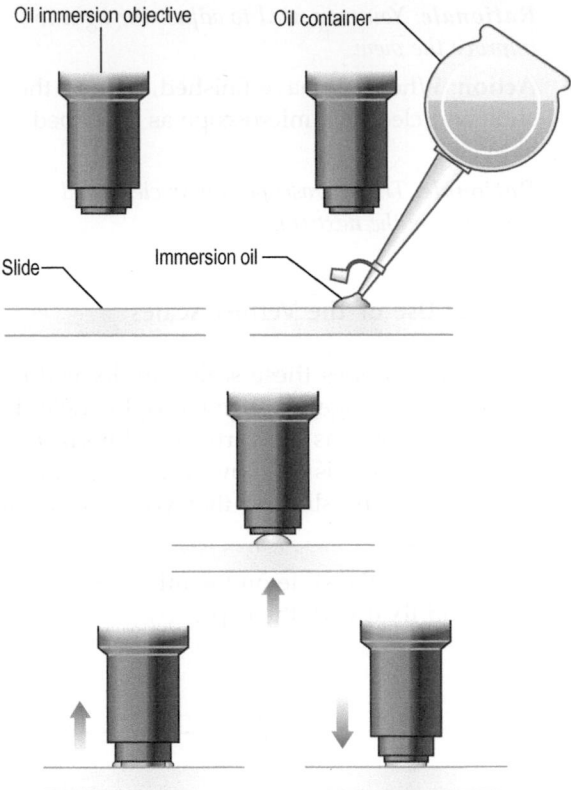

Figure 5.2 Use of the oil immersion objective.

Rationale: This oil is specifically designed for this purpose. Do not use any other type of oil.

4. **Action:** Rotate the nosepiece until the ×100 lens is above the slide and click into position.

   Rationale: This technique can only be done using the ×100 lens.

5. **Action:** Gently adjust the focus so that the lens descends to touch the drop of oil.

   Rationale: Always watch what you are doing. Do not look at the slide through the eyepiece as you will find it impossible to judge the distance and may smash through the slide. The lens must be lying in the oil to avoid distortion of the image and to achieve magnification.

6. **Action:** Looking through the eyepiece, adjust the focus using the fine control. At this point the oil may be seen to spread out (Fig. 5.2).

Rationale: You may need to adjust the light to improve the view.

7. **Action:** When you have finished, remove the slide and clean the microscope as described above.

Rationale: The microscope is now clean and ready to use the next time.

Procedure: Use of the Vernier scales

On most microscopes these scales are located on both sides of the stage, arranged at right angles to each other – known as the vertical and horizontal axes. Their function is to allow location of a particular point on the slide so that you can find it again (Fig. 5.3).

1. **Action:** Place the slide on the microscope stage and fix it with the clips.

Rationale: It is important that the slide does not move around as this will invalidate your scale references.

2. **Action:** Locate the object you wish to identify.

3. **Action:** Look at the scale on the vertical axis of the stage.

Rationale: See Figure 5.3.

4. **Action:** Record the number where the zero mark on the Vernier plate meets the main scale.

Rationale: In Figure 5.3 the zero mark falls between 31 and 32. If it falls between two divisions, record the lower number.

5. **Action:** Make a note of which of the marks on the Vernier plate is exactly opposite a division on the main scale.

Rationale: In Figure 5.3, mark number 6 is exactly opposite a division on the main scale.

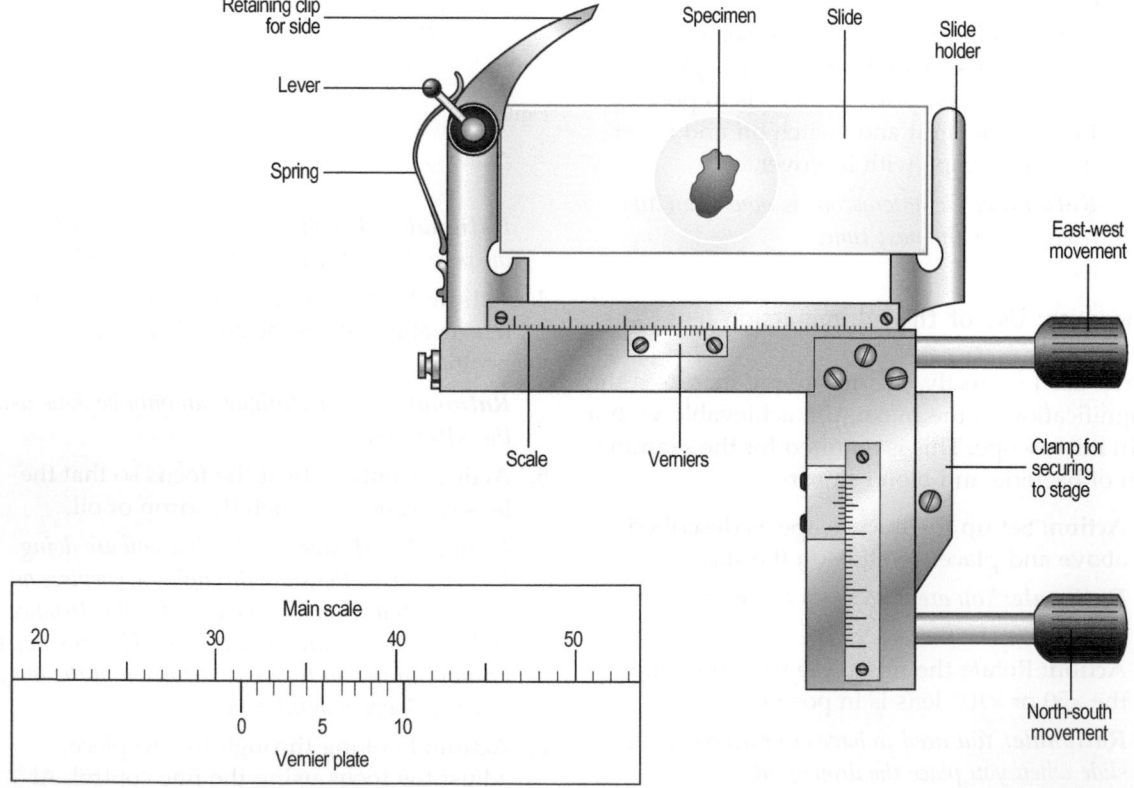

Figure 5.3 The Vernier scale. The zero on the Vernier plate is between 31 and 32 on the main scale, and it is mark number 6 on the Vernier plate that is exactly opposite a division on the main scale. The reading is therefore 31.6.

6. **Action:** Record this reading, placing it after the decimal point.

   Rationale: In Figure 5.3 this will give a reading of 31.6.

7. **Action:** Repeat steps 3–6 using the horizontal scale.

   Rationale: You will now have two readings – always write the horizontal scale first, e.g. 90.1 × 31.6.

8. **Action:** You now have a grid reference for that object on that slide provided that the slide is placed in the same position on the stage.

   Rationale: By tradition, slides are placed on the stage with the label to the right.

9. **Action:** You may now remove the slide, but can return to the same location using the grid reference.

   Rationale: This is useful if you wish to show someone else what you have found. You can locate it quickly and easily.

THE CENTRIFUGE

Centrifuges are an essential piece of laboratory equipment and, although they may vary, they all work on the principle of centrifugal force. Samples enclosed in special containers are spun around at speed, which results in the heavier particles settling at the bottom while the lighter ones go to the top. This would occur naturally in response to gravity if the container was left alone for some time, but the centrifuge accelerates the process.

The use of a centrifuge is required in many tests including:

- Separation of plasma or serum from blood cells
- Urine sedimentation
- Faecal analysis.

There are two main types:

1. **Angle head** – the specimen tubes are held in a fixed position, usually at 25–50° to the vertical. Higher rotational speeds can be achieved because of the aerodynamic shape of the rotor; however, because of the angulation

of the tubes, the sediment settles at this angle making it difficult to remove.

2. **Swing-out head** – the specimen tubes are placed in buckets that swing out from the vertical to the horizontal as the speed of rotation increases. As the machine stops the buckets return to the vertical position. The surface of the sediment is level, which means that the supernatant can be more easily removed with a pipette.

A microhaematocrit centrifuge, which is required to spin down blood samples prior to doing a packed cell volume estimation (PCV), consists of a metal plate on which fixed horizontal grooves carry the microhaematocrit capillary tubes.

Procedure: Care and use of the centrifuge

1. **Action:** Always ensure that the centrifuge is placed on an even, stable surface.

   Rationale: Slight vibration may occur when the centrifuge is switched on, and an uneven or unstable surface may cause the machine to move around and even fall to the ground.

2. **Action:** Use only the tubes recommended by the manufacturer.

   Rationale: These tubes, apart from microhaematocrit tubes, have conical bottoms and are designed to withstand centrifugal force.

3. **Action:** When placing the tubes in the machine, make sure that the top is not protruding above the top of the bucket.

   Rationale: This may affect the way that the machine works and make it unbalanced.

4. **Action:** Make sure that the sample tubes are balanced by placing in diametrically opposite buckets assessed by weight not volume.

   Rationale: If you do not do this then the machine will be unbalanced and may vibrate excessively. Stop the machine and check the tubes – this is the most common cause of vibration and instability.

5. **Action:** When using microhaematocrit tubes, ensure that the Plasticine® end is

placed against the outer ring of the instrument.

Rationale: This prevents the blood inside from escaping as it is subjected to centrifugal force.

6.   **Action:** Vacutainer® tubes may be spun with their stoppers in place.

Rationale: If the tube is opened or broken then aerosol contamination of the environment might occur.

7.   **Action:** Lock the lid of the centrifuge securely.

Rationale: If you do not the lid will fly open; however, most machines will not switch on if the lid is not secured properly.

8.   **Action:** Set the spin speed as appropriate.

Rationale: Different procedures require different speeds; for example, urine requires a lower speed than heparinized blood for biochemistry.

9.   **Action:** Never attempt to open the centrifuge until the head has stopped rotating.

Rationale: If you do this you may damage the machine and yourself.

10.   **Action:** After use, turn off the power supply and clean the machine thoroughly using a mild disinfectant and a soft cloth.

Rationale: To prevent contamination of the next samples.

11.   **Action:** Wear disposable gloves to remove any spillages or broken glass.

Rationale: To prevent any harm to yourself.

ELECTRONIC ANALYSERS

Many veterinary practices now use various types of electronic analyser to assist in the diagnosis of their clinical cases. These include those designed to analyse biochemistry, haematology, electrolytes and hormones. The variety of design makes it impossible to accurately describe their use within this book; however, you should take note of the following:

- Always refer to the manufacturer's instructions when first using the machine or if you encounter any problems.

- Site the machine away from chemicals and centrifuges, which may cause damaging vibrations.
- Run quality control tests at regular intervals to ensure accuracy and validity of the machine. These should be in addition to external quality control tests.
- Switch off and cover when not in use.
- Make sure the machine is regularly serviced.

PRACTICAL TECHNIQUES

HAEMATOLOGY

This is the study of the cellular elements of the blood and its associated clotting factors. Many haematology tests are nowadays done using a haematology analyser which automatically determines red and white cell counts, differential white cell counts, packed cell volume, haemoglobin levels and platelet counts; however, it is important to be able to know how to perform some of the more basic tests.

BLOOD COLLECTION

The sites and methods of restraint for the collection of blood from dogs, cats and rabbits have been described in Chapter 1, but once the sample has been collected it must be put into some form of container to preserve it and, if required, to prevent it from clotting. There are several forms of container:

1. **Screw-topped tubes** – these are usually made of plastic and have lids whose colour conforms to a standard colour code indicating the type of anticoagulant or preservative that they contain. This is shown in Table 5.1. Some brands may have push-on tops.

    These tubes are cheap and require only a small amount of blood to fill them. Remove the needle from the syringe and quickly transfer the blood into the tube. Immediately replace the cap and then mix the contents by repeated inversion unless you require a clotted sample. If you forcefully squirt the blood through a small gauge needle or shake the tube to mix it up you run the risk of breaking the blood cells resulting in a haemolysed sample.

Table 5.1 Standard colour coding for blood sample tubes

Colour of lid	Contents and uses
Pink	EDTA – for routine haematology
Mauve	Citrate – for coagulation tests
Orange	Heparin – plasma can be used for general biochemistry
Yellow	Fluoride – for glucose measurement
White	No additive – these allow the blood to clot so that serum can be extracted; these tubes must be made of glass

2. **Evacuated glass tubes (Vacutainers®)** – these consist of an evacuated glass tube sealed with a colour-coded rubber bung. They require the use of a double-pointed needle, which fits into a special needle holder. One end of the needle is used to penetrate the vein while the other end penetrates the rubber bung. The vacuum within the tube draws blood out of the vein into the tube. These are expensive and are more widely used in large animal practice.

3. **Plastic blood-collecting syringes (Monovette®)** – these are syringes that are designed for aspirating blood and contain anticoagulant. Once blood has been collected the needle is replaced with a cap and the plunger is unscrewed creating a leak-proof container.

PLASMA VS SERUM

Blood consists of the cellular fraction consisting of erythrocytes (red cells), leucocytes (white cells) and thrombocytes (platelets) and the fluid part – the plasma or serum.

- **Plasma** – obtained by centrifugation of a blood sample collected in anticoagulant, for example (e.g. ethylenediaminetetraacetic acid (EDTA) or heparin. Store at 5°C. Contains all the clotting factors. May be used for some biochemical tests, but anticoagulant can interfere in some tests.

- **Serum** – collect blood in glass tubes without anticoagulant and allow to clot. Serum is released as the blood clots; alternatively, it may be separated by serum separator

tubes, which contain a layer of gel that separates the cells from the serum. Store at 5°C. Serum does not contain clotting factors V and VIII or fibrinogen and is used for biochemistry.

Procedure: Packed cell volume

Packed cell volume (PCV) is used to measure the volume of the erythrocytes in whole blood when packed tightly together. It is used to assess the degree of anaemia and of dehydration in a patient.

Equipment list: Blood sample collected in an EDTA tube, plain capillary tubes, microhaematocrit centrifuge and reader, soft Plasticine® or Cristaseal®.

1. **Action:** Collect sample in an EDTA tube and rotate gently to mix the contents.

   Rationale: EDTA is an anticoagulant. Heparin tubes may also be used. Do not shake the tube as you may damage the blood cells.

2. **Action:** Remove the cap and tilt the sample so that a clear surface free of air bubbles can be seen.

   Rationale: If bubbles get into the capillary tube, they may cause an air-lock and slow the rate of filling.

3. **Action:** Place the end of a capillary tube into the blood sample, tilting the sample to at least 55°, and allow blood to run in until the tube is about ¾ full.

   Rationale: Blood will run into the capillary tube by capillary action. The microhaematocrit reader requires at least 5–7 cm of blood.

4. **Action:** Wipe the blood from the outside of the tube with a piece of tissue.

   Rationale: This reduces the risk of spread of infection to you.

5. **Action:** Holding the tube between your finger and thumb, insert the opposite end (from the blood) into the Plasticine® or Cristaseal® block. Twist two or three times and take it out of the Plasticine®.

   Rationale: This creates a plug, which prevents the blood from coming out of the end of the tube. If you use the wrong end of the tube you will contaminate the Plasticine®. The tube can be heat sealed in the flame of a Bunsen burner.

6. **Action:** Hold the tube vertically, sealed end down, and allow the blood column to run down.

   Rationale: Make sure that there is no evidence of a leak.

7. **Action:** Place the tube into one of the grooves of the microhaematocrit with the Plasticine® plug facing outwards towards the rim.

   Rationale: Centrifugal forces will cause the cells and fluid to spin outwards. The sealed end will prevent blood escaping.

8. **Action:** Place a similar tube on the opposite side of the centrifuge.

   Rationale: This balances the centrifuge and reduces vibration, although it is not essential in this type. If you are doing several tubes from a variety of patients then make a note of the number of each groove.

9. **Action:** Screw the safety plate over the tubes and close the lid.

   Rationale: The safety plate holds the tubes in place while they are spun. If you do not do this you will regret it!

10. **Action:** Set the timer for 6 minutes.

    Rationale: A microhaematocrit centrifuge spins at 10 000 r.p.m. and it takes 6 minutes to pack the erythrocytes properly.

11. **Action:** After 6 minutes allow the machine to stop naturally.

    Rationale: Avoid using the brake as this can damage the machine. Never attempt to open the machine while it is still running.

12. **Action:** Remove the capillary tube and check the colour and the thickness of the buffy coat. Write down your observations.

    Rationale: Check the plasma for evidence of haemolysis, jaundice and lipaemia. The buffy coat is made up of the leucocytes.

13. **Action:** Place the tube into the groove on the microhaematocrit reader (Fig. 5.4).

    Rationale: The blood will have separated into three layers (Fig. 5.4A):

» Plasma on the top
» Buffy coat in the middle
» Erythrocytes at the bottom.

14. **Action:** Adjust the tube vertically so that the bottom of the red cell layer is aligned with the 0%.

    Rationale: Make sure that you do not include the Plasticine® plug in your measurement.

15. **Action:** Slide the perspex plate so that the top of the plasma aligns with the 100% mark (Fig. 5.4B).

    Rationale: Use the bottom of the plasma meniscus as your measuring point.

16. **Action:** Adjust the reader handle on the left so that the line passes through the buffy coat / red cell junction.

    Rationale: This can be quite thick and pinpoint accuracy may be difficult.

17. **Action:** Read the measurement from the scale on the right hand side.

    Rationale: The scale on the reader runs from 0 to 100 and this is expressed as a percentage.

18. **Action:** PCV can also be calculated without the use of the reader by measuring the total length of the blood column (B) and the length occupied by the red blood cells (A) (Fig. 5.4A).

    Rationale: Do the following calculation:
    PCV % = A/B × 100%.

NB PCV ranges for the dog, cat and rabbit are shown in Table 5.2, and normal PCV values are shown in Table 5.3.

Total white blood cell count (TWBC) and total red blood cell count (TRBC) are useful diagnostic parameters (Table 5.2), but are nowadays usually done by an electronic haematology analyser. They used to be done using a Neubauer haemocytometer, but this takes time and experience. Commercial labs can get the result back to the practice within 12 hours so manual analysis is rarely done.

Procedure: Preparation of a blood smear

Blood samples can be examined and preserved by smearing a drop of blood onto a glass slide. The skill of preparing a blood smear can be achieved

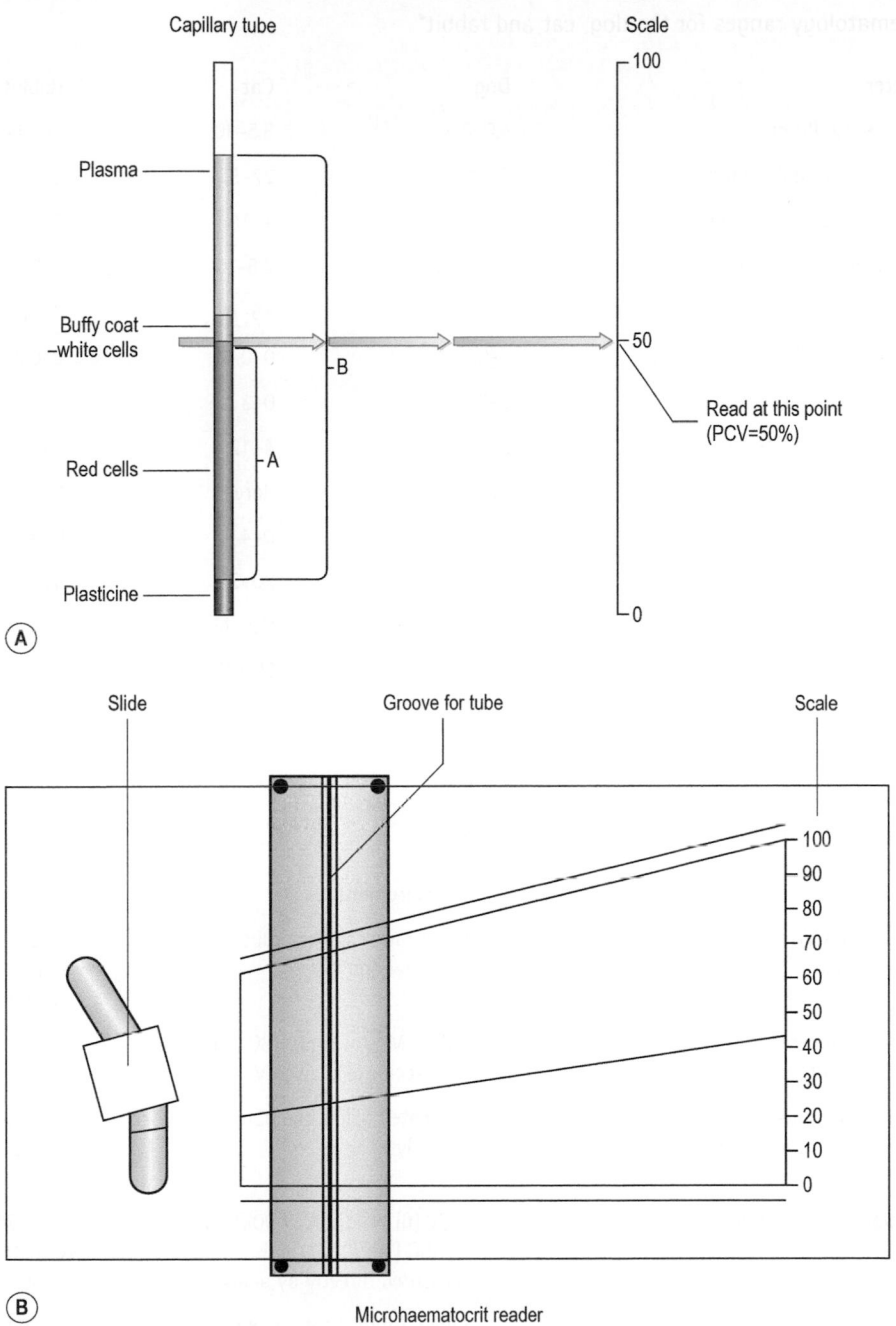

Figure 5.4 Measuring packed cell volume (PCV): (A) Capillary tube; A is the length of the tube occupied by red cells; B is the total length of the column of blood. (B) Microhaematocrit reader.

Table 5.2 Haematology ranges for the dog, cat and rabbit*

Blood parameter	Dog	Cat	Rabbit
Red blood cells ($\times 10^{12}$/litre)	5.0–8.5	5.5–10.0	5–8 ($\times 10^6$/mm^3)
Packed cell volume (%whole blood)	37–57	27–50	34–50
Total white blood cells ($\times 10^9$/litre)	6–15	4–15	5–12
Mature neutrophils ($\times 10^9$/litre)	3.6–10.5	2.5–12.5	3–20
Mature neutrophils (% of all blood cells)	60–70	45–75	34–60
Band neutrophils ($\times 10^9$/litre)	0–0.3	0–0.45	0–0.2
Band neutrophils (% of all blood cells)	0–2	0–3	–
Eosinophils (% of all blood cells)	2–10	4–12	0–2
Basophils (% of all blood cells)	Rare	Rare	0–1
Monocytes (% of all blood cells)	3–10	0–4	0–4
Lymphocytes – small (% of all blood cells)	12–30	20–55	(All) 43–62
Lymphocytes – large (% of all blood cells)	Approx. 8%	Variable	–
Platelets ($\times 10^9$/litre)	200–500	200–600	240–600 ($\times 10^3$/mm^3)

Taken from a range of sources.

Table 5.3 Red blood cell indices in the dog, cat and rabbit*

Name/definition	Measurement	Normal values
Packed cell volume (PCV): percentage of packed red cells in a sample	Centrifuge capillary tube containing blood	Dog: 37–57% Cat: 27–50% Rabbit: 34–50%
Haematocrit (HCT): percentage of blood composed of red cells (often interchanged with PCV)	HCT = MCV × total RBC (10^{12}/l) Less accurate than PCV	–
Haemoglobin (Hb): amount of Hb within red cells – estimation of O_2-carrying capacity	Estimated using haematology analyser	Dog: 12–18 g/dl Cat: 8–15 g/dl Rabbit: 10–17.5 g/dl
Mean corpuscular volume (MCV): measure of red cell size	MCV (fl) = (PCV × 1000)/total RBC (10^{12}/l) Measured directly by analysers	Dog: 70 fl Cat: 45 fl Rabbit: 69 fl
Mean corpuscular haemoglobin concentration (MCHC): average concentration per red blood cell	MCHC (g/dl) = total haemoglobin (g/dl) /PCV	35 g/dl for all species

Taken from a range of sources. fl = femtolitre: 1 fl = 10^{-15}l.

by practice, and it is worth the effort as a smear can provide a great deal of diagnostic information. They may be used to evaluate the relative proportions of the cellular components of blood and even to check the cell counts done by a machine. They may also be used to indicate the presence of cellular abnormalities, provide a rough estimation of platelet numbers and identify the presence of blood parasites.

Blood smears may be fixed by air drying or, if examination is to be delayed, by immersing in 100% methyl alcohol for 1 minute. If the smear is to be sent to an external laboratory, it should be carefully packaged to prevent damage.

Equipment list: blood sample in an EDTA tube, glass microscope slides previously soaked in methanol and dried, glass cutter and marker pen.

1. **Action:** Select a new clean glass microscope slide and wipe it with lint-free tissue. If it has been soaked in methanol, rinse and dry it.

   Rationale: The slide must be as clean as possible to avoid the inclusion of dirt in the smear. Methanol removes grease and stops gaps appearing in the smear.

2. **Action:** Prepare a spreader by chipping the corner off another glass slide (Fig. 5.5). You may use a glass cutter to do this.

   Rationale: The use of the spreader prevents the smear overlapping the sides of the slide.

3. **Action:** Using a chinagraph pencil or an indelible felt pen, label the slide on the underside.

   Rationale: This identifies the slide. Marking it on the underside prevents the label being removed during staining.

4. **Action:** Take the EDTA tube containing the blood sample and gently rotate it between your finger and thumb. The tube must be at room temperature.

   Rationale: This resuspends the cells evenly within the plasma. Do not be overvigorous as this will damage the cells.

5. **Action:** Place the slide flat on the bench, preferably on a white background, with the long edges parallel to the edge of the bench.

   Rationale: The white background will help to show up the blood smear.

6. **Action:** Dip a capillary tube into the blood sample and allow it to collect a small amount of blood.

   Rationale: Blood will move up the capillary tube by capillary action.

7. **Action:** Place a small drop of blood on the right-hand end of the slide about 1 cm from its edge.

   Rationale: If you are left handed place the drop on the left-hand end. Too large a drop of blood will make the smear too thick; too small a drop gives too short a smear and/or 'hesitation lines'.

8. **Action:** Place the spreader to the left of the blood at an angle of 45° to the horizontal and draw backwards to 'pick up' the blood (Fig. 5.5).

   Rationale: The blood will run along the edge of the spreader as soon as it makes contact with the blood. The angle of the spreader helps to determine the thickness of the smear.

9. **Action:** Move the spreader forwards towards the left-hand end of the slide in a single smooth movement so that the blood is smeared along the slide.

   Rationale: The blood is drawn along behind the spreader. If you were to push the blood along the slide without drawing back, as in step 6, you would damage the blood cells. The sides of the smear should be parallel and there should be a feathery 'tail'. It should take up about ⅔ of the slide.

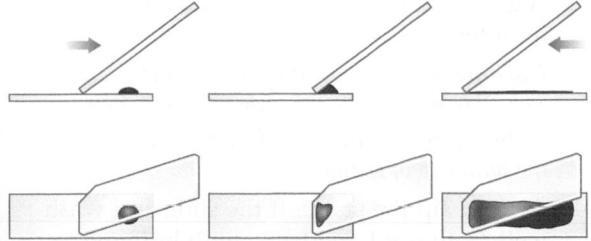

Figure 5.5 Preparation of a blood smear.

10. **Action:** Dry the slide in the air by holding the sides between your finger and thumb and waving it gently.

    Rationale: The use of heat to dry the slide will damage the cells. Instant drying will preserve cell morphology.

11. **Action:** Make another blood smear.

    Rationale: It is always a good idea to make more than one smear in case one is unsatisfactory.

12. **Action:** Assess the quality of your smears.

    Rationale: The quality of the smear affects its use in diagnosis:

    » Thickness – if it is too thick it may be difficult to see the cells and it may take longer to dry, which may damage the cells.

    » Uneven – due to jerky movements during spreading known as 'hesitation marks' – some areas may be unusable.

    » Streaks, gaps and spots – may be caused by dirt or grease on the slide – discard the slide.

    » Narrow smear – smear has been made before the blood has run the full width of the spreader. Limits the use of the smear.

13. **Action:** Stain the most satisfactory smears.

    Rationale: Use an appropriate stain depending on what you need to know from the slide.

STAINING BLOOD SMEARS

In order to see and accurately identify blood cells, the smear must be stained with the appropriate stain. Haematological stains can be used to:

• Perform a differential white cell count.

• Identify the presence of blood parasites such as *Mycoplasma haemofelis* and *Babesia* spp.

• Detect changes in shape, size and staining of the blood cells.

• Perform a rough estimate of platelet numbers.

The most commonly used stains are known as the Romanowsky stains. These employ the combination of two different dyes to achieve their effect. Diff-Quik® is the most popular as it is quick and easy to use. The manufacturer's instructions should always be followed when using it, but there is a tendency for the slides to fade during storage and it gives poor cellular definition.

Leishman's stain is better for differential white cell counts and Giemsa's stain is used to demonstrate blood parasites. Supravital staining, which is used to stain cells before their chemical life ceases (e.g. fresh unclotted blood), is not routinely used in practice, but the use of methylene blue is recommended for reticulocyte counts.

Always wear gloves when staining blood smears as the process is messy and some stains are toxic when inhaled, ingested or when they come into contact with the skin.

Procedure: Leishman's stain

This stain uses a combination of haematoxylin and eosin and is used for differential white cell counts.

Equipment list: Leishman's stain, buffered water pH 6.8, Coplin jar (not essential), tissues or blotting paper, staining rack, filter paper, forceps.

1. **Action:** Place a prepared blood smear with the smear uppermost, on a staining rack across a sink or staining bath.

   Rationale: This is a messy process and you must allow the stain to drain off into a sink or staining bath.

2. **Action:** Pour neat Leishman's stain through a piece of filter paper on to the slide. Leave for 2 minutes.

   Rationale: There must be enough stain to cover the entire slide. Filtering the stain removes sediment, which could be mistaken for blood parasites.

3. **Action:** Do not wash off the stain, but add twice the volume of buffered distilled water (pH 6.8) and mix well. Leave for 15 minutes. A gold film may be seen within a few minutes.

   Rationale: This indicates that the pH is correct. The slide may be placed, using forceps, in a vertical position, in a Coplin jar – this prevents the build-up of sediment.

4. **Action:** Tip the stain off the slide and wash well, both front and back, with buffered water.

Rationale: Do not use tap water as the changed pH will alter the staining characteristics of the cells.

5. **Action:** Wipe the underside of the slide with tissue and air dry.

   Rationale: Avoid touching the smear as you will wipe it off.

6. **Action:** Examine under the microscope using ×100 oil immersion.

   Rationale: This stain is useful for differential white cell counts as it provides good cellular definition.

Procedure: Giemsa stain

This stain uses a combination of methylene blue and eosin and is used to demonstrate the presence of blood parasites.

Equipment list: Giemsa stain – both neat and diluted 1:3 with buffered water (pH 6.8), Coplin jar, filter paper, buffered distilled water (pH 6.8), pipette, staining rack, methanol, forceps.

1. **Action:** Place a prepared blood smear with the smear uppermost, on a staining rack across a sink or staining bath.

   Rationale: This is a messy process and you must allow the stain to drain off into a sink or staining bath.

2. **Action:** Using a pipette, flood the smear with methanol. Leave for 3–5 minutes.

   Rationale: This fixes the smear.

3. **Action:** Drain off the methanol and allow the slide to air dry.

   Rationale: This is essential before using the stain.

4. **Action:** Flood the slide with neat Giemsa stain pouring it through a piece of filter paper. Leave for 30 seconds.

   Rationale: Filtering the stain removes sediment, which may be mistaken for blood parasites.

5. **Action:** Using forceps transfer the slide to a Coplin jar containing Giemsa stain diluted 1:3 with buffered distilled water pH 6.8. Leave for 15–20 minutes.

Rationale: The slide is held in a vertical position in the Coplin jar, which prevents the build-up of sediment on the slide.

6. **Action:** Remove the slide from the Coplin jar and rinse on both sides with buffered distilled water.

   Rationale: Do not use tap water as the changed pH will alter the staining characteristics of the cells.

7. **Action:** Wipe the underside of the slide and allow to air dry. Do not touch the top of the slide.

   Rationale: You may remove the stained smear.

8. **Action:** Examine under the microscope using ×100 oil immersion.

   Rationale: This stain is used to identify blood parasites and can also be used for differential white cell counts.

Procedure: Differential white cell count

1. **Action:** Place a prepared blood smear stained in either Leishman's or Giemsa under a light microscope.

   Rationale: Both Leishman's and Giemsa provide good cellular definition for this procedure.

2. **Action:** Examine under ×10 objective lens.

   Rationale: This enables you to select an area that is one-third of the way from the tail end of the smear on the side edge.

3. **Action:** Scan over the slide and assess the distribution of the white cells.

   Rationale: If the distribution is uneven or clumped then it may be better to make another smear.

4. **Action:** Select an area near to the tail of the smear and apply a drop of immersion oil and move the ×100 objective into the oil.

   Rationale: See Figure 5.2. This increases the magnification.

5. **Action:** Adjust the condenser as described previously.

   Rationale: This provides maximum illumination.

6. **Action:** When focusing use the fine focus knob.

   Rationale: If you use the coarse focus knob the incremental movements mean your view moves out of focus very quickly.

7. **Action:** Move the slide so that it follows the line of a 'battlement' (Fig. 5.6) as follows: scan two fields along the edge of the smear, two fields down into the smear, two fields along, two fields back up towards the edge and so on.

   Rationale: This movement describes the battlement of a castle. By doing this you cover a wide area of the smear and it prevents biased cell distribution on the slide.

8. **Action:** While you are examining the fields count 200 white blood cells.

   Rationale: White blood cells have nuclei, which are stained in varying shades of pink or purple depending on their type (Fig. 5.7).

9. **Action:** Identify each type of white blood cell and record it (Fig. 5.7).

   Rationale: This will form the basis of your blood count. You may record your results manually on paper or by using some form of commercial counter.

10. **Action:** You can also scan the slide by travelling in a straight line along the length of the smear starting at the tail.

    Rationale: The tail is the thinnest part of the smear and the cells may be more clearly seen in this area. This method achieves the same final result as the battlement method.

11. **Action:** Using the records of each type of white blood cell, calculate the percentage of each type. The more cells you count in total the more accurate your results will be.

    Rationale: For example if you have 144 neutrophils in a sample of 200 then the percentage is

    $144/200 \times 100 = 72\%$.

12. **Action:** Compare your results with the normal ranges shown in Table 5.2.

NB If you have trouble finding 200 cells then move to the other side of the smear; in cases of leucopaenia you may have difficulty finding 100 cells, but you should make a note of this. Do not record any unrecognizable or damaged cells, but if they occur in large numbers make a note of the fact. Normoblasts (i.e. immature red cells) should also be noted as if they were among the other nucleated cells.

Procedure: Reticulocyte count

Reticulocytes are immature erythrocytes (red cells) and they are derived from normoblasts. During the production of blood by haemopoietic tissue within the bone marrow, reticulocytes are released into the circulation. Their presence indicates a healthy regeneration of erythrocytes and, in cases of anaemia, blood loss and old age, depending on their numbers, is a good prognostic sign. The final maturation of reticulocytes into erythrocytes takes place in the liver and spleen. Table 5.3 shows a range of indices relating to normal mature erythrocytes.

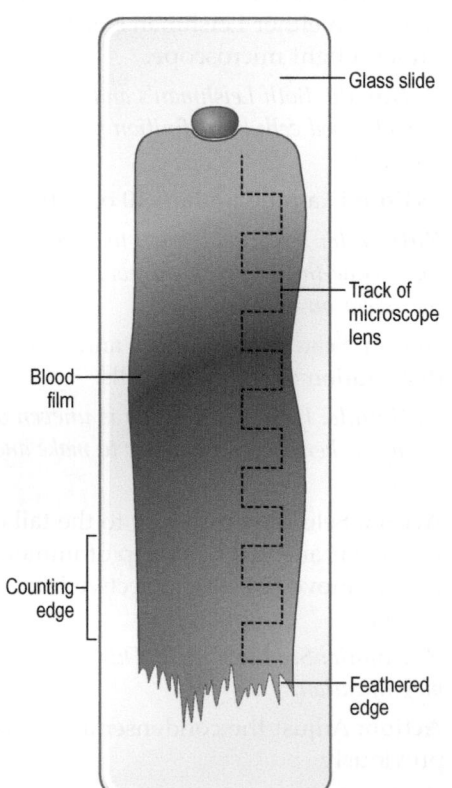

Figure 5.6 The battlement technique for differential blood films.

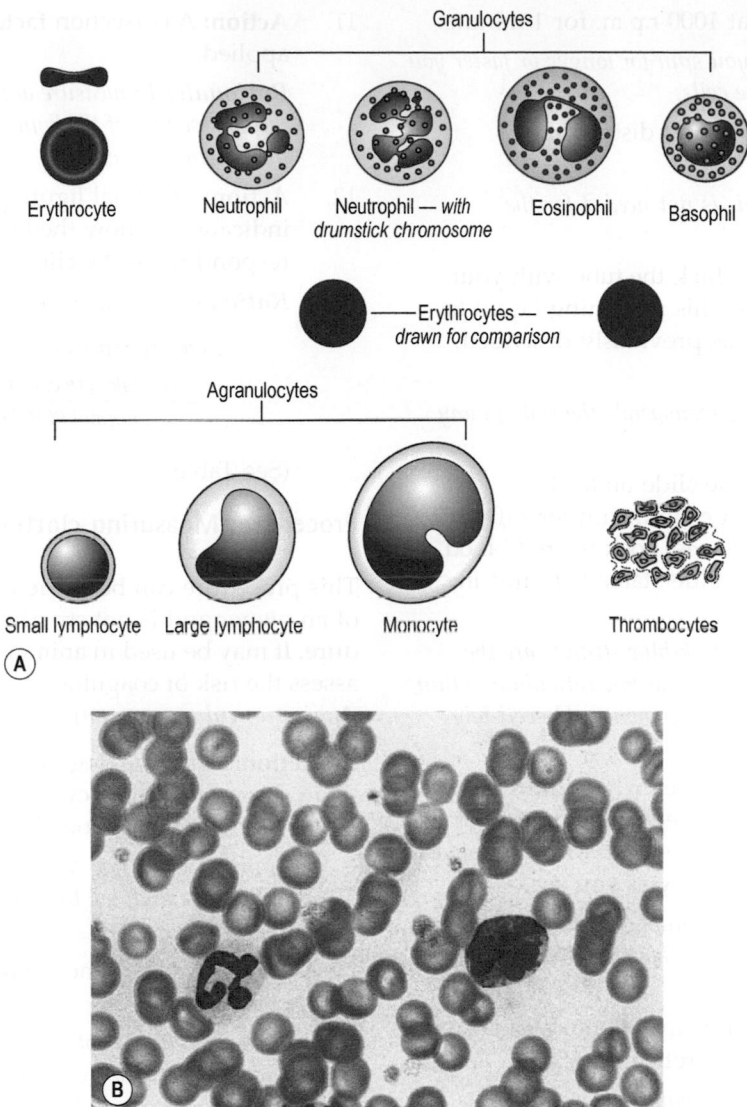

Figure 5.7 (A) The range of blood cells visible in a blood smear. (B) Light micrograph of canine basophil (left) and nearby neutrophil (right).

1. **Action:** Using a pipette, dispense 2 ml of methylene blue stain into a centrifuge tube.

   Rationale: *Ensure that the stain is new methylene blue. McFadyean's methylene blue is used to stain and identify* Bacillus anthracis, *the causal organism of anthrax.*

2. **Action:** Using a pipette, add 4–5 drops from a well-mixed sample of blood in an EDTA tube.

   Rationale: *Do not use heparin for this procedure.*

3. **Action:** Mix the two components gently in the tube and place in an incubator at 37°C for 30 minutes.

   Rationale: *If no incubator is available, the sample can be incubated at room temperature.*

4. **Action:** Remove from the incubator and place in a centrifuge.

   Rationale: *Make sure that you balance the centrifuge with a tube of similar weight as described previously.*

5. **Action:** Spin at 1000 r.p.m. for 1 minute.

 Rationale: If you spin for longer or faster you will damage the cells.

6. **Action:** Remove and discard the supernatant.

 Rationale: This is not needed for the procedure.

7. **Action:** Gently flick the tube with your fingers and use this remaining liquid to make a smear as previously described; allow to air dry.

 Rationale: This resuspends the cells in any remaining liquid.

8. **Action:** Place the slide under the microscope and examine under ×10 and ×40 objective lenses. Look for red blood cells with dark-blue-stained strands in them (Fig. 5.8).

 Rationale: The dark-blue strands are the remnants of the endoplasmic reticulum within the cell and they are known as Howell-Joly bodies (Fig. 5.8).

9. **Action:** Select an area where individual cells can be easily seen and count a total of 500 cells within the smear. Make a note of how many reticulocytes you see.

 Rationale: If individual cells can be seen clearly this indicates that the smear is one cell thick.

10. **Action:** Using this information, calculate the percentage of reticulocytes.

 Rationale: To calculate:

$$reticulocyte\ count = \frac{no.\ of\ reticulocytes \times 100\%}{total\ no.\ of\ cells\ counted}$$

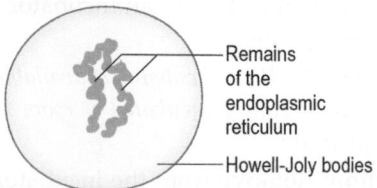

Figure 5.8 A reticulocyte. An immature circulating red cell, it can be stained with a supravital stain, e.g. new methylene blue.

Remains of the endoplasmic reticulum

Howell-Joly bodies

11. **Action:** A correction factor is now applied.

 Rationale: To measure accurately the responsiveness of the bone marrow, the PCV of the patient is used.

12. **Action:** The final figure provides an indication of how the bone marrow is responding to the clinical situation.

 Rationale: To calculate:

$$corrected\ reticulocyte\ count$$
$$= \frac{reticulocyte\ count \times patient's\ PCV}{normal\ PCV\ for\ the\ species}$$

(See Table 5.3.)

Procedure: Measuring clotting time

This procedure can be carried out in the presence of an owner and is not strictly a laboratory procedure. It may be used in animals prior to surgery to assess the risk of coagulopathy (e.g. infection with *Angiostrongylus vasorum*).

1. **Action:** Place the dog in a sitting position or in sternal recumbency on an examination table covered in a non-slip mat.

 Rationale: If the dog feels secure and comfortable it will be less inclined to move or to try and escape.

2. **Action:** Ask the owner to restrain the dog appropriately.

 Rationale: This is not really painful, but the dog should be prevented from jumping off the table during the procedure. Local anaesthetic must not be used.

3. **Action:** Clip the hair from the area of skin to be used. Include a reasonable area around the site.

 Rationale: In dogs the most common site is the ear pinna.

4. **Action:** Gently clean the area with surgical spirit and allow to dry.

 Rationale: Take care to avoid causing hyperaemia of the area by overvigorous rubbing.

5. **Action:** Using a sterile scalpel blade, make an incision about 1 cm long and 2 mm deep and start the stopwatch.

Rationale: This provides a base from which to measure the clotting time.

6. **Action:** After 15 seconds, touch a piece of filter paper to the blood so that it absorbs into the paper.

   Rationale: Avoid touching the skin.

7. **Action:** Repeat 15 seconds later using a fresh area of filter paper.

   Rationale: If using a circular piece of filter paper, move it around 1 cm at a time every time you touch the blood.

8. **Action:** Repeat the action until no more blood oozes from the incision. Stop the stopwatch.

   Rationale: The time on the stopwatch is the bleeding time and it is normally less than 5 minutes.

CYTOLOGY

Cytology is the study of cells. It includes where they have originated from, their structure and their function and also, in clinical cases, their pathology. The techniques are generally non-invasive, quick and easy to perform and have minimal risk to the patient. Cytology may provide a diagnosis or, at least, an indication as to how to proceed with the case. The disadvantage is the limitations of the collector's experience. He / she must know how to harvest the cells correctly, prepare the slides appropriately, and then interpret what is seen under the microscope.

SAMPLE COLLECTION

The equipment required for collecting samples is relatively simple and consists mainly of needles, syringes, sterile scalpel blades, clean glass microscope slides, sterile swabs or cottonwool buds, and blood collection tubes, both EDTA and serum tubes.

The technique used to collect the sample depends on the location of the sampling site and the type of tissue to be collected. Samples from inside the body may be collected during endoscopy (see Ch. 6). Always prepare several samples and use different methods of preparation; for example, if collecting fluid use both EDTA and serum tubes. These must be fixed by adding a couple of drops of formalin if sending to an external lab; if preparing slides, stain some and leave others unstained to use for specialized staining techniques or for sending off to an external lab. It is better to have too many samples than to have to go back and collect more.

The techniques are mainly used to diagnose tumours and can be divided into four main types:

- Imprints or touch impressions
- Fine needle aspiration
- Harvesting cells using swabs
- Collection and examination of fluids (e.g. exudates).

If the technique results in the collection of tumour cells this means that a tumour is present; however, if none are found it simply means that tumour cells were not collected in that sample, and not that there is no tumour.

Procedure: Collection of a sample by an imprint

This is used for assessing the cut surface of deep tissue (e.g. from a tumour or for superficial lesions such as an ulcer or a mast cell tumour).

1. **Action:** The patient will normally be under a general anaesthetic.

   Rationale: This depends on the site and on the degree of pain — if the lesion is superficial the patient may be sedated, or fully conscious and well restrained.

2. **Action:** Preparation of the area must be as aseptic as possible.

   Rationale: To prevent the spread of infection.

3. **Action:** Make a cut across the surface of the tissue.

   Rationale: This will expose fresh uncontaminated cells from deep within the lesion.

4. **Action:** Blot until dry with a piece of paper towel.

   Rationale: If the tissue is too wet the cells may not stick and may run off the glass slide.

5. **Action:** Take a precleaned glass slide and roll the tissue against it.

Rationale: All equipment must be clean and/or sterile to prevent the spread of infection. Rolling the tissue against the slide preserves the shape of the cells.

6. **Action:** Make several imprints on each slide.

   Rationale: This ensures that you obtain the maximum chance of understanding what is happening within the lesion.

7. **Action:** Allow the slides to air dry and stain.

NB If the tissue is hard or very fibrous the yield of cells may be low. This can be overcome by scraping the surface with a scalpel blade and spreading the material on to a glass slide.

Procedure: Collection of a sample by fine needle aspiration

Fine needle aspiration (FNA) is used for fluid-filled (e.g. abdominal viscera) or solid soft tissue masses.

1. **Action:** Place the patient in a comfortable position on the table with the area to be sampled uppermost and accessible.

   Rationale: If the technique is to be performed on a superficial mass then the patient may be either conscious or sedated and firmly restrained. If the area to be sampled is an abdominal mass then the patient may need to be sedated or under general anaesthesia.

2. **Action:** Clip the hair from the selected site and prepare the area aseptically.

   Rationale: To reduce the chance of introducing infection.

3. **Action:** For superficial masses, fix the mass firmly with one hand and insert the needle with the other hand.

   Rationale: Use 21–23G (¾–3″) needles depending on the depth of tissue to be sampled.

4. **Action:** If internal organs such as the liver, spleen and kidney or intra-thoracic or intra-abdominal organs are to be sampled, guidance of the needle by ultrasound may be necessary

   Rationale: It is impossible to fix these organs with one hand and there is a risk of penetrating another organ. Use 21–23G (¾–3″) needles as appropriate.

5. **Action:** If an internal organ such as the liver, spleen or kidney is to be sampled, haemorrhage may be a problem. In such cases use a Tru-cut® needle (Fig. 5.9).

   Rationale: A Tru-cut® needle is used to collect tiny samples. The needle has a small notch cut out of its barrel and a cover that slides down trapping the sample. This can then be removed, fixed and examined by cytology or histopathology.

6. **Action:** For a true FNA, when the needle is inserted attach a 5–10 ml syringe and pull back on the plunger several times while moving the needle to and fro within the lesion. Do not withdraw the needle.

   Rationale: This action helps to exfoliate cells from around the needle so that they can be drawn up into the needle. There is a risk of damaging fragile cells and increasing the amount of blood in the sample.

7. **Action:** When you are satisfied that you have collected enough cells, withdraw the needle and syringe from the site.

   Rationale: This keeps the harvested cells within the needle. Creating too much negative pressure by withdrawing the needle and syringe with the plunger half-way up would cause the cells to rush into the barrel of the syringe as the needle was withdrawn from the lesion. If there were relatively few cells in the sample, you might then lose them within the syringe.

8. **Action:** Detach the syringe from the needle and attach a clean air-filled syringe.

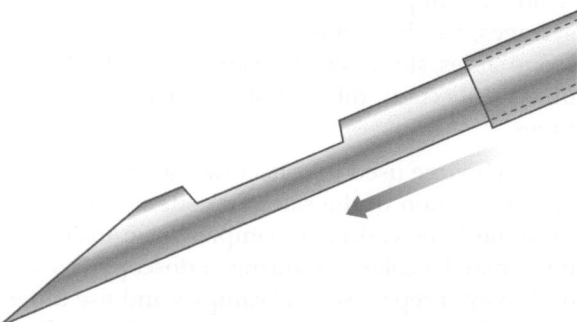

Figure 5.9 Simplified diagram of a Tru-cut® needle.

Rationale: This will ensure that only the contents of the needle are expelled.

9. **Action:** Depress the plunger and expel the contents of the needle onto one or more clean microscope slides.

   Rationale: Ensure that all the cells are expelled.

10. **Action:** Prepare smears as described below and examine under a microscope.

Procedure: Collection of a sample for cytology of the ear

1. **Action:** Place the animal in a sitting position on a stable examination table covered in a non-slip mat.

   Rationale: If the animal feels secure it will be less likely to try and escape.

2. **Action:** Ask the owner or an assistant to restrain the animal so that you have access to the ear.

   Rationale: See Chapter 1. This technique is not painful, but if an animal has an inflamed ear it may resent the procedure.

3. **Action:** Using a clean cotton bud soaked in a little sterile saline, insert it into the external ear canal and move it gently over the surface of the canal.

   Rationale: The aim is to pick up lining cells without further traumatizing the delicate epithelium.

4. **Action:** Roll the cotton bud over the surface of a clean microscope slide.

   Rationale: This deposits the cells harvested from the ear canal on the slide.

5. **Action:** If you have picked up a great deal of material you may have to spread or tease it out.

   Rationale: See the starfish technique below. The aim is to produce a thin layer of cells that can be easily stained and identified.

6. **Action:** Allow the slide to air dry and stain using Diff-Quik®.

   Rationale: Read the manufacturer's instructions.

7. **Action:** Place a drop of microscope oil on the slide and then place a cover slip on top.

   Rationale: This helps to protect and spread the layer of cells.

8. **Action:** Place the slide under the microscope and examine under ×100 oil immersion lens.

   This technique can be used to diagnose the presence of *Malassezia pachydermatis*, although you may also find bacteria and *Otodectes* mites, which will more easily be seen under ×4 or ×10 magnification. Gram stain is used to differentiate between Gram negative and Gram positive bacteria.

Other types of sample used for cytology are shown in Table 5.4.

SMEAR PREPARATION

The samples that have been collected must now be stained and examined under the microscope. The cells may be very fragile and the technique employed to make the smears must take this into account.

Table 5.4 Types of sample used for cytology

Type of sample	Uses
Skin masses	Lipoma, mast cell tumour, histiocytoma, epidermal cysts; examine samples for characteristic and changed cells.
Lymph nodes	Lymphosarcoma and hyperplasia.
Transtracheal washes and bronchoalveolar lavage	Used to assess the airways; may be low in cells – look for evidence of inflammation and bacteria, fungi and parasites.
Joint fluid	Low numbers of cells – look for evidence of inflammation or sepsis.
Effusions	Collected from the abdomen or pleural cavities into EDTA for cytology and total protein – look for neutrophils and other inflammatory cells.

Procedure: Squash preparation – *used where there are few cells in the sample*

1. **Action:** Expel the cells within the needle onto the centre of a clean glass microscope slide.

   Rationale: Ensure that all the cells are expelled.

2. **Action:** Place another clean glass slide (the spreader) at right angles to the first and apply gentle pressure (Fig. 5.10).

   Rationale: This aids spreading, but too much pressure may rupture the cells.

3. **Action:** Draw the spreader quickly and smoothly across the bottom slide.

   Rationale: The underside of this slide will pick up the cells making a useable smear.

4. **Action:** Allow the smear on the spreader to air dry.

   Rationale: Do not use heat because the cells will be damaged.

5. **Action:** Stain appropriately.

   Rationale: Choice of stain depends on what you are looking for.

Procedure: Line smear technique

This technique is used for fluid aspirates (e.g. synovial fluid).

1. **Action:** Expel the aspirate at one end of a clean glass microscope slide.

   Rationale: This gives maximum space on the slide to make the smear.

2. **Action:** Using another glass slide, break off one corner using a glass cutter – this creates a spreader.

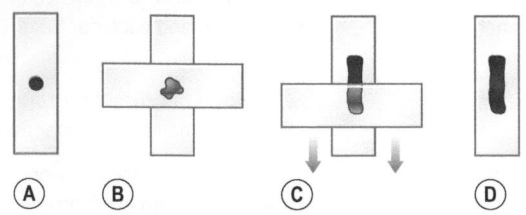

Figure 5.10 (A–D) Preparation of a smear of tissue cells using the squash technique. (After Lane & Cooper 2007, with permission from BSAVA.)

Rationale: The use of this shaped spreader to prepare the smear avoids spreading the cells over the edge of the slide.

3. **Action:** Place the spreader in front of the aspirate at an angle of approx. 30° and draw it backwards until the spreader picks up the aspirate (see Fig. 5.5).

   Rationale: This is the same technique as has been described for preparing a blood smear. The aspirate will flow along the spreader.

4. **Action:** Push the spreader quickly and smoothly along ⅔ of the slide.

   Rationale: The spreader will draw the aspirate, smearing the cells along the slide.

5. **Action:** At this point, abruptly lift the spreader upwards.

   Rationale: This creates a line in which the cells within the smear are concentrated. This is different to the true blood smear technique.

6. **Action:** Allow to air dry and stain appropriately.

   Rationale: Choice of stain depends on what you are looking for.

Procedure: Starfish preparation

1. **Action:** Expel the aspirate onto a clean glass microscope slide.

   Rationale: Ensure that all the cells are expelled.

2. **Action:** Using the point of the needle, drag the aspirate in several directions.

   Rationale: This method tends not to damage the cells. The aim is to draw out the cells to create a thin layer.

3. **Action:** Continue until the shape resembles that of a starfish with many projections (Fig. 5.11).

   Rationale: The thick layer of fluid around the cells may prevent evaluation of the cellular detail.

4. **Action:** Allow to air dry and stain appropriately.

   Rationale: Choice of stain depends on what you are looking for.

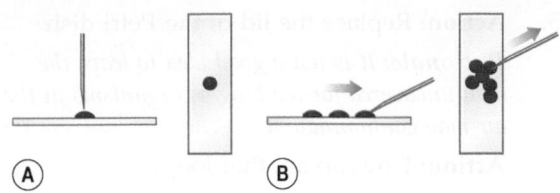

Figure 5.11 (A, B) Preparation of a smear of tissue cells using the starfish technique. (After Lane & Cooper 2007, with permission from BSAVA.)

CYTOLOGY STAINS

Most cytology samples can be stained using Romanowsky stains, which are generally easy to do and do not require special fixatives. They are useful for evaluating both nuclear and cytoplasmic features and can be used to stain fungi and parasites. They will stain bacteria, but they do not differentiate between Gram negative and Gram positive; this requires the use of Gram stain.

- Diff-Quik® – useful, quick and easy to use, but cellular definition may be impaired. Follow the manufacturer's instructions.
- Leishman's – used for blood cells. See previous notes.
- Giemsa – see previous notes.
- New methylene blue – does not stain the cytoplasm, but is good for nuclei. See previous notes.
- Sudan 3 – used to stain fat (e.g. in lipomata).

Procedure: Staining with Sudan 3

1. **Action:** Prepare slide as described above and allow to air dry.
   Rationale: Use of heat may damage the cells.
2. **Action:** Place the slide on a draining rack over a sink or over a staining bath.
   Rationale: This allows the stain to drain away without causing a mess.
3. **Action:** Flood the slide with Sudan 3 stain and leave for 3 minutes.
   Rationale: Sudan 3 binds with the fat in the sample.
4. **Action:** Wash gently with tap water.
   Rationale: This stops the action of the stain and removes any surplus.

5. **Action:** Place a coverslip over the smear.
   Rationale: This prevents the objective lens from being contaminated.
6. **Action:** Examine under the microscope.
   Rationale: Fat globules will stain orange.

When performing cytology in practice, you would be most likely to take several slides from your patient, look at one or two of them and then, if you are still not confident of your diagnosis, you would send them to an external laboratory for confirmation of your diagnosis.

BACTERIOLOGY

Unlike viruses, bacteria do not require living cells on which to grow and as result they can be easily cultivated within the lab. Some practice laboratories have the facilities to cultivate bacteria from samples collected from patients to identify the cause of an infection or to perform an antibiotic sensitivity test. Many other practices rely on external labs to provide this service.

Procedure: Bacterial cultivation

Bacteria can only be cultivated in the lab if they are provided with the appropriate growing conditions, i.e. an incubator, to control the temperature and a suitable type of growing medium that supplies the correct nutrients, water and pH. There are two main types of media: liquids or broths and solid media based on agar gel poured into a Petri dish. Basic or simple media may then be enriched, e.g. by the addition of blood, egg or bile lactose, resulting in selective media designed to differentiate between different species. Although the different types of media can be made up in the practice lab, it is easier to buy them already prepared and sterilized.

Equipment list: Petri dish containing the appropriate agar gel, platinum loop, Bunsen burner, incubator, marker pen, sample from patient.

1. **Action:** Label the Petri dish on the underside with a marker pen using the client's name and the animal's name or the case number.

Rationale: All agar plates look the same and it is important not to mix up the samples.

2. **Action:** Unwrap a single-use disposable loop and dip it into the sample.

   Rationale: These are ready sterilized. The use of platinum loops is discouraged as sterilizing, them by passing them through a Bunsen burner flame may cause aerosol spread of bacteria.

3. **Action:** Pick up the half of the Petri dish containing the agar gel and turn it over so that the surface of the gel is uppermost.

   Rationale: Petri dishes have a base containing the set agar gel and a lid that looks very similar.

4. **Action:** Smear the material on the loop over a small area on the left of the agar (Fig. 5.12).

   Rationale: This 'well' is the start of your inoculation area.

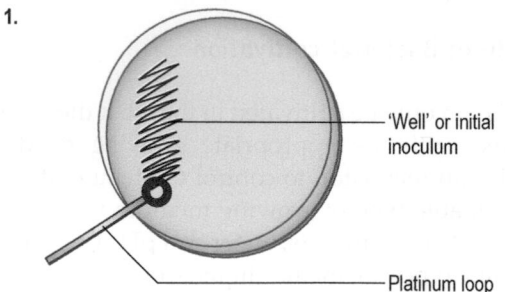

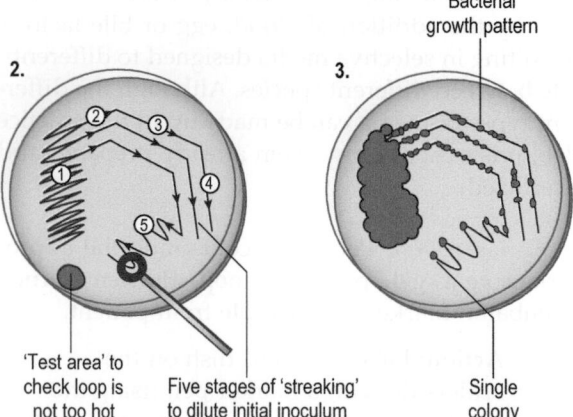

Figure 5.12 Technique for the inoculation of an agar plate.

5. **Action:** Replace the lid of the Petri dish.

   Rationale: It is not a good idea to leave the dish uncovered for too long as organisms in the air may contaminate it.

6. **Action:** Unwrap another loop.

   Rationale: To make sure that the only bacteria on the plate are from the original sample.

7. **Action:** Pick up the Petri dish as before and using the loop, make 3–4 streaks, all in the same direction from the edge of the well. Take care not to tear the agar (Fig. 5.12).

   Rationale: This technique helps to spread the contents of the sample evenly over the plate.

8. **Action:** Continue to spread the sample over the agar as shown in Figure 5.12.

   Rationale: The aim is to spread the sample ever more thinly so that single colonies will grow in the area of the final stroke.

9. **Action:** Place the lid back on the dish and put it in the incubator upside down (i.e. with the agar side on top).

   Rationale: If the lid is uppermost then water droplets, formed by condensation during incubation, will drip onto the agar causing the bacterial colonies to spread.

10. **Action:** Do not stack the agar plates more than two or three high in the incubator.

    Rationale: Overcrowding will prevent free circulation of air within the incubator.

11. **Action:** Incubate at 37°C for 18–24 hours.

    Rationale: Most pathogenic bacteria grow at normal body temperature (i.e. 37°C).

12. **Action:** Remove from the incubator and examine for bacterial colonies.

    Rationale: Colonies of bacteria appear as raised 'bumps' along the streak lines. Take note of their colour and any change in the agar around them as this may help in their identification.

13. **Action:** If there is no visible growth, incubate the plate for another 18–24 hours.

    Rationale: Some bacteria take longer to grow than others.

NB After use, Petri dishes containing bacterial cultures and the used loops must be placed in clinical waste and incinerated.

Procedure: Antibiotic sensitivity testing

This is a method of testing the susceptibility of bacteria to antibiotic therapy. Not all bacteria necessarily succumb to all antibiotics. A sensitivity test is part of a commercial laboratory's routine testing regimen, but in a practice lab, where it may be less common, it may be used in cases where a condition proves intractable (e.g. long-standing osteomyelitis or some bacterial skin conditions). It may also be used to identify the most effective antibiotic in cases of antibiotic resistance.

1. **Action:** Prepare a bacterial culture from the patient's sample as described previously.

   Rationale: This test cannot be done straight from the sample.

2. **Action:** Take a single-use disposable loop from its packaging.

   Rationale: These loops are designed to be used once and are presterilized.

3. **Action:** Holding the Petri dish as described above, use the loop to pick up an isolated colony and transfer it to a buffered peptone broth.

   Rationale: If there appears to be more than one type of colony growing on the plate you will have to test each one separately, but start with the predominant type.

4. **Action:** Incubate the peptone broth at 37°C for 4 hours.

   Rationale: Buffered peptone broth is available commercially and enhances bacterial growth, particularly of more fastidious organisms such as Pasteurella and Corynebacterium.

5. **Action:** Immerse a sterile swab in the broth and use it to completely cover a Mueller Hinton blood agar plate.

   Rationale: Using a swab ensures good coverage of the agar. Mueller Hinton blood agar contains sheep's blood and is available commercially. It is the standard agar for sensitivity tests.

6. **Action:** Pick up the antibiotic assay ring with forceps or tweezers and place it in the centre of the agar (Fig. 5.13).

   Rationale: The ring will have several antibiotic impregnated discs attached to it. Each disc is impregnated with a specific antibiotic (e.g. erythromycin, methicillin, tetracycline, etc.) and is printed with an identifying code. Some tests use individual antibiotic discs that are dropped onto the agar. Avoid handling the ring or discs with your fingers as this may contaminate them.

7. **Action:** Place the lid back on the dish and put it in the incubator upside down (i.e. with the agar side on top).

   Rationale: If the lid is uppermost then water droplets, formed by condensation during incubation, will drip onto the agar causing the bacterial colonies to spread.

8. **Action:** Do not stack the agar plates more than two or three high in the incubator.

   Rationale: Overcrowding will prevent free circulation of air within the incubator.

9. **Action:** Incubate at 37°C for 18–24 hours.

   Rationale: Most pathogenic bacteria grow at normal body temperature (i.e. 37°C).

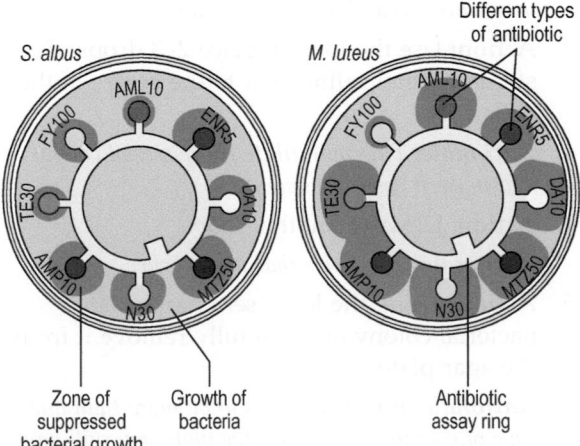

Figure 5.13 Antibiotic sensitivity testing on a bacterial culture. (Adapted with permission from www. Biology.ed.ac.uk The Microbial World – Penicillin and other antibiotics by James Deacon, University of Edinburgh.)

10. **Action:** Remove from the incubator and examine for bacterial growth.

    Rationale: If the bacteria are sensitive to a particular antibiotic, growth will be suppressed, which appears as a clear zone around the relevant disc (Fig. 5.13).

11. **Action:** Record your results.

    Rationale: This information will allow you to prescribe the antibiotic to which the causal organism is most sensitive, thus promoting a rapid recovery.

NB Antibiotic sensitivity testing is more widely used in large animal practice.

Procedure: Preparation of bacterial smears

Equipment list: Petri dish containing bacterial growth, platinum loop, Bunsen burner, glass microscope slide, sterile normal saline.

1. **Action:** Prepare a glass microscope slide by cleaning it with alcohol and allowing it to dry.

    Rationale: This removes any residues or grease that may be sticking to the slide.

2. **Action:** Unwrap a single-use disposable loop and dip it into the saline.

    Rationale: These are ready sterilized. The use of platinum loops is discouraged as sterilizing them by passing them through a Bunsen burner flame may cause aerosol spread of bacteria.

3. **Action:** Use the loop to place 2–3 drops of sterile normal saline near to the centre of the slide.

    Rationale: This will dilute the bacterial colony and make it easier to spread.

4. **Action:** Unwrap another loop.

    Rationale: To ensure that it is sterile.

5. **Action:** Using the loop, select an isolated bacterial colony and carefully remove it from the agar plate.

    Rationale: If there appears to be more than one type of colony growing on the plate you will have to make a smear for each type.

6. **Action:** Place the colony on the slide close to the saline and mix the two together using the loop.

Rationale: Mixing with saline results in a single layer of cells, allowing easier identification.

7. **Action:** Spread the mixture out over the slide to cover 1–2 cm.

    Rationale: A thin layer of cells enables you to see the shape of the cells.

8. **Action:** Dry the bacterial smear by passing the slide with the smear side uppermost through a Bunsen burner flame two or three times.

    Rationale: This fixes the slide. If the slide is stained while it is still wet then some of the bacteria will float off. Be careful not to overheat the slide.

9. **Action:** Stain the smear using Gram's stain or methylene blue.

    Rationale: These stains show up the shape of the bacteria.

Procedure: Staining a bacterial smear using Gram's stain

Gram's stain is used to identify the shape of the bacteria and to differentiate between the pink Gram negative bacteria (e.g. *Escherichia coli, Salmonella*) and the deep purple Gram positive bacteria (e.g. *Staphylococcus, Streptococcus, Clostridium*). The difference in colour is brought about by the bacterial cell wall's reaction to the stain and is the first step towards specific identification.

Equipment list: Prepared bacterial smear, crystal violet stain, Gram's or Lugol's iodine, acetone, carbol fuchsin (dilute) or safranine, staining rack, wash bottle containing tap water, blotting paper or tissue, timer, Pasteur pipettes.

1. **Action:** Place the prepared slide with the smear facing uppermost on a staining rack over a sink or staining bath.

    Rationale: Staining is a messy process and the surplus stain must be able to drain away. You can also stain using upright Coplin jars.

2. **Action:** Using a pipette, flood the slide with crystal violet for 30 seconds.

    Rationale: At this point, both types of bacteria absorb the stain and become purple.

3. **Action:** Wash the slide with tap water.

   Rationale: To remove the crystal violet stain.

4. **Action:** Flood the slide with iodine for 60 seconds.

   Rationale: This acts as a mordant, fixing the stain. Gram's iodine is stronger than Lugol's iodine and is the stain of choice.

5. **Action:** Flood the slide with acetone for 2–3 seconds.

   Rationale: This decolourizes the smear and is very rapid. Gram negative bacteria lose their colour.

6. **Action:** Wash the slide with water.

   Rationale: To remove the acetone.

7. **Action:** Flood the slide with carbol fuchsin for 30 seconds.

   Rationale: This counter-stains the bacteria and Gram negative bacteria become pink.

8. **Action:** Wash the slide with tap water.

   Rationale: To remove the stain.

9. **Action:** Wipe the back of the slide.

   Rationale: Do not wipe the smear off the front of the slide.

10. **Action:** Pass the slide rapidly over the flame of the Bunsen burner.

    Rationale: To dry the slide. Do not overheat the slide as it will shatter.

11. **Action:** Place the slide under the microscope and examine under high power.

    Rationale: Bacteria range in size from 0.5 μm to 5.0 μm so use ×100 oil immersion lens.

NB Never allow a slide to dry between stains. Dispose of all used slides in disinfectant prior to disposal in the sharps bin.

Procedure: Staining a bacterial smear using methylene blue stain

Methylene blue stains all bacteria blue and is used to identify the size and shape of the bacteria (i.e. coccus, bacillus, vibrio, etc.).

Equipment list: Prepared bacterial smear, staining rack, Löffler's methylene blue, tissue or blotting paper, Pasteur pipette, wash bottle containing tap water.

1. **Action:** Place the prepared slide with the smear facing uppermost on a staining rack over a sink or staining bath.

   Rationale: Staining is a messy process and the surplus stain must be able to drain away. You can also stain using upright Coplin jars.

2. **Action:** Using a pipette flood the slide with methylene blue stain and leave for 3 minutes.

   Rationale: This stains the bacterial cells.

3. **Action:** Wash the slide with tap water from the water bottle.

   Rationale: This removes the excess stain from the slide.

4. **Action:** Wipe the back of the slide.

   Rationale: Do not wipe off the smear from the front of the slide.

5. **Action:** Pass the slide rapidly over the flame of the Bunsen burner.

   Rationale: To dry the slide. Do not overheat the slide as it will shatter.

6. **Action:** Place the slide under the microscope and examine under high power.

   Rationale: Bacteria range in size from 0.5 μm to 5.0 μm so use ×100 oil immersion lens.

URINALYSIS

The kidney is responsible for filtering the blood to remove toxic substances from the body and for osmoregulation; 20% of cardiac output flows through the healthy kidney at any one time so it follows that analysis of the resulting urine will provide information about the patient's current health status. Urine tests are easy to perform and it is rarely necessary for urine to be sent to a commercial laboratory for analysis. Table 5.5 shows normal urine values.

Urine collection – urine may be collected by a normally voided mid-stream sample, by catheterization or, if a sterile sample is required, by cystocentesis. If an owner is required to collect a sample from a dog he / she may require instruction about suitable containers; emphasize that these must be clean – a partially cleaned jam jar may affect the results! Impermeable cat litter is useful for obtaining a voided sample from a cat.

Urine preservation – it is always better to examine the urine sample as soon as possible as any crystals present may dissolve, the pH increases with age, bacteria may overgrow and colour changes on dipstick tests may be abnormal.

If a sample cannot be tested immediately it should be stored in the fridge and tested within 24 hours. Collect urine in boric acid tubes for bacteriology and in plain tubes for all other tests. Plain tubes may be used for bacteriology provided that the urine is tested within 20 minutes.

Procedure: Urinalysis using dipstick tests

Dipsticks, consisting of strips of chemical reagents in the form of small pads and designed to test a variety of parameters, are produced by several manufacturers; however, none of them are specifically designed for the veterinary market. They are calibrated for human urine and you should be aware of their inaccuracies for certain parameters in animals (e.g. specific gravity).

1. **Action:** Select the correct type of dipstick test.

    Rationale: Reagent pads vary in number and type according to manufacturer.

2. **Action:** Check the expiry date.

    Rationale: Out of date sticks may give unreliable results.

3. **Action:** Remove the lid of the container, remove one stick and replace the lid.

    Rationale: Avoid contaminating the rest of the sticks with urine.

4. **Action:** Dip the stick in the fresh urine sample until all the pads are wet.

    Rationale: Never perform this test on stale urine as the results may be affected.

5. **Action:** Remove the stick from the sample and gently tap it on the side of the sample pot.

    Rationale: To remove any surplus urine.

6. **Action:** Using a timer or the second hand on your watch, keep to the time specified on the side of the dipstick bottle to take your reading.

Table 5.5 Normal urine values*

Parameter	Dog	Cat	Rabbit
Colour	Pale yellow due to staining with urochrome	Pale yellow due to staining with urochrome	Cream – red; rabbit urine may be stained red with porphyrin pigments – this is normal
Turbidity (**NB** Old urine samples appear cloudy)	Clear	Clear	Cloudy
Smell	Slightly sour smell	Characteristic smell in unneutered tomcats	Little or none
Daily volume (ml/kg bodyweight)	20–100	10–12	20–350
pH	5.2–6.8	6.0–7.0	7.6–8.8
Specific gravity	1.015–1.045	1.020–1.040	1.003–1.036
Protein	Small amounts	Small amounts	Trace
Glucose	None	None	Trace

*Taken from a range of sources.
NB Normal urine contains only water, salts and urea. It should **not** contain any bilirubin, haemoglobin or glucose.

Rationale: Each test pad requires a specific time in contact with the urine before it reacts appropriately.

7. **Action:** Hold the dipstick bottle in one hand and the dipstick in the other and compare the colour of each pad with the correct one on the side of the container.

    Rationale: Each reagent pad will change colour. The range of colour changes is illustrated on the side of the bottle along with the appropriate result.

8. **Action:** Check that you read the results from the correct end of the stick.

    Rationale: If you read from the wrong end you will get results that are incorrect for each test pad.

9. **Action:** Write down your results.

    Rationale: Do not rely on your memory – the results may need to be kept for some time before you use them to assist your diagnosis.

10. **Action:** Dispose of the dipstick in the clinical waste.

    Rationale: There may be pathogens on the stick.

NB Some people recommend placing the dipstick flat on the lab bench and putting a drop of urine onto each pad with a pipette. While this is not completely incorrect it is not the method recommended by the manufacturers – hence they are called dipsticks!

Procedure: Measuring specific gravity of urine using a refractometer

The reagent pad for specific gravity on a dipstick is calibrated for human urine and should not be relied upon. Always measure the specific gravity of animal urine using a refractometer (Fig. 5.14).

1. **Action:** To calibrate the refractometer, wipe the glass prism (Fig. 5.14) with a piece of lint free tissue. Using a pipette place approximately 2 drops of distilled water onto the prism and close the lid.

    Rationale: The refractometer must be calibrated every time you use it to ensure that it measures the specific gravity accurately.

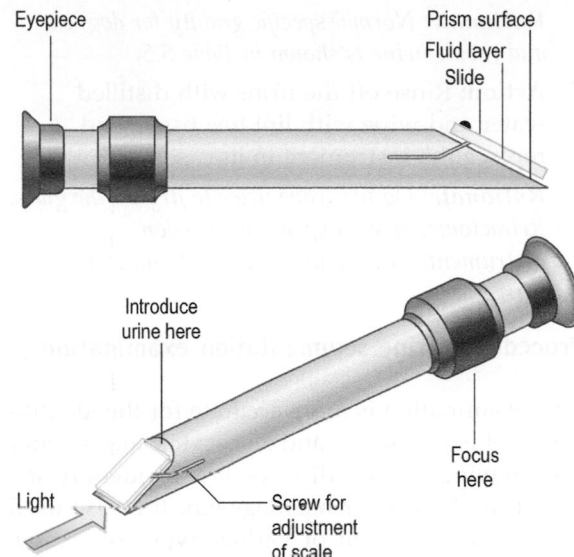

Figure 5.14 Refractometer for measuring the specific gravity of urine.

2. **Action:** Hold the refractometer up to the light and look through the eyepiece. Read the scale visible through the eyepiece.

    Rationale: The reading is taken at the point where there is a boundary between light and dark. As the liquid is pure water it should read 1.000.

3. **Action:** If the reading is not 1.000 then adjust the refractometer using the screw on the top of the instrument and the screwdriver provided. Adjust until the reading is 1.000.

    Rationale: Some instruments have different ways of making the adjustment – read the instruction leaflet.

4. **Action:** Wipe the water off the glass with lint free tissue.

    Rationale: Lint free tissue should not leave any fibres on the glass.

5. **Action:** Using a clean pipette, place 2 drops of the urine sample on to the glass and close the lid.

    Rationale: Using the same pipette may dilute the urine sample. The instrument is now set up to read the specific gravity of urine.

6. **Action:** Hold the refractometer up to the light, look through the eyepiece and read the scale. Record your result.

Rationale: Normal specific gravity for dog, cat and rabbit urine is shown in Table 5.5.

7. **Action:** Rinse off the urine with distilled water and wipe with lint free tissue and replace the instrument in its case.

   Rationale: Do not leave urine to dry on the glass. Refractometers are expensive precision instruments and should be cleaned and stored correctly.

Procedure: Urine sedimentation examination

This examination is more accurate for the identification of erythrocytes and leucocytes and is better than relying on the dipstick test to identify the presence of blood or haemoglobin. It is also used for the identification of various types of crystal, some of which are shown in Figure 5.15. A sedimentation test can be easily done in a practice lab, but a fresh sample is essential.

1. **Action:** Using a pipette, place 3–5 ml of fresh urine in a centrifuge tube.

   Rationale: A conical centrifuge tube helps to separate the sediment from the supernatant.

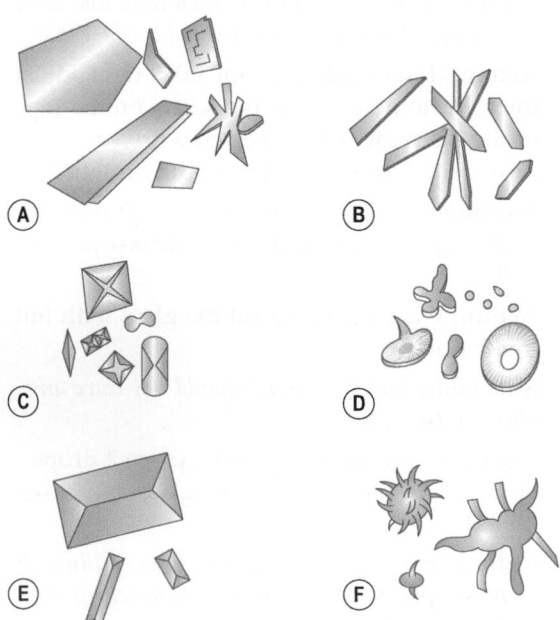

Figure 5.15 Urine crystals: (A) urates; (B) hippuric acid; (C) calcium oxalate; (D) calcium carbonate; (E) struvite; (F) ammonium urate.

2. **Action:** Place the tube in the centrifuge and balance it with a similar tube on the other side.

   Rationale: The machine must be balanced to prevent vibration.

3. **Action:** Set the centrifuge to spin at 1000–2000 r.p.m. for 2–3 minutes.

   Rationale: If you spin for longer you may damage any cells in the urine.

4. **Action:** Use a pipette to remove and discard most of the supernatant. Be careful not to disturb the sediment.

   Rationale: Only the sediment is needed for the examination.

5. **Action:** Flick the test tube with your fingers.

   Rationale: This resuspends the sediment in any remaining liquid and makes a more even smear.

6. **Action:** Add 1–2 drops of Sedistain® to the sediment in the tube.

   Rationale: This is optional, but it helps to make the contents of the sediment more visible and easier to identify. The test can be performed unstained.

7. **Action:** Use a pipette to remove 1–2 drops of the sediment and place them onto the centre of a clean glass slide. Cover with a coverslip.

   Rationale: This makes a uniform layer for examination.

8. **Action:** Place the slide under the microscope and examine using ×10 and ×40 objective lenses.

   Rationale: Look for evidence of blood cells, epithelial cells, crystals (Fig. 5.15), casts, sperm, mucin threads and bacteria.

PARASITOLOGY

Parasites may be:

- **Ectoparasites** – i.e. those living on the surface of the patient (e.g. fleas, lice and the burrowing mites such as *Sarcoptes* and *Demodex* (Fig. 5.16)). Samples are gathered by coat brushings and skin scrapings. For details of the procedure see Chapter 2.

- **Endoparasites** – i.e. those living inside the patient (e.g. roundworms and tapeworms). Samples may be obtained from the faeces or from tracheal washings.

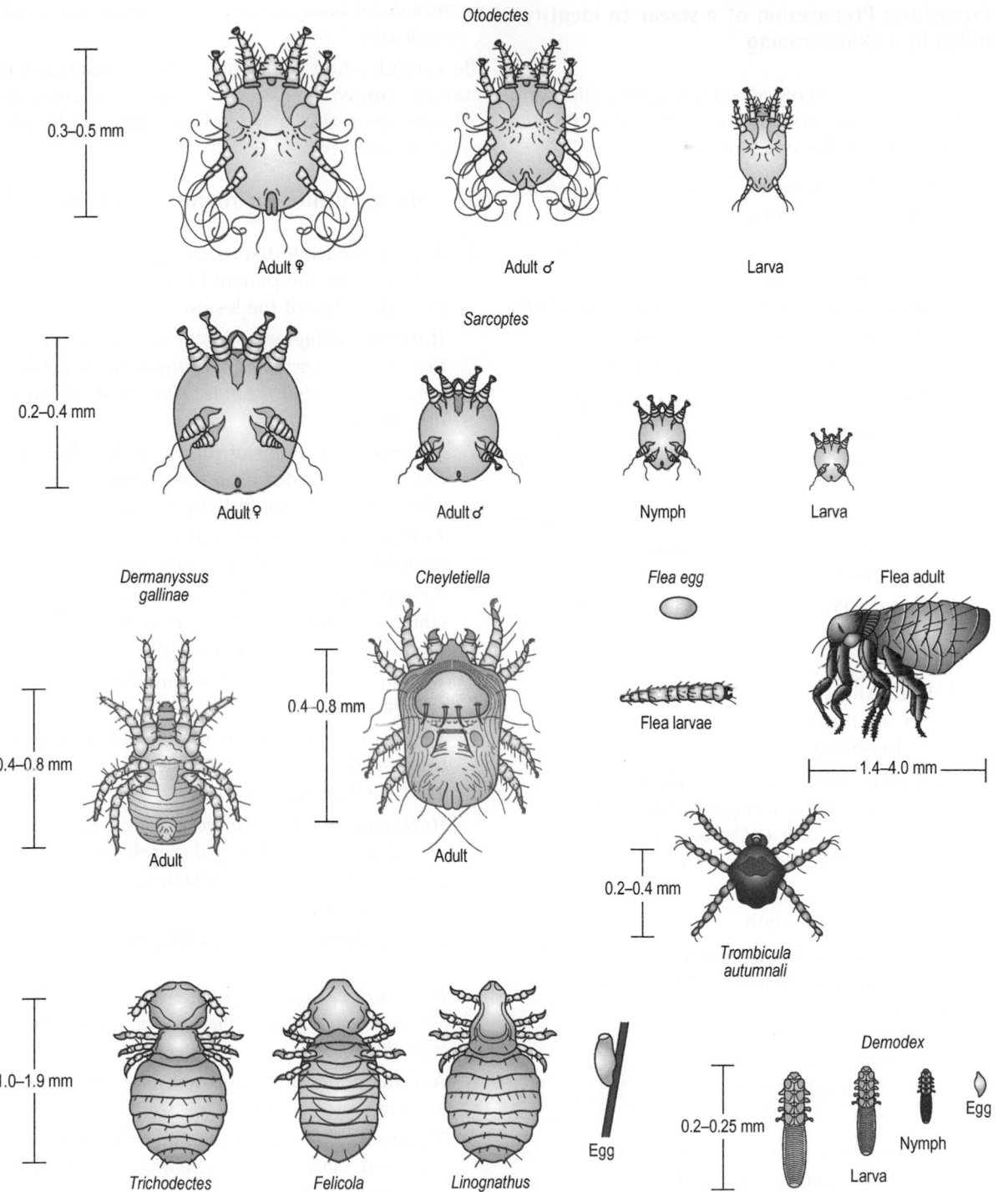

Figure 5.16 Common ectoparasites of companion animals.

Procedure: Preparation of a smear to identify mites in a skin scraping

Equipment list: scraped sample, glass slide and coverslip, 10% potassium hydroxide, Bunsen burner, pipette, forceps, microscope.

1. **Action:** Place some of the skin scraping on to the centre of a clean glass microscope slide.

   Rationale: Do not use too much as the debris may mask the parasites.

2. **Action:** Use a pipette to add 2–3 drops of 10% potassium hydroxide to the debris.

   Rationale: Be careful – this is caustic!

3. **Action:** Place a coverslip over the sample.

   Rationale: This prevents the microscope lens from becoming contaminated and makes a uniform layer to examine.

4. **Action:** Holding the slide with forceps, warm it gently over the Bunsen burner flame – do not let it boil!

   Rationale: Warming the debris breaks it down so that it becomes clear, making the parasites easier to see.

5. **Action:** Allow the slide to cool and place it under the microscope. Examine using the ×4 and ×10 objective lenses.

   Rationale: Larger parasites such as Sarcoptes may be seen with low magnification whereas smaller species such as Demodex require higher magnification (Fig. 5.16).

6. **Action:** It is a good idea to prepare several slides for examination.

   Rationale: Numbers of parasites are likely to be low and they may be missed if you examine only one smear.

RINGWORM

This is caused by a group of fungi known as the dermatophytes that attack keratin. The most significant species in dogs, cats and rabbits are:

- *Microsporum canis* – most common species; 50% of cases will fluoresce under Wood's lamp.
- *Microsporum gypseum* – occasionally seen in dogs and cats.
- *Trichophyton mentagrophytes* – less common in dogs and rare in cats.

Be careful when handling patients suspected of having ringworm as the disease is zoonotic. Always wear gloves when handling samples and warn the owners.

Procedure: Culture for ringworm fungus

1. **Action:** Wearing disposable gloves, collect a sample from the patient by plucking hair from the edge of the lesion.

   Rationale: Ringworm fungi cause circular lesions that spread outwards. The centre of the lesion is dead and scaly but the outer ring should contain live fungus.

2. **Action:** Place a pair of forceps in the flame of the Bunsen burner for a few seconds and then allow to cool to room temperature.

   Rationale: The forceps must be sterilized to reduce the risk of bacterial contamination.

3. **Action:** Remove the lid of a Petri dish containing Sabouraud's agar or a commercial medium such as Dermatofyt®.

   Rationale: Avoid contaminating the agar with your fingers.

4. **Action:** Use the forceps to take 6–8 hairs from the sample and place them in the centre of the agar. Replace the lid.

   Rationale: Avoid contamination from microorganisms, including fungal spores, floating in the atmosphere. Sabouraud's medium is selective for ringworm fungi.

5. **Action:** Incubate at room temperature for 28 days.

   Rationale: Ringworm fungi grow very slowly, although you may see some evidence of growth from the 4th day.

6. **Action:** When fungal growth is visible, examine and identify.

   Rationale: Growth appears as a fluffy white colony on Sabouraud's medium. On commercial media such as Dermatofyt®, an indicator within the agar changes from yellow to red. However, there are some contaminants that may also cause this colour change so it is important to identify the fungus under the microscope.

NB The colony of each species has different identifying characteristics:

- *Microsporum canis* – flat with white silky centre and a bright yellow edge. Underside is yellow.
- *Microsporum gypseum* – flat brown with a powdery yellow fringe. Underside is yellow / brown.
- *Trichophyton mentagrophytes* – flat, granular and tan coloured, or heaped with a white cottony appearance. Underside is yellow / red.

Procedure: Preparation of a slide to identify ringworm fungus

1. **Action:** Culture a colony of fungus from the patient's sample as described.

   Rationale: Infected hairs can be used to make a direct slide, but identification is more difficult and requires experience.

2. **Action:** Take a clean glass microscope slide and, using a pipette, place 2–3 drops of lactophenol cotton blue stain in the centre.

   Rationale: The stain helps to spread the fungal colonies over the slide. The phenol in the stain inactivates the fungal spores and the blue stain aids visualization of the spores and the mycelia. You can use Quink® ink instead of the stain.

3. **Action:** Using a single-use loop, pick up a small amount of fungal colony and mix it with the stain on the slide. Discard the loop in the clinical waste.

   Rationale: To prevent contamination by the fungus on the loop.

4. **Action:** Place a coverslip over the material on the slide.

   Rationale: This provides a layer of uniform thickness for examination.

5. **Action:** Place the slide under the microscope and examine under the ×10 and ×40 objective lenses.

   Rationale: Microscopic examination will confirm the identification of the species.

NB The arthroconidia or spores of the fungus differ according to the species (Fig. 5.17):

- *M. canis* – spores are thick walled, boat shaped and have knob-like structures at the end.
- *T. mentagrophytes* – spores are cigar shaped and thin walled and the hyphae are spiral.

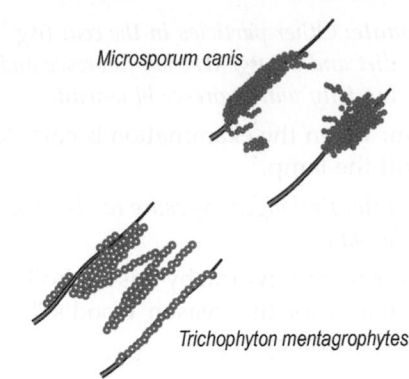

Microsporum canis

Trichophyton mentagrophytes

Figure 5.17 Fungal spores or arthroconidia along a hair shaft.

Procedure: Use of Wood's lamp to identify ringworm infection

Wood's lamps emit ultraviolet (UV) light at a wavelength of 365–366 nm. When this light is directed onto infected hair or claws, the tissue will fluoresce bright apple green. Only 60% of cases infected with *M. canis* will fluoresce. The remaining 40% and ringworm caused by other species will not fluoresce, so a negative result does not mean that the animal does not have ringworm.

1. **Action:** Place the animal on a stable examination table in a darkened room.

   Rationale: The darkened room will enhance the fluorescent effect.

2. **Action:** Put on some form of eye protection.

   Rationale: UV light can cause damage to the conjunctiva and the retina.

3. **Action:** Switch on the Wood's lamp and allow it to warm up for 5–10 minutes.

   Rationale: To ensure that it is emitting the correct wavelength of light.

4. **Action:** Ask the owner or an assistant (who should be wearing eye protection) to restrain the animal appropriately.

   Rationale: This is not a painful procedure, but the animal may try to escape.

5. **Action:** Hold the lamp over the suspect area and then screen the rest of the body thoroughly looking for signs of apple-green fluorescence.

Rationale: Other particles in the coat (e.g. skin flakes, dirt and detergent) may fluoresce and petroleum jelly will fluoresce blue-white.

6. **Action:** When the examination is complete turn off the lamp.

   Rationale: Prolonged exposure to UV light can burn the skin.

NB Diagnosis of ringworm by this method requires experience and for this reason Wood's lamps are rarely used nowadays.

FAECAL ANALYSIS

The faeces of a dog or cat may contain worm eggs (e.g. *Toxocara canis*, *Uncinaria stenocephala*), larvae (e.g. *Oslerus osleri*, *Angiostrongylus vasorum*) or coccidial oocysts (e.g. *Isospora* or *Eimeria* species). A faecal sample may be collected direct from the animal's rectum using a gloved finger or a swab, or by picking it up from the floor of the kennel or the ground. Make sure that the sample has come from the animal in question and that it is not contaminated by grass, soil or cat litter. The sample should be placed in a clean wide-mouthed container filled as full as possible to prevent it drying out.

Storage – faeces should be analysed as soon as possible after collection as any eggs present may hatch, larvae may crawl away and bacterial growth may overrun the sample. If analysis cannot be done quickly then place the sample in a fridge.

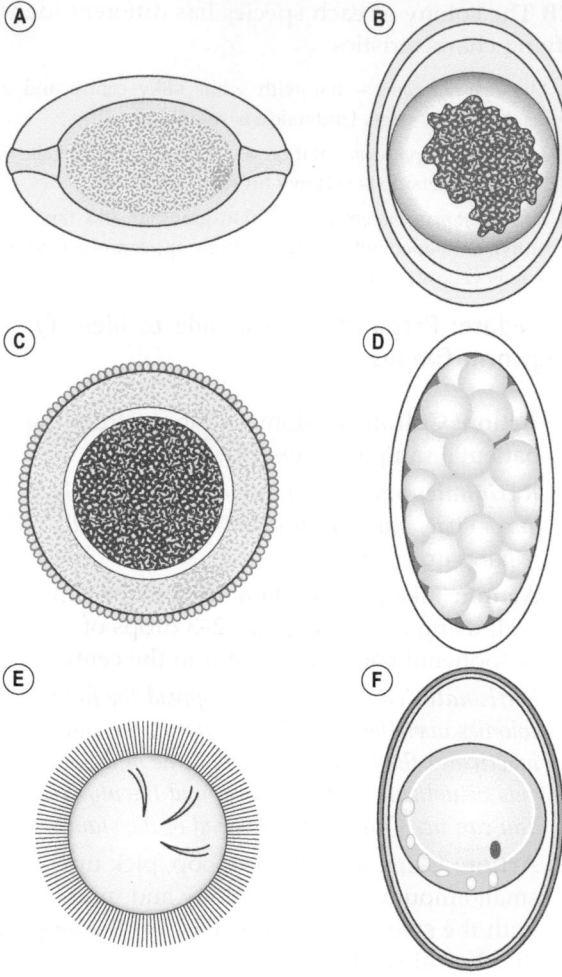

Figure 5.18 Worm eggs and oocysts: (A) *Trichuris* spp.; (B) *Toxascaris* spp.; (C) *Toxocara* spp.; (D) *Uncinaria* spp.; (E) *Taenia* spp.; (F) *Isospora* spp.

Procedure: Direct faecal smear

This may be used to confirm the presence of eggs in the sample (Fig. 5.18), but as only a small amount of faeces is examined the absence of eggs in the smear does not confirm the absence of parasites in the patient. Prepare and examine several smears to be sure of your diagnosis. This is a qualitative analysis that indicates parasites are present but does not indicate the severity of the infection.

1. **Action:** Take a small amount of faeces and place it in the centre of a clean glass microscope slide.

   Rationale: If the smear is too thick then it is difficult to see the eggs. The ideal smear should appear almost clear to the naked eye.

2. **Action:** Place 2–3 drops of water on the slide and mix with the faeces using a glass rod or a mounted needle. Keep the material as close to the centre of the slide as possible.

   Rationale: The water helps to dilute the faeces and makes a thinner solution.

3. **Action:** Remove any large pieces of material from the mixture.

Rationale: These are likely to be undigested fibrous material, which will interfere with the coverslip.

4. **Action:** Carefully place a coverslip over the area of the sample. Try to avoid trapping bubbles under the slip.

   Rationale: Bubbles may be mistaken for eggs. Use a mounted needle to lower the edge of the slip onto the faeces.

5. **Action:** Make sure that the coverslip lies as flat as possible.

   Rationale: This forms a uniform layer to examine under the microscope. Any large pieces of debris will prevent the slip lying flat.

6. **Action:** Place the slide under the microscope and examine systematically under ×10 and ×40 objective lenses.

   Rationale: Systematic examination of the slide will ensure that you examine the whole slide. Air bubbles appear as black circles.

Procedure: Quantitative analysis of a faecal sample using the modified McMaster method

This method is used to evaluate the severity of the infection.

1. **Action:** Weigh 3 g of faeces into a glass beaker.

   Rationale: The faeces should be fresh and moist.

2. **Action:** Measure 45 ml of saturated sugar solution into a measuring cylinder, pour into the beaker and mix with a spatula.

   Rationale: Saturated sugar solution helps the eggs to float out of the faeces. The addition of several glass beads may help to break up the faecal matter – cat faeces are particularly hard to break up.

3. **Action:** Pour the solution through a sieve into a second beaker. Discard the debris in the sieve.

   Rationale: This removes any large particles but allows the eggs to go through.

4. **Action:** Mix the solution gently and allow to stand at room temperature for 5–10 minutes.

Rationale: This enables the worm eggs to float to the top of the saturated sugar solution.

5. **Action:** If using a single chamber McMaster slide, prepare it by placing the coverslip grid side down on the slide.

   Rationale: Some chambers have a single chamber and use a coverslip grid whereas others have two chambers and an integral grid (Fig. 5.19).

6. **Action:** Using a pipette, withdraw approximately 2 ml of the solution and fill the counting chamber.

   Rationale: Make sure that you have enough fluid to completely fill the chamber. If there is insufficient fluid then bubbles may form over the grid.

7. **Action:** Apply the coverslip.

   Rationale: To avoid the inclusion of bubbles, which may distort the image, make sure that the coverslip makes contact with the chamber.

8. Leave the counting chamber on the bench for 5–10 minutes.

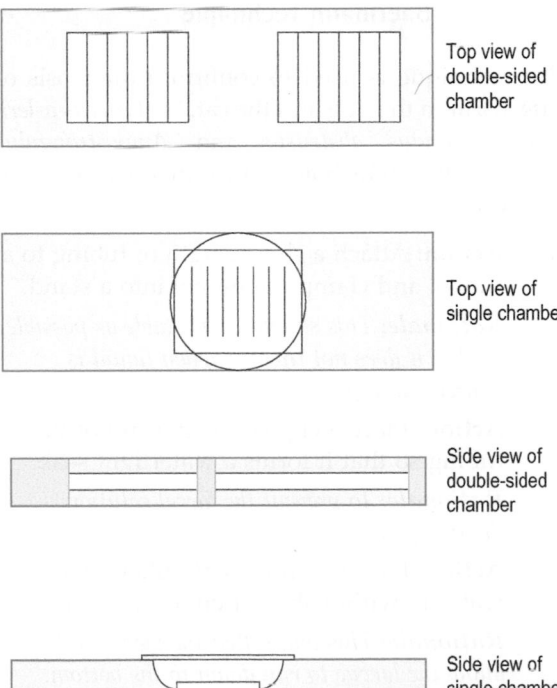

Top view of double-sided chamber

Top view of single chamber

Side view of double-sided chamber

Side view of single chamber

Figure 5.19 McMaster worm egg counting chambers.

Rationale: This allows any worm eggs or coccidial oocysts to float to the top, making them visible.

9.   **Action:** Place the chamber under the microscope and examine using the ×10 objective. Focus on the grid and count all the eggs seen over the grid area.

     Rationale: Count eggs that lie over the lines and between the lines. If there is more than one type of egg then repeat the count for each type separately (Fig. 5.18). Air bubbles will appear as black circles.

10.   **Action:** Calculate the number of eggs as follows:

     • For a single counting chamber, multiply the number of eggs by 100.

     • For a double-sided chamber, count the eggs in both chambers, add them together and multiply the total by 50.

     Rationale: This gives you the number of eggs per gram of faeces.

NB This technique is not suitable for tapeworm segments as they do not float – use direct smear.

Procedure: Baermann technique

This technique is used to confirm a diagnosis of lungworm in the dog and the cat, i.e. *Oslerus osleri*, *Aleurostrongylus abstrusus* and *Angiostrongylus vasorum*, all of which are transmitted by larvae in the faeces.

1.   **Action:** Attach a short length of tubing to a funnel and clamp the funnel into a stand.

     Rationale: This should be as stable as possible so that it does not tip over when liquid is poured through.

2.   **Action:** Place a clip across the end of the tubing so that it forms a watertight seal.

     Rationale: To prevent the faecal solution dripping out.

3.   **Action:** Fill the funnel with lukewarm water to within about 1 cm of the rim.

     Rationale: This will soften the faeces and allow the larvae to run down to the bottom.

4.   **Action:** Take a small piece of muslin and thread a strong wire through each side.

     Rationale: The loops will suspend the muslin across the top of the water.

5.   **Action:** Place the muslin across the top of the funnel so that the wires lie across the top to suspend it.

     Rationale: The muslin forms a 'lid' that is held in place by the wires.

6.   **Action:** Place about 10 g of faeces onto the muslin, which will now dip down into the water.

     Rationale: Make sure that the faeces sample is completely covered by the water.

7.   **Action:** Leave the apparatus overnight.

     Rationale: This gives enough time for the larvae to migrate to the bottom of the funnel and enter the tubing.

8.   **Action:** In the morning draw off a centrifuge tube of liquid by releasing the clip on the tubing.

     Rationale: If larvae are present they should accumulate in the tubing.

9.   **Action:** Allow the tube to stand for 4 hours, or centrifuge at 1500 r.p.m. for 1 minute.

     Rationale: As the larvae are heavier than water, gravity or centrifugal force will pull them down to the bottom of the tube.

10.   **Action:** Using a pipette, remove the supernatant fluid from the tube.

     Rationale: This should not contain anything significant.

11.   **Action:** Place the sediment on a clean glass microscope slide, add a drop of Lugol's iodine and cover with a coverslip.

     Rationale: Lugol's iodine will kill the larvae and stop them moving. It also stains them brown, which increases visibility.

12.   **Action:** Place the slide under the microscope and examine under ×10 and ×40 objective lenses.

     Rationale: Look for the presence of nematode larvae.

CHAPTER 6
Diagnostic imaging

CHAPTER CONTENTS

There is no doubt that the use of 'pictures' makes it much easier to confirm a diagnosis and nowadays there are several methods of taking this 'picture'. The majority of practices have facilities for radiography and most have ultrasound. This chapter will describe the basic use of both techniques, but it is not the brief of the book to describe the more complicated ways of creating an image such as magnetic resonance imaging (MRI), computed tomography (CT) or nuclear scintigraphy. These three imaging techniques are advanced and require expensive, and in some cases cumbersome, equipment making them currently unavailable to all but the most sophisticated referral practices.

RADIOGRAPHY

Radiography may be defined as all the procedures involved in the production of a radiograph of diagnostic quality and is very often carried out by a veterinary nurse. It involves cleaning and maintenance of the equipment, whatever its type, and the vital correct positioning of the patient. In many practices, positioning is the responsibility of the nurse and the veterinary surgeon acts as a supervisor checking that everything is as he / she wants it before an exposure is made; in other practices it is the vet who positions the patient. Whichever applies in your practice, it is important that you understand the recommended methods of positioning to achieve the optimal image.

Radiology is the interpretation of the radiograph and it is recommended that you refer to specific textbooks for guidance on this subject.

Whatever your role in the production of an image, it is important to remember that radiation is potentially hazardous and the use of x-rays should never be taken lightly. The legislation concerning the use of radiation is embodied in the Ionizing Radiation Regulations (IRR) 1999 and all practices are required to have a copy. Practices are also recommended to have a copy of the guidance notes, which provide a more digestible form of the regulations. Remember that it is scatter that is the unseen and unpredictable hazard; wearing a dosemeter at all times, wearing protective clothing when appropriate and avoiding the use of manual restraint are three rules that should prevent you developing problems in later life. Screen films and grids should be used as often as possible.

When positioning the patient, manual restraint should be avoided if possible as this increases the risk of exposure to scatter even if you are wearing protective clothing. Chemical restraint necessitates the use of sedation or general anaesthesia and when reading the instructions for the following procedures you should assume that the patient is anaesthetized. When you are examining the chest, the condition of the patient may be such that general anaesthesia is considered to be dangerous and each patient must be assessed in the light of the individual clinical signs.

Procedure: Preparing the patient for a radiographic examination

1. **Action:** Make sure that there is a valid clinical reason for the examination.

   Rationale: All radiographic examinations must be clinically justified and exposures must be kept to a reasonable minimum.

2. **Action:** Use some form of chemical restraint (i.e. sedation or general anaesthesia as appropriate to the patient).

   Rationale: Manual restraint should be used only in extreme circumstances to reduce the risk of radiation to personnel.

3. **Action:** Remove any potential artefacts from the patient (e.g. collar, clips, matted hair, etc.).

   Rationale: An artefact may overlie the area of interest, may distract from the main point and may lead to an incorrect diagnosis.

4. **Action:** If required for the procedure, make sure that the patient is properly prepared (e.g. use of an enema, emptying the bladder, starvation).

   Rationale: In some views the presence of food in the stomach, faeces in the colon, or urine in the bladder may restrict the view of some diagnostic points.

5. **Action:** Position the patient correctly for the radiograph.

   Rationale: Following the correct procedure will ensure that the appropriate area is visible on the radiograph and is not obscured by an overlying part of the anatomy. This reduces the numbers of repeat exposures.

PRACTICAL POSITIONING
(Tables 6.1 and 6.2)

Correct positioning is vital if you are to produce a radiograph of diagnostic quality at the first attempt. If you have to repeat an exposure you have doubled the amount of scatter produced, which is bad for all personnel involved, and you have increased the time for which the patient is anaesthetized. It goes without saying that you have also added to the cost of the procedure.

1. SPINE

Imaging of the spine may be used to investigate prolapsed discs, spinal tumours, traumatic injuries and in conjunction with a myelogram.

Procedure: Lateral spine (Fig. 6.1)

1. **Action:** Place the patient in right lateral recumbency.

   Rationale: It is traditional to have the head to the left on the radiograph.

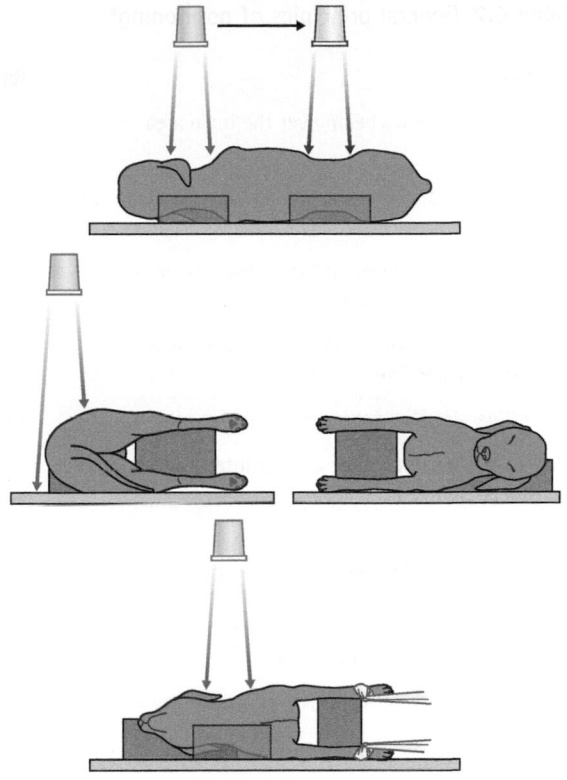

Figure 6.1 Positioning for lateral spine. (With permission from Lee R (ed) (1995) Manual of Small Animal Diagnostic Imaging 2e, BSAVA Gloucester, p 137.)

Table 6.1 Positioning aids*

Type	Use	Effect on the radiograph
Troughs – range of sizes	To restrain the animal on its back and prevent rotation of the trunk	Radiolucent – can be placed over the cassette if necessary
Foam wedges – range of sizes. Often covered in wipeable fabric	To provide support of trunk and limbs; can be used to prevent rotation of the spine and to maintain it in a horizontal plane	Radiolucent
Sandbags – loose filling allows bending and twisting. Covered in wipeable fabric	Can be wrapped around limbs to hold them in place or placed over the neck	Radio-opaque – do not place in the primary beam
Tapes or ties – range of lengths	Looped around limbs to pull them into position and then tied to the cleats on the table	Radiolucent
Wooden blocks	For raising the cassette closer to the x-ray tube head	Radio-opaque – do not place over the cassette

After Aspinall 2003a, p 216, with permission of Elsevier Butterworth-Heinemann.

Table 6.2 General principles of positioning*

Action	Rationale
Centre the primary beam over the main area of interest	To prevent distortion of the area by an oblique view
Place the area of interest as close as possible to the film	If there is an excessive object–film distance the part in question may be magnified and blurred
Ensure that the centre of the primary beam is at right angles to the film	To avoid distortion of the image; this is important when examining joints or intervertebral spaces
Collimate the beam to as small an area as is realistically possible	To reduce the amount of scattered radiation and thus improve the sharpness of the image
Take two views at right angles to each other	To assist in location of a lesion and to visualize the area completely
Try to contain the whole area of interest on a single film	To reduce the number of exposures; however, if this means that important parts are viewed obliquely (e.g the whole spine) then it is better to take views of several smaller areas
When imaging the spine, the body must be supported in areas which may drop down or rotate (e.g. neck and lumbar spine) so that the entire vertebral column is in the same horizontal plane	To prevent distortion and magnification of individual vertebrae and of the intervertebral discs

*After Aspinall 2003a, p 216, with permission of Elsevier Butterworth-Heinemann.

2. **Action:** Place supporting pads under the natural curves of the spine (i.e. the neck and lumbar spine).

   Rationale: This support prevents these areas dropping down towards the table and keeps the spine in a level horizontal line.

3. **Action:** Place pads under the sternum and between the limbs.

   Rationale: These prevent rotation, which will pull the spine out of its horizontal position.

4. **Action:** If the lower cervical spine is to be examined, pull the limbs caudally (Fig. 6.1).

   Rationale: This ensures that the musculature of the shoulder does not overlie C6 and C7.

5. **Action:** If the cervical spine as a whole is to be examined, place a pad under the nose.

   Rationale: This prevents rotation of the head. This should also be done if the whole spine is to be examined.

6. **Action:** Centre the primary beam (as indicated by the cross wires in the light-beam diaphragm) over the point of interest. Include muscle mass, but not fat and skin.

   Rationale: Centring must be accurate and care must be taken to avoid covering too large an area in one view because divergence of the beam at the edges of the field will cause artificial narrowing of the intervertebral spaces. Aim to cover 3–4 intervertebral spaces in each view.

7. **Action:** If the entire spine is to be examined, ensure that each image overlaps with the ones on either side.

   Rationale: By ensuring overlap a complete study of each vertebra and its associated intervertebral spaces can be achieved with a minimum of distortion.

8. **Action:** If the first film fails to identify an abnormality, take repeat films on either side of the initial film.

   Rationale: To ensure that you have thoroughly examined the area of the spine.

NB Centring points for the whole spine are as follows:

- Upper cervical – C2/3
- Lower cervical – C5/6
- Mid-thoracic – T8

- Thoraco-lumbar – T13/L1
- Mid-lumbar – L4/5
- Sacrum.

Fewer films may be sufficient for cats and small dogs.

Procedure: Ventro–dorsal spine (Fig. 6.2)

1. **Action:** Place the dog in dorsal recumbency supported in a trough or by foam pads or sandbags.

   Rationale: The spine must be positioned so that the sternum and spine are in the same vertical plane. It may be difficult to prevent rotation, particularly in deep-chested dogs. Remember that sandbags are radio-opaque.

2. **Action:** Extend the hind- and forelimbs and secure with ties.

   Rationale: This prevents rotation and flexion of the lumbar spine.

3. **Action:** Extend the neck and hold in place with tape or a sandbag overlay. It may help to place a pad under the neck.

   Rationale: This ensures that the spine is fully extended.

4. **Action:** Centre the primary beam (as indicated by the cross wires in the light-beam diaphragm) over the point of interest.

   Rationale: Try to select the areas radiographed in the lateral view so that you have two planes per area of the spine, which makes location of the lesion much easier.

5. **Action:** If the entire spine is to be examined, ensure that each image overlaps with the ones on either side.

   Rationale: By ensuring overlap a complete study of each vertebra and its associated intervertebral spaces can be achieved with a minimum of distortion.

6. **Action:** If the first film fails to identify an abnormality, take repeat films on either side of the initial film.

   Rationale: To ensure that you have thoroughly examined the area of the spine.

NB Centring points for the whole spine are as follows:

- Upper cervical – C2/3
- Lower cervical – C5/6
- Mid-thoracic – T8
- Thoraco-lumbar – T13/L1
- Mid-lumbar – L4/5
- Sacrum.

Fewer films may be sufficient for cats and small dogs.

2. HEAD AND NECK

Imaging of the skull may be required for the investigation of trauma or of swellings related to infection or neoplasia, and of neurological signs associated with the CNS and the cranial nerves. The anatomy of the skull is complex and the interpretation of radiographs relies on accurate positioning.

Procedure: Rostro-caudal view – open mouth

This is used to demonstrate the tympanic bullae, the foramen magnum, C1 and C2 and the atlanto-occipital joint.

1. **Action:** Place the animal in dorsal recumbency with the hard palate vertical to the cassette. Tip the nose backwards slightly past the vertical.

   Rationale: This position ensures that the tympanic bullae are as close as possible to the cassette. Tilting the head ensures that the bones of the skull do not obscure the view of the bullae.

2. **Action:** Hold the mouth open to form a V shape (Fig 6.3) using tapes, or place an old needle case (with one end cut off to form a hole) between the teeth of the upper and lower jaws.

   Rationale: This removes the mandible and maxilla from the area of interest.

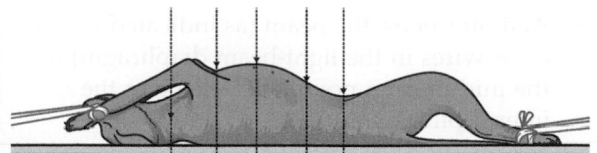

Figure 6.2 Positioning for ventro-dorsal spine.

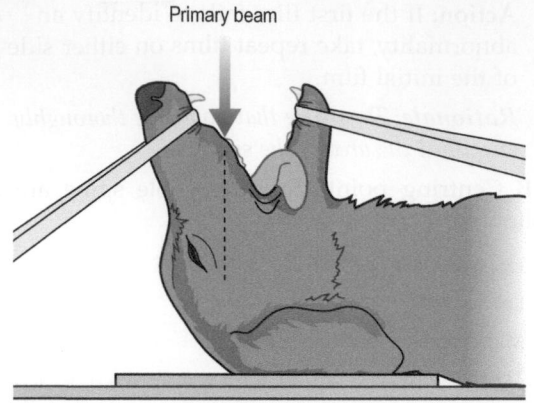

Primary beam

Figure 6.3 Positioning for open mouth – rostro-caudal view.

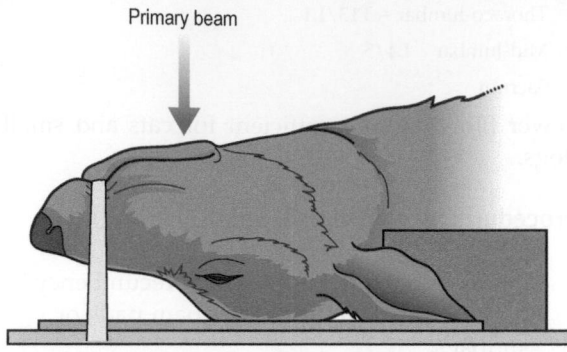

Primary beam

Figure 6.4 Positioning for ventro-dorsal skull to show the position of the hard palate.

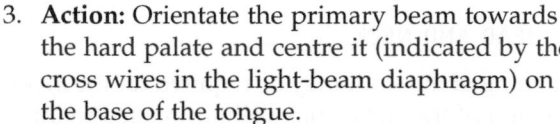

3. **Action:** Orientate the primary beam towards the hard palate and centre it (indicated by the cross wires in the light-beam diaphragm) on the base of the tongue.

   Rationale: In this position the tympanic bullae are located directly behind the base of the tongue.

4. **Action:** If the animal is intubated, remove the endotracheal tube just before exposure.

   Rationale: The tube may be superimposed on the tympanic bullae.

Procedure: Rostro–caudal view – closed mouth

This is used to demonstrate the frontal sinuses, zygomatic arch and temporal region, and the sagittal crest. It is of less use in the cat as the conformation of the skull is different.

1. **Action:** Place the animal in dorsal recumbency with the hard palate vertical to the cassette.

   Rationale: This position ensures that the frontal sinuses, zygomatic arch and temporal region, and the sagittal crest are all in line on the cassette.

2. **Action:** Wind a tape around the nose.

   Rationale: To hold the jaw closed.

3. **Action:** Direct the primary beam at an angle of 5–10° to the vertical in a rostro-caudal direction.

   Rationale: This enables an image of the structures to be seen on the radiograph.

Procedure: Ventro–dorsal view

The ventro-dorsal (VD) view is used for the examination of the tympanic bullae and the external auditory meatus on either side.

1. **Action:** Place the animal in dorsal recumbency.

   Rationale: This ensures that the skull is as close as possible to the film.

2. **Action:** Extend the neck (Fig 6.4).

   Rationale: Extension makes sure that the head is horizontal. This position may be quite difficult to hold because the sagittal crest tends to tilt the head to one side or the other.

3. **Action:** Place a pad under the neck.

   Rationale: This forces the head back so that the hard palate is parallel to the cassette.

4. **Action:** Secure a tape around the upper canines and tie it to the table top (Fig. 6.4).

   Rationale: This ensures that the hard palate remains in a horizontal plane.

5. **Action:** Place a right or left marker on the cassette beside the head as appropriate.

   Rationale: It is important to be able to identify the location of a lesion or mass.

6. **Action:** Centre the beam (as indicated by the cross wires in the light-beam diaphragm) in the midline at a point halfway along the interpupillary line.

   Rationale: This point may vary with the area to be examined.

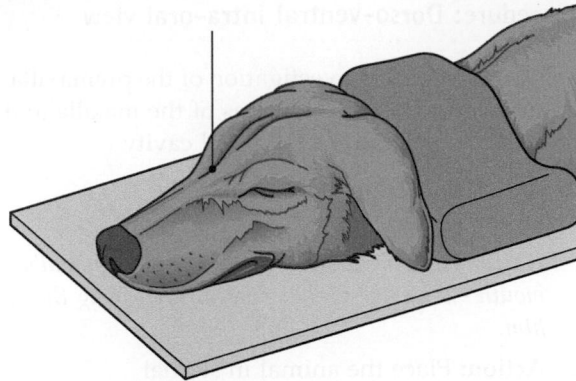

Figure 6.5 Dorso-ventral view of the skull. (With permission from Lee R (ed) (1995) Manual of Small Animal Diagnostic Imaging 2e, BSAVA Gloucester, p 17.)

7. **Action:** Collimate the beam to include the entire skull.

   Rationale: If necessary, collimate more tightly over the area of interest.

Procedure: Dorso–ventral view

The dorso-ventral (DV) view is used for examination of the ear and the temporo-mandibular joint.

1. **Action:** Place the animal in sternal recumbency with the neck extended (Fig. 6.5).

   Rationale: The head is now in a stable position. This is preferred to the VD position even though there is some magnification because of the distance of the skull from the cassette.

2. **Action:** Place a sandbag over the neck.

   Rationale: This keeps the hard palate parallel to the cassette especially in deep-chested dogs.

3. **Action:** Place a right or left marker on the cassette beside the head as appropriate.

   Rationale: It is important to be able to identify the location of a lesion or a mass.

4. **Action:** Centre the beam (indicated by the cross wires in the light-beam diaphragm) on a line midway between the eyes.

   Rationale: This point may vary according to the point of interest.

Procedure: Lateral view of the skull

This is of limited value especially in visualizing the oral cavity as one side of the jaw is superimposed on the other.

1. **Action:** Place the animal in lateral recumbency.

   Rationale: The animal will be completely stable in this position.

2. **Action:** Place foam pads under the nose and the mandible.

   Rationale: This ensures that the sagittal plane of the skull is parallel to the cassette.

3. **Action:** Centre the primary beam (indicated by the cross wires in the light-beam diaphragm) midway between the ear and eye.

   Rationale: This will provide a view of most structures on the head.

Procedure: Lateral oblique view

This is used to show masses or lesions identified in other views and to view the tympanic bullae or temporo-mandibular joints. It is also used to view the dental arcades (e.g. for the diagnosis of a malar abscess).

1. **Action:** Place the animal in lateral recumbency.

   Rationale: This is the most stable position for this view.

2. **Action:** Tilt the head along its long axis and support with foam pads.

   Rationale: This will separate each side of the head.

3. **Action:** Alternatively tilt the animal's nose up by about 15° and support with pads.

   Rationale: The aim of this view is to raise the lesion or mass so that it is on the 'skyline'; the position will vary according to the location of the lesion.

4. **Action:** If viewing the teeth, place foam wedges under the appropriate arcade.

   Rationale: Remember to keep the mandible or maxilla in a horizontal plane parallel to the cassette; foam wedges will help to do this. The side under investigation should be closest to the cassette.

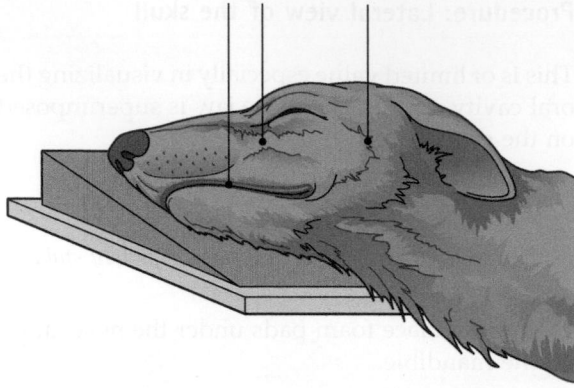

Figure 6.6 Lateral view of the skull. (With permission from Lee R (ed) (1995) Manual of Small Animal Diagnostic Imaging 2e, BSAVA Gloucester, p 17.)

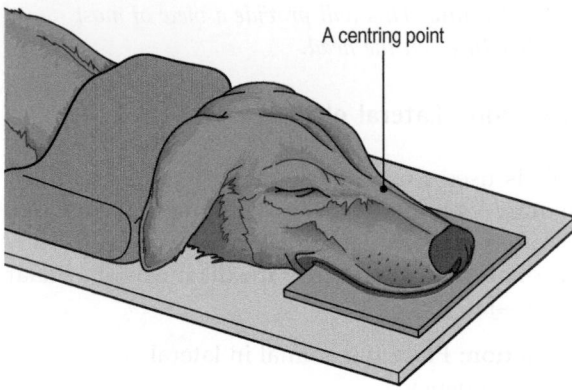

A centring point

Figure 6.7 Positioning for dorso-ventral intra-oral view of the nasal chambers.

5. **Action:** If necessary, open the mouth and hold it open with a dental gag or needle case between the teeth.

   Rationale: This will prevent the mandible from obscuring the view of the upper arcades.

6. **Action:** Centre the beam (indicated by the cross wires in the light-beam diaphragm) on the point of interest (Fig. 6.6).

   Rationale: This will vary according to the case. If viewing a dental arcade, centre the beam half way along it.

NB This view can be varied according to what you want to investigate in more detail having identified a lesion in other positions.

Procedure: Dorso-ventral intra-oral view

This is used for the investigation of the premaxilla, upper incisors, rostral portions of the maxilla and premolar teeth, and for the nasal cavity.

1. **Action:** The animal must be fully anaesthetized.

   Rationale: The cassette is placed in the animal's mouth – anaesthesia will prevent it chewing the film.

2. **Action:** Place the animal in sternal recumbency and extend the neck. Support with foam pads (Fig. 6.7).

   Rationale: The position of the head is straighter if the neck is extended.

3. **Action:** Place a sandbag over the neck.

   Rationale: To prevent rotation of the head.

4. **Action:** The endotracheal tube should be tied to the lower jaw.

   Rationale: To keep it in place and to allow correct placement of the cassette.

5. **Action:** Place a non-screen film above the tongue and the tube as far as possible into the mouth.

   Rationale: Non-screen film will provide better definition, particularly of the maxillary arcades, but screen film in flexible oral cassettes may be used for the incisors.

6. **Action:** Place a left or right marker beside the head as appropriate.

   Rationale: It is important to be able to identify the location of any lesions.

7. Centre the beam as follows:

   - **Action:** Visualization of the nasal chambers – place on a line between the external nares and the interpupillary line.

     Rationale: This is the most useful view for examination of the nares as it allows comparison of both sides.

   - **Action:** Incisor teeth – angle the beam at 20° to the vertical.

     Rationale: Angulation prevents foreshortening of the area.

Procedure: Ventro–dorsal intra–oral view

This is used for investigation of the body of the mandible, the rostral parts of the horizontal rami of the mandibles and the mandibular incisor teeth.

1. **Action:** The animal must be fully anaesthetized.

    Rationale: To enable accurate positioning and to prevent the animal chewing on the cassette placed in its mouth.

2. **Action:** Place the animal in dorsal recumbency and support it.

    Rationale: Use a plastic trough and/or foam wedges to keep the body from tilting.

3. **Action:** Push the tongue firmly to one side or place it symmetrically in the centre of the oral cavity.

    Rationale: To avoid any confusion when evaluating the radiograph.

4. **Action:** Use only radiolucent gags in the mouth.

    Rationale: To prevent the image appearing on the radiograph.

5. **Action:** Position the endotracheal tube away from the point of interest.

    Rationale: To prevent it interfering with the image.

6. **Action:** Place the cassette as far as possible into the mouth between the tongue and hard palate.

    Rationale: Flexible oral cassettes (screen film) are used to enable the film to be pushed as far back in the mouth as possible. Non-screen film will provide better definition.

7. Centre the beam as follows:

    *   **Action:** The incisor teeth – at an angle of 20° to the vertical (Fig. 6.8) – i.e. aiming rostro-caudally.

        Rationale: To prevent foreshortening and to allow full evaluation of the dental roots and alveoli.

    *   **Action:** The horizontal rami of the mandible – over the mid-point of a line drawn from the mandibular symphysis to the larynx (Fig. 6.8).

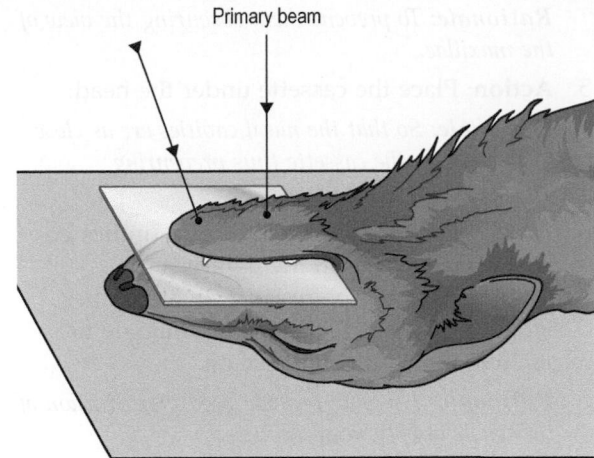

Figure **6.8** Ventro-dorsal intra-oral view. (With permission from Lee R (ed) (1995) Manual of Small Animal Diagnostic Imaging 2e, BSAVA Gloucester, p 24.)

Rationale: The centring point will vary according to the point of interest.

Procedure: Ventro–dorsal open mouth oblique rostro–caudal view

This is used to investigate the nasal passages and allows better visualization of the more caudal regions than the dorso-ventral intra-oral view.

1. **Action:** The animal must be fully anaesthetized.

    Rationale: To allow adequate relaxation and thus accurate positioning.

2. **Action:** Place the animal in dorsal recumbency with the head as straight as possible. Use a trough or wedges to hold the body in position without tilting to one side.

    Rationale: If the body tilts it will tilt the head. This will lead to inequalities in the nasal cavities and may lead to a misdiagnosis.

3. **Action:** Open the mouth as widely as possible and prop open with a dental gag or a needle case between the caudal molars or the carnassials.

    Rationale: This prevents the mandibles obscuring the view of the maxillae.

4. **Action:** Pull the tongue and the endotracheal tube to one side.

Rationale: To prevent them obscuring the view of the maxillae.

5. **Action:** Place the cassette under the head.

   Rationale: So that the nasal cavities are as close as possible to the cassette thus preventing excessive magnification.

6. **Action:** Centre the primary beam (indicated by the cross wires in the light-beam diaphragm) on a point halfway along the length of the hard palate and collimate to include the whole hard palate.

   Rationale: This will provide good visualization of the whole of both nasal cavities.

3. THORAX

Radiography of the thorax provides a guide to the diagnosis of many conditions because it allows examination of the lower respiratory tract, the lung tissue and the pleurae, the heart, the mediastinum, the diaphragm and the thoracic wall. Problems may occur because the chest wall and diaphragm are always moving and steps must be taken (e.g. reducing the exposure time) to minimize movement blur.

Procedure: Lateral thorax

1. **Action:** Place the animal in right lateral recumbency.

   Rationale: This is the conventional position for a thoracic radiograph because the heart lies in a more consistent position, there is more air-filled lung between the heart and the chest wall, which gives better cardiac detail, and the diaphragm obscures less of the caudal lung field.

2. **Action:** Extend the forelegs and secure with ties tied to cleats on the table or with sandbags.

   Rationale: Extending the forelegs prevents the soft tissue mass of the shoulder girdle impeding the view of the thoracic contents.

3. **Action:** Place a pad under the sternum.

   Rationale: To prevent rotation of the chest and ensure that it remains in the same horizontal plane as the spine. This prevents distortion of the thoracic structures.

4. **Action:** Place sandbags over the neck and the hindlegs.

   Rationale: The hindlegs should be secure, but should not be tied as this leads to rotation of the chest.

5. **Action:** Centre the beam (as indicated by the cross wires on the light-beam diaphragm) midway between the sternum and spine and level with the caudal border of the scapula (approximately the 5th rib).

   Rationale: This ensures that the primary beam coincides with the base of the heart.

6. **Action:** Collimate the beam to include the cranial thoracic inlet, the edge of the sternum, the thoracic spine and the full extent of the diaphragm.

   Rationale: All parts of the lung will be included. In large breeds it may be necessary to cover the area with two overlapping films.

7. **Action:** Expose on inspiration.

   Rationale: This ensures that the diaphragm is flattened, creating maximum space in the cavity for the organs. The lungs are fully inflated, which provides better contrast between the air in the lungs and the soft tissues.

NB It is good practice to take both right and left lateral views. A lesion may appear on one side only, masked by a lung lobe and may be missed on the other view.

Forced inspiration is preferable to natural inspiration as it provides better contrast. This can be achieved only in the anaesthetized patient and requires someone to squeeze the reservoir bag at the appropriate moment, necessitating his / her exposure to radiation. Consider the IRR 1999 and make sure the assistant is wearing protective clothing and a dosemeter and that it is not always the same person!

Procedure: Dorso–ventral thorax

This view is recommended for animals in respiratory distress but is less comfortable for animals with hindlimb injuries.

1. **Action:** Place the animal in sternal recumbency with the elbows symmetrically

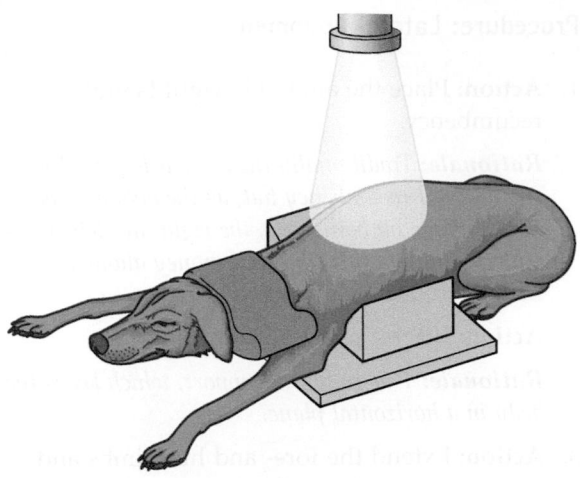

Figure 6.9 Positioning for dorso-ventral view of the thorax. (With permission from Lee R (ed) (1995) Manual of Small Animal Diagnostic Imaging 2e, BSAVA Gloucester, p 46.)

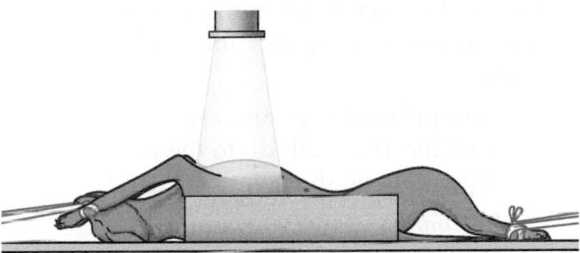

Figure 6.10 Positioning for ventro-dorsal view of the thorax. (With permission from Lee R (ed) (1995) Manual of Small Animal Diagnostic Imaging 2e, BSAVA Gloucester, p 46.)

drawn outwards and gently pulled forwards – you may find it easier to place the animal in a trough (Fig. 6.9).

Rationale: This view allows the heart to lie in its normal position and is used for heart investigations. It is also used for conscious or sedated animals in respiratory distress as this allows them to breathe more easily. Drawing the elbows outwards prevents the muscles of the shoulder girdle from overlying the thoracic cavity.

2. **Action:** Support the chin on a foam pad.

   Rationale: This keeps the head, neck and spine in a horizontal plane. If the animal is conscious it will be more comfortable.

3. **Action:** Place a sandbag over the neck (Fig. 6.9), making sure that it does not obscure the edge of the collimated area.

   Rationale: To prevent movement. Sandbags are radio-opaque.

4. **Action:** Place a left or right marker as appropriate.

   Rationale: To assist in the location of any lesions.

5. **Action:** Centre the beam (as indicated by the cross wires in the light-beam diaphragm) in the midline on the caudal border of the scapula.

   Rationale: This ensures that the heart is in the centre of the image.

6. **Action:** Collimate the beam to include the skin edges, the thoracic inlet and the diaphragm.

   Rationale: The image should include the caudal and cranial lung fields.

7. **Action:** Expose on inspiration.

   Rationale: This ensures that the diaphragm is flattened, creating maximum space in the cavity for the organs. The lungs are fully inflated, which provides better contrast between the air in the lungs and the soft tissues (see additional notes above).

NB The radiographic image should be symmetrical and show the spine superimposed on the sternum in the midline.

Procedure: Ventro-dorsal thorax

This should be avoided in animals that are in respiratory distress because breathing may be made even more difficult. Animals with hindlimb injuries may be more comfortable.

1. **Action:** Place the patient in dorsal recumbency supported in a trough or by foam wedges (Fig. 6.10).

   Rationale: Care must be taken to avoid rotation. In this view the heart may rotate to one side and its size and shape may be distorted.

2. **Action:** Extend each foreleg separately and secure with a tie attached to cleats under the

table or with a sandbag placed over each carpus.

Rationale: This prevents rotation. Do not place sandbags over the axillae as this is uncomfortable.

3. **Action:** The hindlegs may be extended or allowed to remain in a flexed position.

   Rationale: Take care that the pelvis does not rotate to either side as this will tilt the thorax out of its central position.

4. **Action:** Place a left or right marker on the cassette as appropriate.

   Rationale: It is important to be able to locate a lesion.

5. **Action:** Centre the primary beam (as indicated by the cross wires in the light-beam diaphragm) midway along the sternum and collimate to include the cranial thoracic inlet and the diaphragm / cranial abdomen.

   Rationale: This should ensure that you include the whole thoracic cavity.

6. **Action:** Expose on inspiration.

   Rationale: This ensures that the diaphragm is flattened, creating maximum space in the cavity for the organs. The lungs are fully inflated, which provides better contrast between the air in the lungs and the soft tissues (see additional notes above).

NB The radiographic image should be symmetrical and show the spine superimposed on the sternum in the midline.

4. ABDOMEN

There are many indications for radiography of the abdomen, including investigation of the various parts of the alimentary tract, the kidneys and urinary tract, the reproductive tract and the associated parenchymatous organs such as the liver. The positioning of the patient is fairly simple, but accurate collimation and centring of the primary beam will provide your main guides to diagnosis. It is good practice to take two views of the abdomen (i.e. lateral and VD in particular); this will help you to identify the location of air within the abdomen – if it moves it is free in the peritoneal cavity; if it does not it is trapped within an organ.

Procedure: Lateral abdomen

1. **Action:** Place the animal in right lateral recumbency.

   Rationale: Traditionally the animal is placed in right lateral recumbency but, as the abdomen is not the same on both sides, the right and left views will vary slightly. If time and money allow, you should take radiographs of both sides.

2. **Action:** Place a pad under the sternum.

   Rationale: This provides support, which keeps the body in a horizontal plane.

3. **Action:** Extend the fore- and hindlimbs and secure them with sandbags or ties.

   Rationale: To prevent movement. Remember to keep the sandbags out of the primary beam as they are radio-opaque.

4. Centre the primary beam (as indicated by the cross wires in the light-beam diaphragm) as follows:

   - **Action:** Small dogs and cats – on a line from the 11th/12th rib to the iliac crest depending on the point of interest.

     Rationale: The whole abdomen can be included on one film.

   - **Action:** Large dogs – for the cranial abdomen, centre over the costal arch; for the caudal abdomen, centre midway between the last rib and the pelvic inlet.

     Rationale: Take two overlapping films to radiograph the whole abdomen.

5. **Action:** Collimation should include the dorsal and ventral skin edges and the appropriate boundaries depending on size of patient and point of interest.

   Rationale: The cranial border of the liver should always be included if the whole abdomen is to be examined.

6. **Action:** Expose on expiration.

   Rationale: During expiration the diaphragm relaxes into a dome shape, providing the maximum amount of space for the abdominal organs.

Procedure: Ventro-dorsal abdomen

This is the preferred view for the examination of the abdomen. A DV may sometimes be used for contrast studies of the stomach.

1. **Action:** Place the patient in dorsal recumbency supported in a trough or with pads or sandbags (Fig. 6.11).

   Rationale: Use of positioning aids prevents rotation of the body. The sternum and spine should be aligned vertically.

2. **Action:** Extend each foreleg cranially and secure with a tie attached to the cleats under the table or with a sandbag placed over each carpus.

   Rationale: This prevents rotation. Avoid placing sandbags over the axillae as this will be uncomfortable.

3. **Action:** Extend the hindlimbs and secure with ties or sandbags.

   Rationale: The hind limbs can be left untied but the body may rotate, especially in deep-chested breeds.

4. **Action:** Place a left or right marker on the cassette under the body.

   Rationale: It is important to be able to locate any abnormalities.

5. Centre the primary beam (as indicated by the cross wires in the light-beam diaphragm) as follows:

   - **Action:** Small dogs and cats – in the midline at the level of the umbilicus.

     Rationale: The whole abdomen can be included on one film.

   - **Action:** Large dogs – for the cranial abdomen, in the midline level with the last rib; for the caudal abdomen, midway between the last rib and the pelvic inlet.

     Rationale: Take two overlapping films to radiograph the whole abdomen.

6. **Action:** Collimation should include the lateral skin edges and the appropriate boundaries depending on the point of interest.

   Rationale: The cranial border of the liver should always be included if the whole liver is to be examined.

7. **Action:** Expose on expiration.

   Rationale: During expiration the diaphragm relaxes into a dome shape, providing the maximum amount of space for the abdominal organs.

NB A VD view is useful to show the presence of air in the colon.

5. APPENDICULAR SKELETON

Radiography of the limbs and their girdles has always been the main use of x-rays in veterinary practice and there is a wide range of clinical indications for its use (e.g. fractures, lameness, deformities and the monitoring of inherited conditions

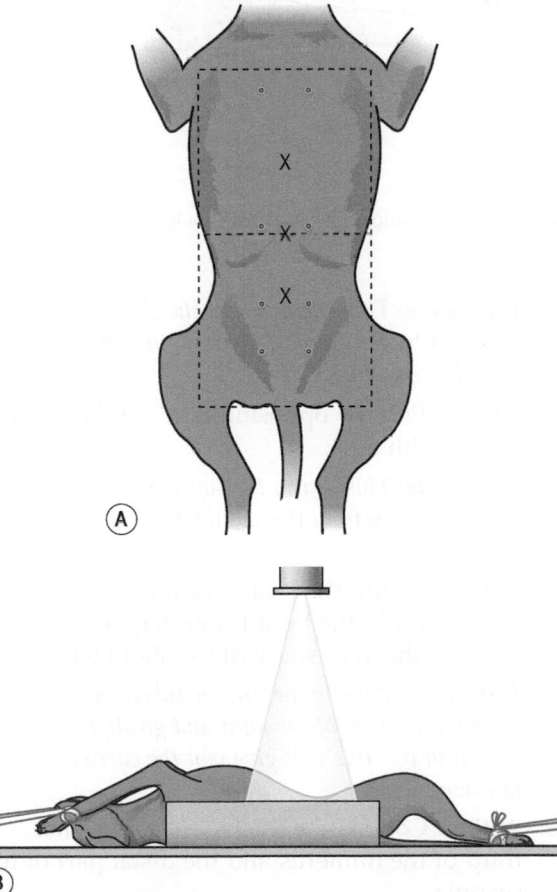

Figure 6.11 (A, B) Positioning for ventro-dorsal abdomen.

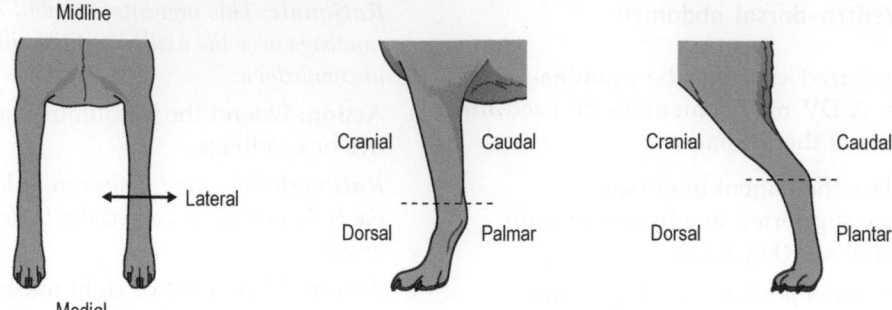

Figure 6.12 Correct nomenclature for identifying radiographic planes of the limbs.

such as hip dysplasia). As with other areas of radiography, to locate an abnormality accurately it is important to take at least two views of an area. Collimation should be as tight as possible and it is rarely necessary to include the whole limb.

To describe the planes in which limb radiographs are taken, remember that views are described in the direction the beam enters and then leaves the limb and also remember to use the correct nomenclature: e.g above the carpus and tarsus – use the terms cranial and caudal (Cr/Cd); below the carpus – use the terms dorsal and palmar (D/Pa); below the tarsus – use the terms dorsal and plantar (D/Pl) (Fig. 6.12).

A. The forelimb

Procedure: Shoulder – medio–lateral view

By centring correctly, this may be used to examine both the shoulder joint and the scapula.

1. **Action:** Place the animal in lateral recumbency making sure that the limb to be examined is closest to the cassette.

    Rationale: This prevents magnification of the joint.

2. **Action:** Extend the head and neck and secure by placing a sandbag over the neck. Be careful not to interfere with normal respiration.

    Rationale: This ensures that an endotracheal tube lying within the larynx and trachea is pulled away from the area of the shoulder. You may still have to partially withdraw the tube for a short period.

3. **Action:** Pull the affected leg cranially and ventrally and secure with a tie (Fig. 6.13).

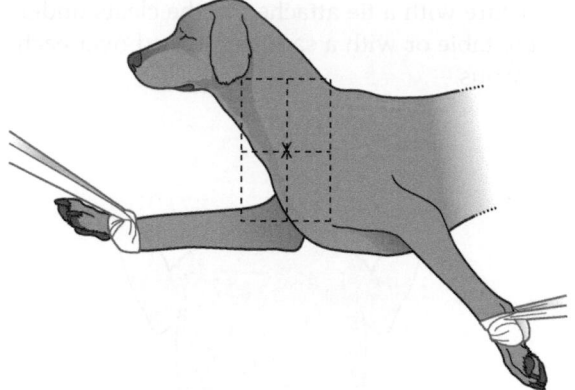

Figure 6.13 Positioning for lateral shoulder.

Rationale: This ensures that the shoulder is not obscured by the cervical spine or the soft tissues of the other shoulder.

4. **Action:** Pull the opposing limb caudally and secure with a tie.

    Rationale: This draws the soft tissues of the shoulder away from the shoulder under examination.

5. **Action:** Centre the beam (as indicated by the cross wires in the light-beam diaphragm) through the joint space of the shoulder.

    Rationale: Palpate the greater tuberosity on the lateral aspect of the joint and go slightly caudal to it – this will give you the correct location.

6. **Action:** Collimate to include the proximal third of the humerus and the distal part of the scapula.

    Rationale: This will cover the entire joint.

NB To view the whole scapula, centre the beam midway along the spine of the scapula. To view the humerus, centre midway between the shoulder and the elbow.

Procedure: Shoulder – cranio–caudal view

This is the best position for examining the shoulder joint or the scapula.

1. **Action:** Place the animal in dorsal recumbency and support in a trough or with sandbags (Fig. 6.14).
   Rationale: This allows extension of the limb while preventing obstruction of the chest wall.
2. **Action:** Fully extend the limb to be examined cranially and secure with a tie.
   Rationale: This will demonstrate the joint without the elbow overlying the area.
3. **Action:** Rotate the thorax until the limb is in the cranio-caudal position.
   Rationale: This enables a true cranio-caudal position to be achieved.
4. **Action:** Centre the beam (as indicated by the cross wires in the light-beam diaphragm) over the acromion of the scapula.
   Rationale: The acromion can be palpated on the lateral aspect of the shoulder joint. The joint should be in the centre of the radiograph and demonstrated without distortion.
5. **Action:** Collimation should include the proximal third of the humerus and distal part of the scapula.
   Rationale: This will cover the entire joint.

NB To view the scapula, centre the beam midway between the acromion and the caudal part of the scapula blade.

Elbow – one of the reasons for examination of the elbow may be to screen for elbow dysplasia. This is a multifactorial condition manifesting as a variety of developmental disorders that may eventually progress to osteoarthritis. It may appear in a wide range of breeds, e.g. Basset Hound, Great Dane, Labrador and Golden Retriever, and, as there is a strong genetic component, the British Veterinary Association / Kennel Club (BVA / KC) have a scheme for screening dogs intended for breeding and their progeny.

Radiographs are submitted to a panel for grading and must be labelled with the KC number, the date and a left / right marker. Each elbow must be examined and the positioning is as described below. Radiographs that are positioned or labelled incorrectly will be returned by the scrutinizing panel.

Procedure: Elbow – medio–lateral view

By changing the centring of the primary beam, this position can also be used to achieve a medio-lateral view of any part of the distal extremity (Fig. 6.15).

1. **Action:** Place the animal in lateral recumbency with the limb to be radiographed closest to the cassette; for example, for the right elbow – place in right lateral recumbency (Fig. 6.15).
   Rationale: This prevents distortion and magnification of the image.
2. **Action:** Pull the upper leg caudally and dorsally and secure with a tie.
   Rationale: This pulls the limb and its associated tissue away from the area of interest.
3. **Action:** Extend the lower limb and, if necessary, place a foam pad under the olecranon, carpus and foot. The angle between the humerus and lower forelimb should be 110°.
   Rationale: The pad will prevent rotation, allowing the limb to lie parallel to the cassette and producing a true medio-lateral view.
4. **Action:** Place a left or right marker on the cassette.
   Rationale: It is important to identify which limb is being examined.
5. **Action:** Centre the primary beam (as indicated by the cross wires in the light-beam

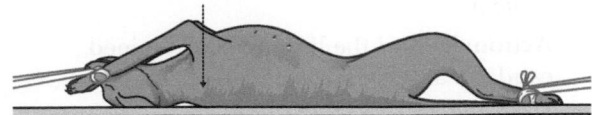

Figure 6.14 Positioning for cranio-caudal shoulder.

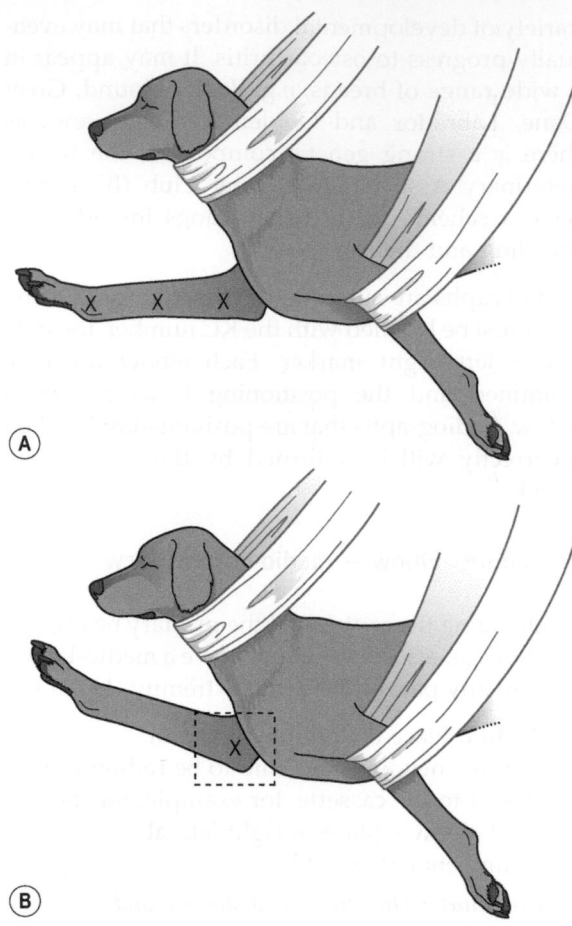

(A)

(B)

Figure 6.15 Positioning for medio-lateral view of the distal forelimb.

diaphragm) over the medial humeral condyle.

Rationale: This extended view is used to evaluate the cranial aspect of the radial head and the humero-radial joint space.

6. **Action:** Collimate to include the lower third of the humerus and the upper third of the lower forelimb.

Rationale: This will include the whole joint.

NB The elbow should also be examined in flexion so that the angle between the humerus and lower forelimb is 45°. Centre on the medial humeral condyle and collimate as above. This view is used to show the anconeal process and the humeral epicondyles.

You may be able to include both elbows on one film, remembering to cover one side with a lead sheet while exposing the other side. This is acceptable for the BVA / KC scheme.

Procedure: Elbow – cranio–caudal view

This is a difficult position to achieve and steps must be taken to prevent rotation. It is no longer required as part of the BVA / KC scheme for elbow dysplasia.

Method 1

1. **Action:** The animal is placed in sternal recumbency supported by sandbags under the chest on the side not under examination.

Rationale: It is important to stop the animal from slipping sideways – deep-chested breeds may need more support. Sandbags are radio-opaque so take care not to obscure the image.

2. **Action:** Extend the forelimb to be examined and secure with ties.

Rationale: You may need to slightly tilt the thorax towards the limb to keep the latter comfortably extended. You may also need to turn the head and neck away from the limb under examination, which allows a clearer view of the elbow.

3. **Action:** Centre the primary beam (as indicated by the cross wires in the light-beam diaphragm) on the radio-humeral joint at an angle of approximately 15° to the vertical.

Rationale: Palpate the humeral condyles to locate the distal end of the humerus (Fig. 6.16).

Method 2

1. **Action:** Place the animal in dorsal recumbency with its body supported in a trough or with sandbags.

Rationale: It is important to keep the animal straight.

2. **Action:** Extend the limb to be examined caudally and secure with a tie.

Rationale: This will bring the elbow joint into the correct plane for examination.

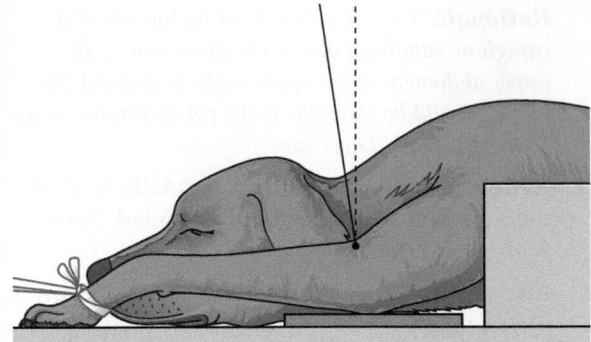

Figure 6.16 Positioning for the cranio-caudal view of the elbow in sternal recumbency. (With permission from Lee R (ed) (1995) Manual of Small Animal Diagnostic Imaging 2e, BSAVA Gloucester, p 117.)

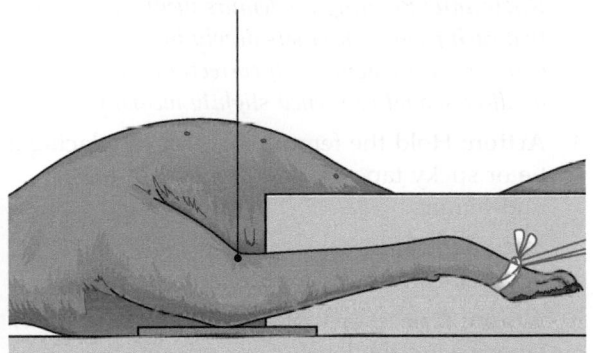

Figure 6.17 Positioning for the cranio-caudal view of the elbow in dorsal recumbency. (With permission from Lee R (ed) (1995) Manual of Small Animal Diagnostic Imaging 2e, BSAVA Gloucester, p 117.)

3. **Action:** Centre the primary beam (as indicated by the cross wires in the light-beam diaphragm) vertically over the radio-humeral joint.

   Rationale: See Figure 6.17.

NB This position is not recommended for use in the BVA / KC scheme.

Procedure: Dorso–palmar view of the forefoot

1. **Action:** Place the animal in sternal recumbency so that the foot under investigation is parallel to the cassette.

   Rationale: The animal will need some form of support (e.g. sandbags), but unless the dog is deep

chested it should be relatively stable in this position.

2. **Action:** Extend the forelimb so that it is straight.

   Rationale: There may be a tendency for the limb to rotate inwards so, to prevent this, rotate the trunk slightly towards the limb being examined.

3. **Action:** Centre the primary beam (as indicated by the cross wires in the light-beam diaphragm) at the level of the carpal joint or the metacarpus or digits.

   Rationale: Positioning is the same but the different areas can be examined by centring over the point of interest.

4. **Action:** Collimation should be as tight as possible and centred on the point of interest.

   Rationale: Tight collimation reduces scatter, but including the joint above and below or a small area of bone above and below may aid your diagnosis.

NB It is not a good idea to radiograph both distal forelimbs at the same time as there is often a degree of rotation in one limb or both.

Medio-lateral view of the carpus and forefoot – this can be achieved by following the guidelines described under medio-lateral view of the elbow (Fig. 6.15). Using the same positioning the carpus can also be examined in the following positions:

- Flexed position – used to check for articular fractures. Hold the limb in flexion using a tie around the joint.

- Extended stressed position (i.e. as it would be when weight bearing) – used to assess ligamentous damage. This requires manual positioning and attention must be paid to radiation safety.

B. The hindlimb

Procedure: Pelvis – lateral view

1. **Action:** Place the animal in right or left lateral recumbency as appropriate.

   Rationale: This is the only way of providing a true lateral projection of the pelvis.

2. **Action:** Place pads between the hindlimbs.

   Rationale: This prevents rotation of the pelvis.

3. **Action:** Centre the primary beam (as indicated by the cross wires in the light-beam diaphragm) on the greater trochanter of the femur.

   Rationale: This ensures that the wings of the ilium and the acetabulum are visible.

Procedure: Pelvis – ventro–dorsal view

This is the standard view for the assessment of the hips and pelvis and is the view required by the BVA / KC scheme for the assessment of hip dysplasia. It is important to make sure that the radiograph is correctly positioned as those that are not will be returned. The radiograph must also be correctly labelled with the dog's KC number, the date of radiography and a right and / or left marker.

1. **Action:** Place the animal in dorsal recumbency, ensuring that the body is straight (Fig. 6.18).

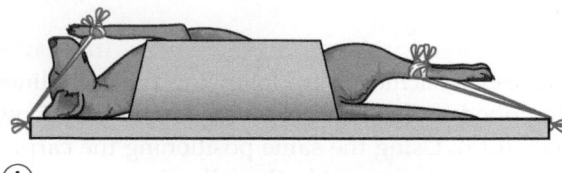

(A)

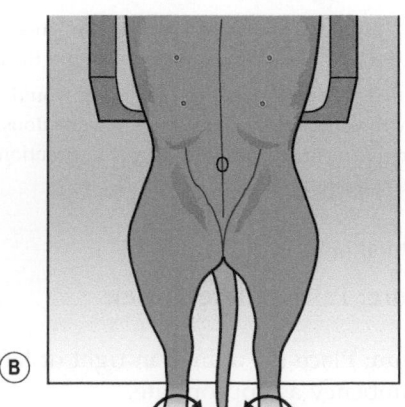

(B)

Figure 6.18 (A, B) Positioning for ventro-dorsal pelvis for assessment of hip dysplasia. (Part B with permission from Lee R (ed) (1995) Manual of Small Animal Diagnostic Imaging 2e, BSAVA Gloucester, p 124.)

Rationale: This may be helped by the use of a trough or sandbags placed on either side of the upper abdomen. If the upper body is straight the pelvis should be straight. If the pelvis rotates, place a pad under the lower hip.

2. **Action:** Extend the hindlegs caudally so that the hips and hocks are fully extended. Secure with ties at the hocks.

   Rationale: This will further ensure that the pelvis is straight.

3. **Action:** Holding the hindlegs separately, one in each hand, rotate medially so that the femurs lie parallel to each other and the patellae are centred over the distal femurs, pointing to the ceiling (Fig. 6.18).

   Rationale: Rotating the femurs medially ensures that each femoral head sits deeply in the appropriate acetabulum. If correctly positioned the hindfeet should be turned slightly medially.

4. **Action:** Hold the femurs together by placing a tie or sticky tape around the level of the mid-femurs.

   Rationale: This ensures that the limbs remain in this position.

5. **Action:** If necessary place another tie or sticky tape around the level of the mid-tibia.

   Rationale: This may be necessary in larger dogs.

6. **Action:** Place a left / right marker as appropriate on the cassette.

   Rationale: This is a requirement of the BVA/KC scheme and it is important to be able to locate any abnormality.

7. **Action:** Centre the primary beam (as indicated by the cross wires in the light-beam diaphragm) in the midline over the pubic symphysis, which can be palpated.

   Rationale: This should provide equal detail on either side of the midline.

8. **Action:** Collimate the beam to include the wings of the ilium and the proximal half of the femurs.

   Rationale: This should demonstrate the entire pelvic girdle and both hip joints.

9. **Action:** Make sure that your label falls within the collimated area.

Rationale: The scrutineers of the radiographs must be able to identify the owner/animal under examination.

NB If the animal is positioned correctly then the obturator foramina will be of equal size on the resulting radiograph; if the animal is lying crookedly then one will appear larger than the other – the animal will be tilted towards the smaller side.

When radiographing an animal with a suspected pelvic fracture, allow the legs to relax in a normal abducted position – this is known as the 'frog leg' position.

Procedure: Stifle – medio-lateral view

1. **Action:** The animal is placed in lateral recumbency with the stifle to be examined lying closest to the cassette.
   Rationale: This prevents distortion and magnification of the image.

2. **Action:** Draw the upper limb cranially and secure with ties.
   Rationale: This prevents the bones and soft tissues of the limb obscuring the limb under examination.

3. **Action:** Allow the lower limb to lie in a neutral position on the cassette – that is, neither flexed nor extended (Fig. 6.19).
   Rationale: This position will provide enough diagnostic detail.

4. **Action:** If the leg begins to rotate, place a foam pad under the caudal aspect of the hock.
   Rationale: This should provide sufficient support to prevent rotation.

5. **Action:** Place a left / right marker as appropriate.
   Rationale: It is important to be able to locate any abnormalities.

6. **Action:** Centre the primary beam (as indicated by the cross wires in the light-beam diaphragm) over the distal femoral condyle.
   Rationale: This can be palpated.

NB To view the femur, centre the primary beam midway between the hip and stifle.

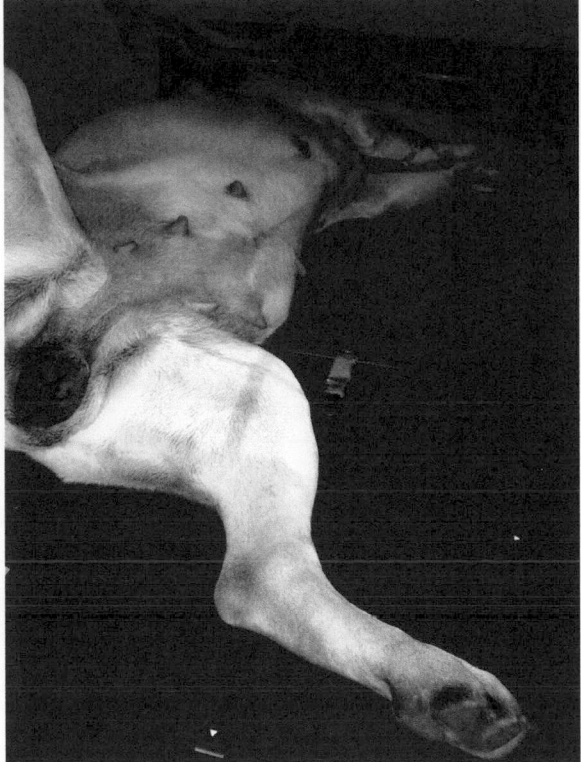

Figure 6.19 Positioning for medio-lateral view of the stifle.

To view the hock, centre the primary over the tibio-tarsal joint.

Procedure: Stifle – cranio-caudal view

1. **Action:** Place the animal in dorsal recumbency supported in a trough or with sandbags.
   Rationale: To prevent the animal tipping over to one side or the other.

2. **Action:** Rotate the body slightly away from the side under examination.
   Rationale: This will put slight tension on the limb when it is balanced by the tie around the limb to be examined.

3. **Action:** Extend the limb caudally and secure with a tie (Fig. 6.20).
   Rationale: This will keep the limb in the correct position.

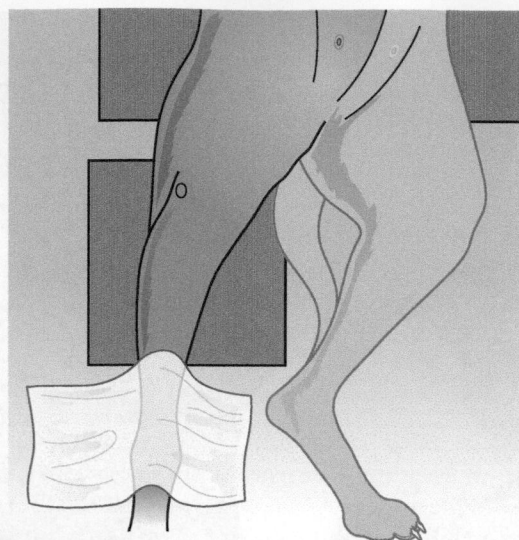

Figure 6.20 Positioning for cranio-caudal view of the stifle. (With permission from Lee R (ed) (1995) Manual of Small Animal Diagnostic Imaging 2e, BSAVA Gloucester, p 128.)

4. **Action:** Place a left / right marker on the cassette.

   Rationale: It is important to be able to locate any abnormality.

5. **Action:** Centre the primary beam (as indicated by the cross wires in the light-beam diaphragm) over the patella and collimate to include half of the femur and half of the tibia.

   Rationale: This will cover the whole stifle joint.

NB A caudo-cranial view of the stifle can be achieved by placing the animal in sternal recumbency and reduces magnification of the joint.

To view the tibia, centre the primary beam midway between the stifle and the hock.

To achieve a dorso-plantar view of the hock, centre the primary beam over the tibio-tarsal joint.

Procedure: Hindfoot – medio–lateral view

1. **Action:** The animal is placed in lateral recumbency with the foot to be examined lying closest to the cassette.

   Rationale: This prevents distortion and magnification of the image.

2. **Action:** Draw the upper limb cranially and secure with ties.

   Rationale: This prevents the bones and soft tissues of the limb obscuring the limb under examination.

3. **Action:** Place the foot to be examined on the cassette and secure on its side using a tie.

   Rationale: The beam is to enter on the medial side and exit laterally.

4. **Action:** If the leg begins to rotate place a foam pad under the caudal aspect of the hock.

   Rationale: This should provide sufficient support to prevent rotation.

5. **Action:** Place a left / right marker as appropriate.

   Rationale: It is important to be able to locate any abnormalities.

6. **Action:** Centre the primary beam (as indicated by the cross wires in the light-beam diaphragm) over the metatarso-phalangeal joints.

   Rationale: These can be located by bending the toes.

Dorso-plantar view of the hindfoot – follow positioning guidelines for the cranio-caudal view of the hock, but centre the beam over the metatarso-phalangeal joints.

USE OF CONTRAST MEDIA

Contrast media are substances that will enhance the radiographic contrast in areas that would otherwise be difficult or impossible to see on a normal plain radiograph. Their use allows the assessment of size, shape and position of an organ and in some cases they may be used to monitor the function as well.

Contrast media can be divided into two groups:

1. **Positive contrast** – these contain elements that have a high atomic number and are able to absorb x-rays, thus creating a white image on the resulting radiograph. The substances commonly used in veterinary medicine are:

- **Barium sulphate** – this is a white inert, non-toxic, tasteless substance that is available as a powder, a colloidal suspension or a paste. It is not absorbed by the body so must be used only by the oral route where it is excreted in the faeces. If it reaches the peritoneum (e.g. through a perforation) or is inhaled accidentally during administration it will result in the formation of granulomatous lesions that remain for life.
- **Water soluble iodine preparations** – these are the most common types of contrast media and come in many forms designed for different clinical situations. They are presented as clear liquids, but appear white on a radiograph. As they are water soluble they may be administered intravenously and they are rapidly excreted by the kidneys – one of their main uses is in urography. They are less commonly used in the digestive tract as they are bitter to taste and produce poorer contrast than barium; however, iodine is recommended if a perforation is suspected as it will be absorbed by the blood stream if it reaches the peritoneum.

2. **Negative contrast** – this involves the use of gases (e.g. atmospheric air, carbon dioxide). These have a low specific gravity and absorb very few x-rays therefore appearing black on a radiograph. They are commonly used to highlight hollow organs such as the stomach and bladder, but mucosal detail is poor. The gas is physically excreted or is absorbed by the blood stream.

Double contrast – this is a technique that combines both types of contrast media and is used to visualize the lining mucosa of hollow organs such as the bladder. It also avoids the masking of filling defects, such as may be caused by a foreign body in the stomach or calculi in the bladder, by dense positive contrast media.

A. ALIMENTARY TRACT

Investigation of the alimentary tract requires the use of barium sulphate in its appropriate form.

With the exception of barium enemas, the patient should not be anaesthetized as this will interfere with normal gut physiology. If the patient is difficult, sedation with acepromazine may be used as this has the least effect on intestinal motility and it may make positioning easier.

If the procedure is elective the patient should be starved for 24 hours to empty the tract as much as possible and an enema should be administered, particularly if a barium enema is to be performed. Starvation is not essential and barium may be used in non-elective procedures.

Care must be taken to avoid the patient aspirating barium during its administration. This is a particular risk when investigating swallowing disorders and may lead to aspiration pneumonia. *Never* use barium in a patient suspected of having a gastric or intestinal perforation.

Procedure: Use of barium in the examination of the alimentary tract (Fig. 6.21)

1. **Action:** Prepare the barium away from the preparation room and the patient. Ready-made barium may be used.

   Rationale: Barium may be administered as a sticky paste (e.g. for oesophageal studies), as a liquid (e.g for a barium series) or mixed with a small amount of food to encourage the patient to eat it. Do not prepare the mixture close to

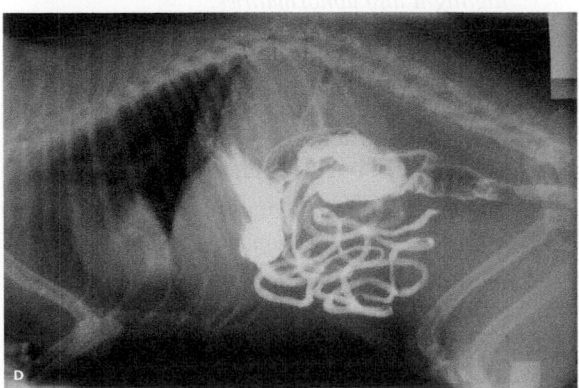

Figure 6.21 Use of barium to highlight the alimentary tract. Barium is visible in the stomach, the small intestine and has begun to reach the colon and rectum – taken 6.5 hours after administration.

the x-ray table as it may contaminate the table or the patient.

2. **Action:** Ensure the patient is prepared appropriately.

   Rationale: This will save time when the patient is presented. Good preparation prevents artefacts on the radiograph.

3. **Action:** Take plain radiographs before the barium is administered.

   Rationale: These can be used for comparison with the contrast studies. In some cases the barium may mask some diagnostic features.

4. **Action:** Entice the animal to eat the barium preparation. Mixing it with food is easier, but if it is in liquid form it may have to be syringed into the mouth. Avoid getting barium on the fur.

   Rationale: Use of food allows the natural eating and swallowing process to be observed. Barium on the fur creates a 'paintbrush' affect or spots on the resulting radiograph.

5. **Action:** If performing a barium swallow for examination of the oesophagus, use food mixed with barium and make an exposure of the oesophageal / thoracic area in right lateral recumbency within 2–3 minutes.

   Rationale: Food takes 15–30 seconds to pass down the oesophagus into the stomach so an exposure must be made quickly. Any barium left in the oesophagus will line the mucosa and highlight any abnormalities.

6. **Action:** If you are performing a barium series (i.e. several radiographs taken at intervals) to follow the barium through the alimentary tract, give approximately 5 ml/ kg of liquid barium (Fig. 6.21).

   Rationale: A large volume is needed to prevent dilution as it passes down the tract.

7. **Action:** If performing a barium enema, the barium must be as liquid as possible. Introduce the barium into the rectum using a catheter by retrograde filling (Fig. 6.22). Air can be introduced to achieve double contrast.

   Rationale: Barium is used to outline the mucosa of the colon and the image can be

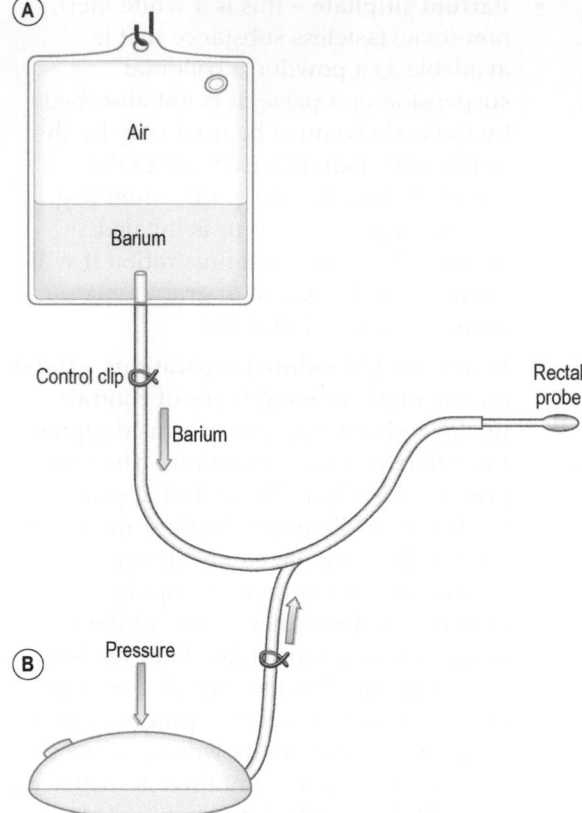

Figure 6.22 Barium enema bag. In position A, the barium flows under gravity into the colon. In position B, barium empties from the colon into the bag and then pressure on the bag will distend the colon with air for the double contrast effect.

enhanced by air. This is a messy procedure – avoid contaminating the fur.

8. **Action:** Position the patient correctly to examine the appropriate part of the alimentary system, centring the primary beam and collimating accurately.

   Rationale: The most common positions will be lateral and VD/DV views of the thorax and abdomen. Incorrect positioning may miss the abnormality or alter the pathology of an organ.

9. **Action:** Increase the kilovoltage above that used for a plain radiograph.

   Rationale: This ensures that the edges of the barium are clearly delineated which aids interpretation of the radiograph.

10. **Action:** Always take four views for a full evaluation – these should be right and left lateral and DV and VD. Remember to use a left / right marker.

    Rationale: This enables accurate location of the abnormality. The appearance of these radiographs will vary as barium will follow gravity and flow into the dependent areas and any gas will rise into the non-dependent areas.

11. **Action:** If examining the stomach, use air to achieve a double-contrast gastrogram.

    Rationale: A thin layer of barium will highlight the gastric mucosa.

12. **Action:** If performing a barium series, take radiographs every 15 minutes until barium enters the colon.

    Rationale: This is used to study gastric motility and emptying time and to identify the presence and location of foreign bodies or tumours. Gastric and intestinal motility can be truly assessed only using fluoroscopy.

13. **Action:** It may be necessary to make an exposure 24 hours after the original administration of barium.

    Rationale: Remaining barium may stick to and highlight any abnormalities not previously identified.

B. URINARY TRACT

Water soluble iodine preparations are used to study the upper urinary tract. As these are administered intravenously, taste bitter and may cause nausea the patient should be deeply sedated or anaesthetized, which also aids more accurate positioning. Perivascular iodine may also be irritant.

Procedure: Intravenous urography for examination of the kidneys and ureters (Fig. 6.23)

1. **Action:** The patient should be anaesthetized and given an enema.

   Rationale: The presence of faeces in the colon may mask the view of the kidneys and ureters and may push the kidney into an abnormal position.

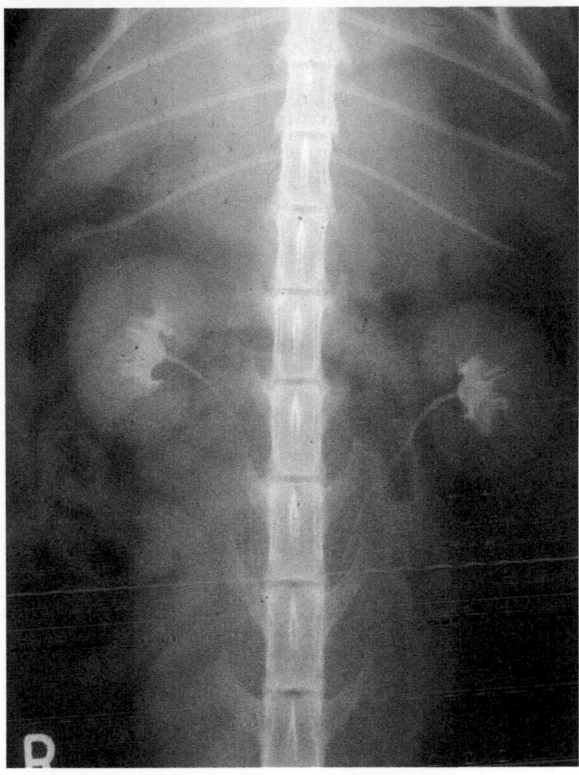

Figure 6.23 Use of water soluble iodine to highlight the urinary tract – taken 5 minutes after i.v. administration.

2. **Action:** Take plain radiographs in right lateral and ventro-dorsal recumbency, centred on the umbilicus.

   Rationale: These views will demonstrate all of the urinary tract and can be used for comparison with the contrast radiographs.

3. **Action:** Using a urinary catheter, empty the bladder. Introduce a small amount of air into the bladder.

   Rationale: It is always a good idea to collect a urine sample while you are emptying the bladder as you may need to analyse it later. Urine must be removed as it will dilute the contrast medium. Air in the bladder produces a clearer view of the ureters and the neck of the bladder.

4. **Action:** Place the animal in dorsal recumbency supported in a trough.

   Rationale: This enables serial radiographs to be taken without disturbing the animal. Lateral radiographs can be taken when adequate opacification of the kidneys and tract has taken place.

5. **Action:** Administer the iodine preparation, which has been previously warmed, via the cephalic vein.

   Rationale: The preparation is warmed to reduce the viscosity, which makes intravenous injection much easier.

6. There are two techniques for the administration of iodine and they depend on the reason for the contrast study:

   • **Action:** Rapid bolus of a low volume.

     Rationale: Rapid bolus – used for examination of the kidneys and ureters.

   • **Action:** Slow infusion of a high volume.

     Rationale: Slow infusion – used for incontinence and for ureteric problems.

7. **Action:** Bolus administration: using 300–400 mg iodine/ml conc. at a dose of 850 mg/kg body weight (approximately 1 ml/kg). Administer as rapidly as possible and take radiographs as soon as the injection is completed. Take serial radiographs at 1, 5, 10, 15 and 20 minutes.

   Rationale: The iodine is excreted by the kidneys and will appear within the renal parenchyma within a few minutes (Fig. 6.23). Opacity increases as the process continues and iodine enters the bladder.

8. **Action:** Infusion administration: using 150–200 mg/ml iodine concentration at a dose of 1200 mg/kg body weight (approx. 8 ml/kg); may be diluted with dextrose or saline and given via an intravenous catheter over a period of 10–15 minutes. Take radiographs at 5, 10 and 15 minutes after the start of the infusion. Both VD and lateral views can be taken.

   Rationale: The iodine is excreted by the kidneys and will appear within the renal parenchyma within a few minutes. Opacity increases as the process continues and iodine enters the bladder.

NB The rapid bolus technique may be used to investigate the bladder when radiographs may be taken 30 minutes after administration of the iodine. Rolling the patient from side to side will ensure thorough mixing of the contrast with any urine in the bladder. The results are not as informative as retrograde methods.

Procedure: Cystography – examination of the bladder using contrast material

1. **Action:** The patient should be anaesthetized or deeply sedated and given an enema.

   Rationale: The presence of faeces in the colon may alter the position of the bladder. A general anaesthetic will aid positioning and ensure radiation safety. The technique can be performed in conscious animals as it is not necessarily painful, but catheterization may cause the urethra to constrict and this should be noted when the radiograph is evaluated.

2. **Action:** Place the patient in right lateral recumbency and take a plain radiograph centred on the neck of the bladder and collimated to include the entire bladder.

   Rationale: This can be used to compare with the contrast radiographs.

3. **Action:** Introduce a urinary catheter into the bladder and drain the urine. Leave the catheter in place.

   Rationale: Do not use a rigid catheter in bitches as this distorts the neck of the bladder and may cause damage during positioning. It is a good idea to save some of the urine for analysis.

4. There are three techniques for visualizing the bladder using contrast media. Each has advantages and disadvantages:

   • **Action:** Pneumocystogram – using room air.

     Rationale: Overinflation may cause damage. Maintaining inflation may be difficult. Inadequate inflation and thickening of the bladder wall may mimic pathological changes. Used to detect the presence of calculi.

   • **Action:** Positive contrast – using 20% contrast iodine.

     Rationale: Good mucosal detail, but contrast may obscure lesions or calculi.

   • **Action:** Double contrast – using air and iodine.

Rationale: Good for mucosal detail, for assessing the thickness of the bladder wall and for highlighting lesions or calculi.

5. **Action:** Pneumocystogram – with patient in right lateral recumbency introduce room air into the empty bladder using a syringe attached to the catheter and a three-way tap at a rate of approximately 10 ml/kg.

    Rationale: The bladder should feel moderately distended when the abdomen is palpated. Take care not to overinflate. The bladder will appear as a dark mass in the caudal abdomen.

6. **Action:** Positive contrast – introduce dilute iodine at a rate of 10 ml/kg body weight into the empty bladder. Total volume will be between 50 and 300 ml depending on the size of the animal.

    Rationale: The bladder appears as a white mass in the caudal abdomen.

7. **Action:** Double contrast – using 150 mg/ml iodine concentration, introduce 2–15 ml into the empty bladder. Gently roll the patient from side to side. Inflate the bladder with air until it feels taut.

    Rationale: Rolling ensures that the mucosa is coated by the contrast material. The bladder mucosa will appear as a thin white line whereas the lumen appears black with a shadow of residual contrast in the centre.

8. **Action:** In all cases a lateral radiograph should be taken as soon as the contrast material has been introduced.

    Rationale: There is a risk that the contrast will leak out.

Procedure: Retrograde urethrography for examination of the urethra using positive contrast in the male

1. **Action:** The patient should be anaesthetized or sedated and given an enema.

    Rationale: The presence of faeces in the colon may mask the view of the kidneys and ureters and may push the kidney into an abnormal position. Sedation may be used in more cooperative animals. The procedure can be done in conscious animals, but it may cause the urethra to constrict and this

should be taken into consideration when assessing the radiograph.

2. **Action:** Place the patient in right lateral recumbency and take a plain radiograph centred on the neck of the bladder and collimated to include the entire bladder.

    Rationale: This may indicate any lesions that are later masked by the contrast material.

3. **Action:** Using a urinary catheter, empty the bladder and remove the catheter.

    Rationale: The presence of urine in the bladder will dilute the contrast material. It is a good idea to save some of the urine for analysis.

4. **Action:** Select a Foley catheter of an appropriate size and flush it with contrast material before it is inserted.

    Rationale: This flushes air out of the catheter. If air is present in the catheter when it is inserted the air may appear to be in the urethra and affect the diagnosis.

5. **Action:** Place the patient in right lateral recumbency.

    Rationale: This is the most comfortable position for the patient and provides easy access to the penis and urethra.

6. **Action:** Gently insert the Foley catheter into the proximal part of the penile urethra and inflate the cuff.

    Rationale: Inflating the cuff prevents backflow of contrast material out of the urethra.

7. **Action:** Using 150 mg/ml iodine conc. inject 5–15 ml slowly up the catheter.

    Rationale: The addition of K-Y® jelly to the contrast material will increase the degree of urethral distension and may produce a better image.

8. **Action:** While you continue to inject the iodine take a lateral radiograph – take two radiographs, one with the hindlimb pulled caudally to show the penile urethra and the other with the hindlimb pulled cranially to show the ischial arch.

    Rationale: Taking the radiograph while you inject the contrast ensures that not too much escapes into the bladder. Leakage of contrast from the opening of the penis may be prevented by occluding the end with your hands. Remember to protect yourself from scattered radiation by wearing a lead apron and either covering your hands with a lead sheet or wearing lead gloves.

NB If the prostatic urethra is to be examined, use a urinary catheter to introduce the contrast material further up the urethra – the tip should lie just distal to the prostate gland. This technique can also be used to identify the presence of ectopic ureters.

Procedure: Retrograde vaginourethrography for examination of the vagina and urethra using positive contrast in the female

1. **Action:** The patient should be anaesthetized and given an enema.

   Rationale: The use of Allis tissue forceps later on in the procedure is painful. The presence of faeces in the colon may alter the position of the bladder or urethra.

2. **Action:** Place the patient in right lateral recumbency and take a plain radiograph centred on the neck of the bladder and collimated to include the entire bladder.

   Rationale: This may indicate any lesions that are later masked by the contrast material.

3. **Action:** Using a urinary catheter, empty the bladder and remove the catheter.

   Rationale: The presence of urine in the bladder will dilute the contrast material. It is a good idea to save some of the urine for analysis.

4. **Action:** Select a Foley catheter of an appropriate size and flush it with contrast material before it is inserted.

   Rationale: This flushes air out of the catheter. If air is present in the catheter when it is inserted the air may appear to be in the vestibule and affect the diagnosis.

5. **Action:** Place the patient in right lateral recumbency.

   Rationale: This is the most comfortable position for the patient and provides easy access to the vagina and vestibule.

6. **Action:** Insert the Foley catheter through the vulval lips and into the vestibule and inflate the cuff.

Rationale: Inflating the cuff prevents backflow and leakage of the contrast material.

7. **Action:** Hold the catheter in place and attach a pair of Allis tissue forceps across the vulval lips.

   Rationale: This prevents loss of the contrast material but can be painful in a conscious bitch.

8. **Action:** Using 150 mg/ml iodine concentration, inject 1 ml/kg body weight slowly up the catheter.

   Rationale: The contrast will fill the vagina as far cranially as the cervix as well as the urethra. The contrast material enters the vagina under pressure and care must be taken not to overfill the vagina and urethra as rupture can occur.

9. **Action:** Stand away from the patient and take a lateral radiograph.

   Rationale: If it is necessary to prevent further leakage of contrast material, you can occlude the vulval lips with your hands. Remember to protect yourself from scattered radiation by wearing a lead apron and either covering your hands with a lead sheet or wearing lead gloves.

DIAGNOSTIC ULTRASOUND

Diagnostic ultrasound uses sound waves with a frequency of 2–10 MHz, which is much higher than the normal range audible to the human ear (20 kHz) and those used for therapeutic ultrasound (1 MHz).

The sound waves are produced from and received by a transducer containing crystals. These have piezo-electric properties so that when a voltage is applied to them they deform and emit characteristic high frequency sound waves – this is the **inverse piezo-electric effect.** The transducer produces regular short pulses of sound that pass through the body tissues. The returning sound or **echoes** are picked up by the same crystals, which deform again producing electrical signals – this is the **piezo-electric effect**. The signals are analysed according to their strength and the depth of tissue from which they have originated and this is displayed as an image on the screen.

When the transducer is applied to the skin, the ultrasound waves pass through the tissues. Each tissue has a different **acoustic impedance** or resistance to the sound waves and when the sound waves reach a boundary or **acoustic interface** between two tissues they may respond in one of two ways depending on the type of tissue. They may:

- Be reflected back again to be picked up by the transducer – this occurs when the acoustic impedance is great (e.g. air / soft tissue or bone / soft tissue).
- Continue deeper into the tissues – this occurs when the acoustic impedance is small (e.g. soft tissue / soft tissue).

As the sound waves travel through the tissues they become weaker or **attenuated** owing to a combination of reflection, absorption and scatter.

IMAGE DISPLAY MODES

- **A mode** (amplitude mode) – this is rarely used nowadays as it provides limited information about the tissue boundaries. It uses a single fixed beam of ultrasound and the returning echoes are shown as peaks along a horizontal line (Fig. 6.24).
- **B mode** (brightness mode) – this is the most common type. Uses multiple beams of ultrasound and the returning echoes from each beam are analysed. Each dot on the screen represents a returning echo, its position indicates its origin and its brightness its strength. This information allows a two-dimensional cross section to be produced, which represents a slice through the tissues under examination. The image is constantly updated so that movement (e.g. the heart beating) can be observed – known as real-time scanning (Fig. 6.24).
- **M mode** (motion mode) – this shows movement of structures on a frozen image and is mainly used for echocardiography. A single scan-line is selected from the B-mode image. Echoes are represented as a vertical line on the left of the screen as dots. The distance of the dot along the line represents the depth of origin and the brightness represents the strength. The image is constantly updated (Fig. 6.24).

TYPES OF TRANSDUCER

- **Linear array** – 60–256 crystals are arranged in a line and are activated sequentially. It produces a wide rectangular field of view but requires a relatively large area of contact, which is difficult when examining thoracic and cranial abdominal structures in small animals.
- **Curved linear array** – this has a convex scanning surface so requires a smaller area of contact.

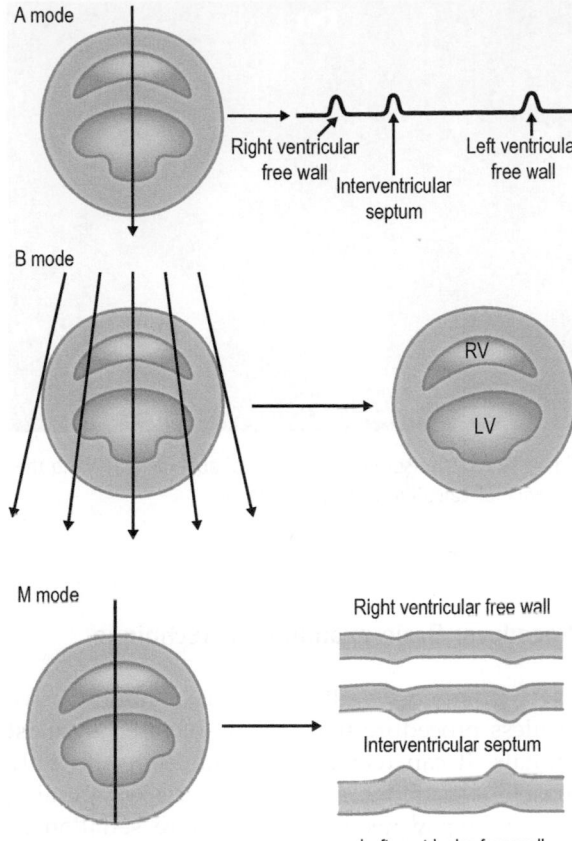

Figure 6.24 Image display modes.

- **Sector** – this is a single or a small number of crystals producing a fan-shaped field of view. Does not allow good visualization of superficial structures, but it requires only a small area of contact so is most likely to be used in small animals (Fig. 6.25).

Other types of transducer are being developed.

TERMINOLOGY

- **Hyperechoic or echogenic** – bright echoes that appear white. These are produced by highly reflective acoustic interfaces (e.g. gas, collagen and bone).
- **Hypoechoic or echopoor** – sparse echoes that appear grey. These are produced by acoustic interfaces that have intermediate reflection or transmission (e.g. soft tissues).
- **Anechoic or echolucent** – no returning echoes so they appear black. These represent complete transmission of ultrasound through the tissue (e.g. fluid).

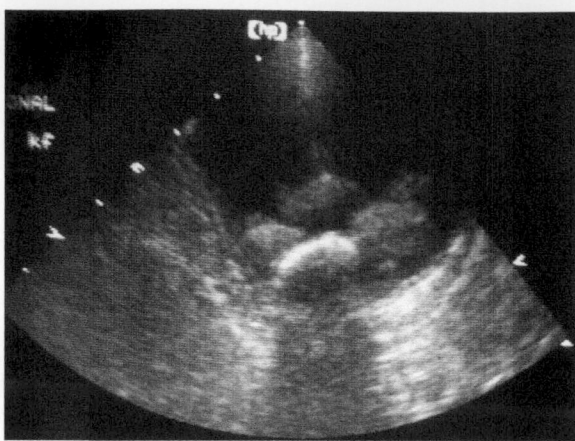

Figure 6.25 Ultrasound of the caudal abdomen showing the presence of calculi in the canine bladder.

Procedure: Basic examination technique

Use of diagnostic ultrasound is a non-invasive painless procedure that is well tolerated by most animals. It can usually be administered to fully conscious patients, although its use for guiding fine or biopsy needles may require sedation or general anaesthesia. There have been no reports of adverse clinical effects in the patient or in the personnel involved in its use.

1. **Action:** Place the patient on an examination table in a position that provides sufficient access to the area under examination.

   Rationale: This may mean that the patient may remain standing or lying in lateral or dorsal recumbency. If the patient feels secure and comfortable it will be less likely to struggle.

2. **Action:** Select an appropriate part of the body for examination.

   Rationale: Choose an area of skin over the point of interest and where the depth of tissue that has to be crossed is minimal.

3. **Action:** Avoid choosing a site where bone or gas-filled structures lie between the skin and the point of interest.

   Rationale: Both bone and gas will block the ultrasound beam and may affect image quality or impair visualization of deeper tissues.

4. **Action:** Clip the skin and clean with surgical spirit.

   Rationale: Fur must be removed to ensure good contact between the transducer and the skin. Surgical spirit is used to remove grease and dirt.

5. **Action:** Apply liberal quantities of acoustic or coupling gel to the transducer and the skin.

   Rationale: This ensures that there is good contact between the transducer and the skin; it is more important to apply gel to the skin than it is to apply it to the transducer. Any other material (e.g. air or dirt) will create another acoustic interface, which may affect the image. Concentric white lines on the resulting image indicate poor contact and the site should be prepared again.

6. **Action:** Apply the transducer to the skin in the prepared area moving it around as necessary.

   Rationale: The strength of the returning echo depends on the nature of the tissues and the angle of the interface relative to the sound beam.

ENDOSCOPY

Endoscopy was originally developed as a technique for looking inside body cavities, but modern equipment also allows the recording of findings, the gathering of biopsy samples and performing minor surgical procedures.

There are two types of endoscope, rigid and flexible, which refer to their relative ability to bend within cavities. Both use a light source, which illuminates the cavity, and the resulting image is transmitted back to the operator. Endoscopes are expensive, delicate pieces of equipment and they should be treated with care.

- **Rigid endoscopes** – use is limited to sites lying in a straight line (e.g. nasal cavity, urethra, joints, ears) and are particularly used in large animals such as horses. Rigidity aids insertion and they consist of a relatively simple hollow insertion tube with a light source and a facility for viewing the image.

- **Flexible endoscopes** – of more use in small animals. They make use of fibreoptic technology, which relies on the fact that light can travel down a bendable fibre by repeated total internal reflection (TIR) exiting as a single spot of light. The fibre tubes are grouped together in image bundles that have the individual fibre faces fixed in an identical pattern (i.e. they are coherent). This ensures that the image transmitted is the same in each fibre, creating an accurate picture of the area under examination. Breakage of any of the tubes creates a black dot or area, which ruins the image. They produce a satisfactory image quality that is limited by the diameter and thus number of fibres in the bundle – narrower endoscopes have a limited amount of illumination. They are more portable and of moderate cost.

Video endoscopes are now available that allow the image to be relayed on a screen. The image quality is excellent and is improving all the time. The system allows several people to observe the process, but the equipment is less portable and is expensive.

Endoscopy is minimally invasive but there is the risk of harm to the patient (e.g. perforation leading to peritonitis, mediastinitis or a tension pneumothorax, airway irritation, infection, haemorrhage) or damage to the equipment (e.g. broken fibres, biting by patient, which may damage the insertion tube cover).

Common endoscopic procedures include:

- Examination of the upper and lower gastrointestinal tracts (proctoscopy or colonoscopy) (Fig. 6.26)
- Rhinoscopy
- Examination of the respiratory tract.

The endoscopic image can be difficult to interpret and it is possible to miss lesions. As with many techniques, practice makes perfect!

Procedure: Patient preparation and general points to consider when performing endoscopy

1. **Action:** Starve the patient for 12 hours and withhold water for 1 hour prior to the procedure.

   Rationale: This is the standard procedure prior to a general anaesthetic.

2. **Action:** If performing *endoscopy of the gastrointestinal tract*, take plain lateral radiographs.

   Rationale: To check that the tract is empty.

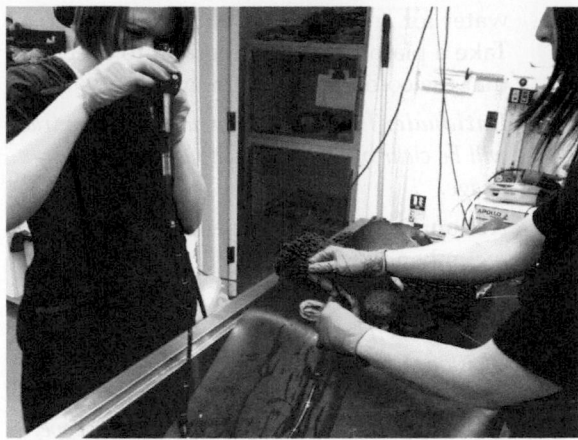

Figure 6.26 Examination of the colon of a dog using a flexible endoscope.

3. **Action:** Administer a general anaesthetic to the patient, regardless of which endoscopic examination is to be performed.

   Rationale: This provides a means of restraint and analgesia. Some practitioners may perform proctoscopy under deep sedation.

4. **Action:** Place a mouth gag between the upper and lower jaw.

   Rationale: To keep the mouth open and to prevent damage to the endoscope.

5. **Action:** Tie the endotracheal tube to the mandible not the maxilla. When performing *rhinoscopy* the tube should be cuffed.

   Rationale: To facilitate the introduction of the endoscope. A cuffed tube will prevent water getting into the respiratory tract during rhinoscopy.

6. **Action:** Avoid the use of atropine if possible.

   Rationale: Atropine affects the motility and secretions of the gastrointestinal tract.

7. **Action:** When performing *proctoscopy* or *colonoscopy* (Fig. 6.26) an oral laxative should be given 24 hours before the procedure. Follow this with two warm-water enemas on the morning of the procedure – the final one should be given 2 hours before the procedure. Withhold

water for an hour prior to the procedure. Take a plain lateral radiograph to check that the colon and rectum are empty.

Rationale: This protocol ensures that the tract will be clear of faeces, which may affect the image.

8. **Action:** Position the patient in left lateral recumbency with the head and neck extended.

   Rationale: The body is in a stable comfortable position. Extending the head and neck straightens the oesophagus and trachea, facilitating the introduction of the endoscope.

9. **Action:** If performing *rhinoscopy*, place the patient in sternal recumbency.

   Rationale: Sternal recumbency provides easier access to the nose or to the trachea.

10. **Action:** When collecting *biopsy samples*, position the biopsy forceps at right angles to the mucosa.

    Rationale: This ensures that you collect the optimal sample and reduces the risk of unnecessary damage to the mucosa.

11. **Action:** When collecting samples from the gastrointestinal tract, avoid overinflating the stomach as this stretches the mucosa.

Rationale: This will lead to smaller samples being collected.

12. **Action:** Avoid collecting samples from a site that you cannot see.

    Rationale: It is permissible to take one sample, but never take repeated samples as you will not be able to see the damage you have caused or deal with it.

13. **Action:** In most cases, samples should always be taken even if there are no apparent lesions. Take samples from multiple sites.

    Rationale: The visual appearance of a site may not always indicate a specific abnormality.

14. **Action:** To remove the sample from the biopsy forceps, immerse it in 10% buffered formalin or remove the sample carefully using a needle and place it into the formalin.

    Rationale: Treat all samples with care to prevent artefactual damage to the tissue.

15. **Action:** After collecting the sample, rinse the biopsy forceps in saline before reinserting them into the endoscope.

    Rationale: To make sure that there is no tissue remaining from the previous sample.

CHAPTER 7

Medical diagnostic and treatment techniques

This chapter describes many of the fundamental techniques used in the diagnosis and / or treatment of animals. They have been included under the heading of 'medical' but some procedures, especially those such as the placing of feeding tubes, may have a surgical element within them. Understanding how to perform these procedures is a vital part of everyday work as a veterinary surgeon.

FLUID THERAPY

BASIC THEORY

The normal healthy body contains 60% to 70% water. Its function is to maintain homeostasis so that the normal metabolic processes can work effectively. If fluid balance is disrupted for any reason the patient will become ill – restoring fluid balance may be the single most important factor in returning the patient to normal health.

Body water is divided into two fluid compartments:

Extracellular fluid (ECF):

- makes up 33% of the total body water and lies outside the cells
- includes the **plasma** within the blood, **interstitial fluid** between the cells and the **transcellular fluid,** which is formed by active secretory membranes (e.g. synovial fluid, cerebrospinal fluid and lymph)
- contains electrolytes (e.g. sodium, potassium, calcium, and magnesium, chloride, bicarbonate and phosphate) – sodium chloride is the predominant electrolyte
- plasma also contains proteins (e.g. albumin, globulin, fibrinogen, prothrombin) whose function is to maintain blood volume and blood pressure by exerting an effective osmotic pressure keeping fluid within the blood vessels. There is no protein in interstitial fluid as the molecules are too large to pass through the capillary walls under normal conditions.

Intracellular fluid (ICF):

- makes up 66% of the total body water and lies within all the cells
- contains electrolytes (e.g. potassium, magnesium and sodium, phosphate, bicarbonate and chloride) – potassium phosphate is the predominant electrolyte

- also contains proteins; these are non-diffusible and maintain an effective intracellular osmotic pressure.

Fluid constantly moves around the body and this is influenced by the osmotic pressure of that fluid. There are three terms used to define the osmotic pressure of a fluid in relation to that of plasma, and this property affects what happens to the fluid within the body and therefore the choice of replacement fluid. Isotonic fluid is the most commonly used:

- **Isotonic** – fluid has the same osmotic pressure of plasma and will remain within the plasma when administered intravenously (e.g. 0.9% saline (normal saline)).
- **Hypotonic** – fluid has a lower osmotic pressure than that of plasma. Fluid will be drawn into the cells resulting in swelling and the risk of cell lysis (e.g. sterile water, 0.45% saline).
- **Hypertonic** – fluid has a higher osmotic pressure than that of plasma, which will draw water out of the cells (e.g. 7.2% saline, 10% dextrose).

SELECTION OF FLUIDS

Many medical and surgical conditions upset the fluid balance within the body; if nothing is done to correct this the patient will become dehydrated or, if severe, go into shock and possibly die. The aim of fluid therapy is to replace the deficit so that the circulating blood volume is restored, tissue perfusion and renal function return to normal and the patient recovers.

There are many types of fluid used in fluid therapy and the replacement fluid must be as close as possible, in terms of its chemical constituents and its volume, to that lost from the circulation. Fluids broadly fall into three classes:

- **Blood, plasma and oxyglobin** – contain blood products used in cases of haemorrhage
- **Colloids or plasma expanders** – contain large molecules of inert substances that are too big to pass through the capillary walls and are used to improve circulatory balance
- **Crystalloids** – contain water, electrolytes and / or glucose.

Table 7.1 describes the principal constituents of replacement fluids.

ADMINISTRATION OF FLUIDS

Most replacement fluids are administered via the parenteral route (i.e. into the space between the

Table 7.1 Main constituents of common replacement fluids

Solution	Type	Contents	Indications	Comments
0.9% Saline (normal saline)	Crystalloid Isotonic	Na, Cl	Vomiting, urinary obstruction, hypoadrenocorticism	This is an acidifying solution
Hartmann's solution or lactated Ringer's solution	Crystalloid Isotonic	Na, K, Ca, Cl, lactate	Diarrhoea, prolonged anorexia, pyometra, prolonged vomiting	Lactate is converted into bicarbonate; do NOT add bicarbonate as it will precipitate out as chalk (i.e. alkalinizing solution)
Ringer's solution	Crystalloid Isotonic	Na, Cl, Ca, K	Pyometra, severe vomiting, intestinal foreign bodies	Contains potassium chloride and calcium chloride in addition to sodium chloride
5% glucose	Crystalloid Isotonic	Glucose	Hyperthermia, water deprivation, hypoglycaemia	Equivalent to isotonic water
0.18% sodium chloride + 4% dextrose (dextrose or glucose saline)	Crystalloid Isotonic	Na, Cl, dextrose	Primary water losses and to replace maintenance losses	If used long term, need to use potassium supplementation
Potassium chloride	Crystalloid Isotonic	K, Cl	To supplement a crystalloid fluid	If being added to a fluid bag, make sure it is clearly labelled to avoid overadministration
7.2% sodium chloride (hypertonic saline)	Crystalloid Hypertonic	Na, Cl	Rapid intravascular volume resuscitation; only in small volumes (e.g. 4–7 ml/kg in dogs)	Contraindicated in simple dehydration, cardiac disease and uncontrolled haemorrhage
Haemaccel®/ Gelofusine®	Colloid Isotonic	Gelatins, Na, Cl, K, Ca	Rapid intravascular volume replacement, hypotensive resuscitation, ongoing haemorrhage	Will not improve oxygen carrying capacity in cases of blood loss; remains in the intravascular space for longer and so helps intravascular fluid volume
Hetastarch	Colloid	Waxy species of maize and sorghum	Rapid intravascular volume replacement, hypotensive resuscitation, ongoing haemorrhage, hypoproteinaemia	Remains in the intravascular space for longer and so helps intravascular fluid volume
Dextrans	Colloid	Dextran	Rapid intravascular volume replacement, hypotensive resuscitation, ongoing haemorrhage	Remains in the intravascular space for longer and so helps intravascular fluid volume

integument and the gut) and the most common route is intravenous. Other routes of administration include:

- **Subcutaneous** – used where dehydration is mild and there is adequate peripheral circulation. Any crystalloid fluid can be given by this route.
- **Intraperitoneal** – used where dehydration is mild and fluids cannot be administered orally. Larger volumes can be given as the peritoneal space is potentially large and is often used in neonates and exotics (see Ch. 1).
- **Intraosseus** – often used in small exotics whose veins are fragile and easily damaged by needles and catheters. If the catheter is dislodged, haemorrhage from the site is unlikely to occur (see Ch. 1).
- **Oral** – used when the animal is willing to drink, not vomiting and in the absence of an intestinal obstruction. It is usual to use hypotonic electrolyte drinks or plain water. This uses the enteral route.

Procedure: Assessing the level of dehydration

1. **Action:** Obtain an accurate history from the owner asking questions about eating and drinking, urination, vomiting and diarrhoea, wounds, etc.

   Rationale: To provide you with an idea of the severity and cause of the problem. The facts will also guide you as to how best to replace the fluid loss.

2. **Action:** Weigh the animal.

   Rationale: This provides a measurement on which to base evidence of recovery or deterioration.

3. **Action:** Check for skin elasticity by tenting the skin and also check the eyes to assess whether or not they are sunken. Box 7.1 shows how to calculate the fluid deficit using clinical signs to estimate percentage dehydration.

   Rationale: Loss of skin elasticity and sunken eyes do not appear until the animal is approximately 5% dehydrated (Table 7.2). Older and wasted animals have reduced elasticity even though they may not be dehydrated; overweight animals only lose their skin elasticity when severely dehydrated.

4. **Action:** Check the mucous membranes.

   Rationale: These become tacky as a result of dehydration.

Box 7.1 Calculation of fluid deficit using percentage dehydration obtained as a result of a clinical examination

A 25 kg Labrador is found to be 8% dehydrated. The total fluid deficit is:

$$bodyweight\,(kg) \times \%\,dehydration \times 10$$
$$= 25 \times 8 \times 10$$
$$= 2000\,ml\,of\,fluid\,deficit$$

Table 7.2 Clinical signs associated with dehydration

Percentage dehydration	Clinical signs	Fluid deficit (ml/kg bodyweight)
<5	No detectable signs Increasing urine concentration	–
5–6 i.e. mild	Subtle loss of skin elasticity Slightly dry mouth	50
6–8 i.e. moderate	Definite loss of skin elasticity Slight increase in CRT Cold extremities Dry mucous membranes Slightly sunken eyes	80
10–12	Skin remains tented when pulled up Prolonged CRT Sunken eyes and protrusion of the 3rd eyelid Dry mucous membranes	100
12–15	Signs of shock Moribund Death imminent	120

5. **Action:** Check the capillary refill time (CRT) by applying gentle pressure to the gum and observing the return to normal colour.

   Rationale: Capillary refill time is prolonged as a result of reduced circulating blood volume.

6. **Action:** Assess responsiveness of the animal by observing its response to the goings on around it – try calling it by name.

Box 7.2 Calculation of fluid deficit using packed cell volume (PCV)

A 15 kg spaniel has a PCV of 54%. (Assume normal PCV = 45%)
The total fluid deficit is:

bodyweight (kg) ×10 ml for every 1% increase in PCV
= 15 kg × (54% − 45%) ×10 ml
= 15 × 9% ×10 ml
= 1350 ml of fluid deficit

Rationale: Severely dehydrated animals become moribund.

7. **Action:** Collect a blood sample and carry out a packed cell volume (PCV) assessment (see Ch. 4). Box 7.2 shows how to calculate fluid deficit using PCV.

   Rationale: PCV will be raised in a dehydrated patient. Every 1% increase in PCV corresponds to a 10 ml/kg fluid loss. PCV is reduced in cases of anaemia and if this is also present the result is unreliable.

8. **Action:** Collect a urine sample and measure the specific gravity (SG) using a refractometer (see Ch. 4).

   Rationale: Dehydration should cause an increase in urine concentration – the SG will rise – however, if there are underlying problems such as renal or hormonal disease the animal may be unable to concentrate its urine.

EQUIPMENT FOR INTRAVENOUS ADMINISTRATION

Replacement fluids are administered by means of giving or infusion sets. There are four types and the choice depends on the individual case:

1. Standard giving set – delivers fluid at a rate of 15–20 drops/ml. Used for larger patients being given crystalloids or colloids (Fig 7.1A).

2. Paediatric giving set – delivers fluid at a rate of 60 drops/ml – this faster rate is useful to administer small volumes more accurately. Used for small patients and incorporates a burette which limits the total amount of fluid received by the animal (Fig 7.1A).

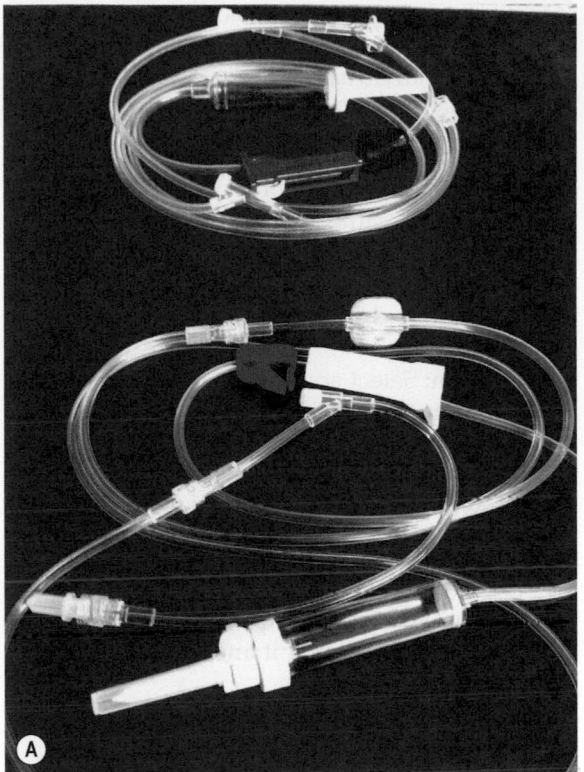

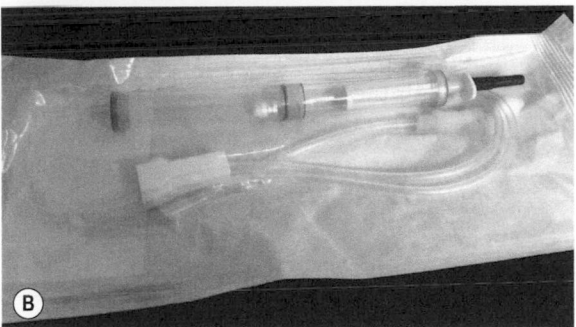

Figure 7.1 (A) Giving sets – standard set above and paediatric giving set below (note burette, which limits the total volume of fluid given to the patient). (B) Blood giving set. Note presence of a double chamber.

3. Blood administration set – a filter is incorporated into the double chamber to prevent any small clots getting into the circulation. Used for plasma, serum or whole blood (Fig 7.1B).

4. Flowline balloon infusers – deliver a very small amount (e.g. a few milliliters). Used for small exotic patients.

Many practices also use infusion pumps to ensure that the correct volume is given at the appropriate rate for the individual patient.

The giving set is attached to an intravenous catheter inserted into an appropriate vein, usually the cephalic vein. For details of restraining the patient and placing the catheter see Chapter 1.

Procedure: Setting up and attaching an intravenous drip

1. **Action:** Select and prepare the equipment (i.e. a bag of appropriate fluid, giving set, clippers, surgical scrub solution, swabs, disposable gloves, intravenous catheter and bowl).

   Rationale: Preparing all equipment in advance ensures a smooth efficient procedure.

2. **Action:** Check the expiry date on the fluid bag before opening it and check for any evidence of damage.

   Rationale: Any sign of damage and/or an out-of-date bag indicates that sterility may be broken and that there is a risk of infection.

3. **Action:** Warm the fluid bag by placing in a microwave or in a pan of hot water for a few minutes.

   Rationale: Prewarming the fluid prevents cold shock when the fluid enters the vein. Drip line warmers and drip bag cosies are available commercially.

4. **Action:** Wash your hands and put on a pair of disposable gloves.

   Rationale: It is important that this whole process is carried out as cleanly as possible to prevent the entry of infection through the vein.

5. **Action:** Remove the fluid bag from its outer covering and identify the outlet port. Hang the bag on a drip stand.

   Rationale: This facilitates handling and administration.

6. **Action:** Remove the giving set from its outer wrappings and switch off the flow control.

   Rationale: This prevents loss of fluid when you insert the giving set into the fluid bag.

7. **Action:** Remove the cover from the infusion spike and introduce it into the bag by pushing it through the outlet port.

   Rationale: Careful handling will avoid puncturing the bag resulting in fluid escaping from the bag.

8. **Action:** Squeeze the fluid chamber so that it fills by one-third.

   Rationale: To aid control of the fluid during administration and avoid the formation of bubbles.

9. **Action:** Remove the cap from the end of the line taking care to avoid touching a non-sterile surface.

   Rationale: It is important to maintain sterility at all times.

10. **Action:** Open the flow control and allow a small volume of fluid to run out into a bowl. At the same time check for air bubbles in the line – if necessary flick them with your finger to encourage them to disperse.

    Rationale: Take care to avoid loss of too much fluid as this will affect the volume that enters the patient. No air bubbles should be allowed to enter the circulation.

11. **Action:** When you are satisfied that everything is ready, close off the flow control, replace the cap on the end of the line and hang the flow line over the drip stand (some giving sets include small plastic clips).

    Rationale: The fluid is now ready to use and the flow line is kept out of risk of falling on the floor.

12. **Action:** Place the patient on a stable table and ask an assistant to restrain in sternal recumbency (see Ch. 1).

    Rationale: If the patient feels secure and comfortable it is less likely to try and escape.

13. **Action:** Select an appropriate vein and ask the assistant to raise it (see Ch. 1).

    Rationale: The cephalic vein is usually the easiest route of administration in dogs, cats. In rabbits the ear vein is useful.

14. **Action:** Clip the vein and prepare the area aseptically using a surgical scrub

    Rationale: It is vital to prevent the entry of infection into the vein.

15. **Action:** Insert an appropriate intravenous catheter into the vein and secure it with tape (see Ch. 1).

    Rationale: To ensure that the catheter does not come out of the vein and to protect it from damage by the patient.

16. **Action:** Remove the cap from the end of the flow line and attach the line to the end of the catheter.

    Rationale: This allows the fluid to run into the vein once the flow control is released.

17. **Action:** Release the flow control and observe the drip rate in the chamber. If necessary adjust the drip rate by manipulating the flow control. Box 7.3 shows you how to calculate the drip rate to correct a given fluid deficit.

    Rationale: Intravenous fluid should flow into the patient at a preset rate according to the requirements of the patient's condition.

18. **Action:** Secure the lower part of the flow line to the paw with tape.

    Rationale: To prevent the line or catheter being torn out by the patient or by catching on objects.

19. **Action:** Instigate a monitoring routine by yourself or the nursing staff (Box 7.4).

    Rationale: A patient on a drip should never be left unattended for long periods. Monitor at regular intervals depending on the severity of the case and keep records on a fluid chart.

MONITORING

Any patient undergoing fluid replacement therapy, by whatever route, should be closely monitored. Box 7.4 lists the parameters that should be checked. Critical care cases should be checked every 5–10 minutes whereas those of lesser severity, or as the patient begins to improve, should be checked at least every 30 minutes. Fluid charts should be kept as a record of treatment and as a way of informing other staff who may take over the care later on.

BLOOD TRANSFUSIONS

As with any form of fluid replacement therapy, the aim is to replace the missing fluid with fluid that is as close as possible to that which has been lost. If a patient has lost blood it follows that you should try to replace it with whole blood. The indications for blood transfusion are:

- Haemorrhage – acute or chronic; internal or external
- Anaemia – acute or chronic
- Clotting problems – associated with deficiencies of platelets or clotting factors.

Box 7.3 Calculation of drip rate to correct a given fluid deficit

A 25 kg Labrador requires 2000 ml of fluid over a 6 hour period at a rate of 5 ml/kg/h. A standard giving set is used delivering 20 drops/ml.
The drip rate should be set at:

$$flow\ rate: 5\ ml \times 25\ kg = 125\ ml/h$$

$$ml/min: 125\ ml \div 60\ min = 2.08\ ml/min$$

$$Drops/min: 2.08 \times 20\ drops/min = 41.6 = 42\ drops/min$$

$$Seconds/drop: 60\ s \div 42\ drops/min = 1.43\ seconds\ (2)$$

– i.e. 1 drop every 2 seconds.

BLOOD COLLECTION

Selection of a donor – the animal must be healthy and fully grown. The owner must be aware of what is involved and have given permission for blood to be collected. Collection of large samples of blood for commercial use requires a licence under the Animals (Scientific Procedures) Act 1986 and the blood products must be supplied under the Veterinary Medicines Regulations. Table 7.3 describes the selection criteria in dogs and cats.

Many practices keep a list of owners who are willing to allow their animals to donate blood and this is particularly useful in an emergency

Box 7.4 Monitoring factors during fluid therapy

Cardiovascular system

- Peripheral pulse rate, rhythm and quality – to check circulatory volume and tissue perfusion.
- Heart rate, rhythm and character – to check heart function.
- Capillary refill time – to assess effectiveness of the circulation.
- Mucous membrane colour and feel – to check levels of oxygenation and hydration; excess moisture and lacrimation may indicate overinfusion.
- Jugular distension – may indicate overinfusion.
- Central venous pressure – normal CVP is 3–7 cm H_2O; below this indicates dehydration; above indicates overinfusion.
- Thoracic auscultation – lung sounds should be clear; laboured, rapid or noisy respiratory sounds may indicate overinfusion or cardiac arrhythmias.

Respiratory system

- Respiratory rate, depth and pattern – should be within normal range and patient should be breathing easily and quietly; laboured, rapid or noisy respiratory sounds may indicate overinfusion.
- Thoracic auscultation – to check for pulmonary oedema; lung sounds should be clear; overinfusion will prevent adequate oxygenation of the blood.

Temperature

- Core temperature – to check for hypothermia or systemic infection.

- Feel the extremities – to check for vasoconstriction or vasodilation.

Other observations

- Skin turgor (elasticity) – to assess pliability of skin; skin tenting may indicate dehydration.
- Peripheral oedema – check distal limbs, ventral body wall and prepuce; presence of oedema could indicate overinfusion; check distal limb below the infusion site as bandage may be too tight.
- Bodyweight – assess over a period of hours or days; marked increase may indicate overperfusion.
- Urine output – to assess renal function and associated circulatory volume; minimum output = 1–2 ml/kg/h; less than this may indicate renal problems.
- Demeanour – any signs of distress or discomfort may indicate a problem (e.g. infection, overinfusion, deterioration of existing problem); overinfusion of the brain results in the patient becoming 'spaced out' and unresponsive.

Equipment checks

- Catheter site – look for leakage of fluid or blood, particularly under the skin, and for evidence of phlebitis.
- Check the fluid flow rate – make sure that the drip rate within the fluid chamber is as it should be; make sure tubing is neither kinked nor blocked.
- Bandages – check that these are clean and not too tight; check for evidence of self mutilation or interference; observe comfort of the patient.

Table 7.3 Criteria for the selection of blood donors

Dogs	Cats
Fully adult but not elderly – ideal age 1–8 years	Fully adult but not elderly – ideal age 1–8 years
Fully vaccinated and not receiving any medication except normal preventative treatment (e.g. anthelmintics)	Fully vaccinated and not receiving any medication except normal preventative treatment (e.g. anthelmintics)
Bodyweight within normal range for the breed	Lean to normal bodyweight – preferably less than 4 kg
Docile temperament – must be able to tolerate procedure	Docile temperament – must be able to tolerate procedure
Normal PCV	Normal PCV
Blood type DEA 1.1 negative	Blood type A, B or AB
No history of travel outside the UK	No history of travel outside the UK
No previous blood transfusion	No previous blood transfusion
Nulliparous	Negative for FeLV, FIV and *Mycoplasma haemofelis*

situation. Blood can be collected as often as every 4–6 weeks without prescribing iron supplementation, but the Home Office recommendation under the Animal (Scientific Procedures) Act 1986 is that you must not take more than 10% of the animal's total blood volume within a 28-day period without holding a personal / project licence under the Act. (Total blood volume of a dog is taken to be 76–107 ml/kg body weight. A 25 kg Labrador would therefore contain approximately 2–2.5 litres of blood so 10% = 200–250 ml.)

Procedure: Cross matching blood

Blood groups – there are over 13 recognized blood groups in the dog. The most important type is DEA 1.1 (dog erythrocyte antigen). Those with DEA 1.1 positive (33–45% of the canine population) are considered to be universal recipients; those with DEA 1.1 negative are considered to be universal donors. Blood groups in cats are A, B and AB.

Testing for compatibility can be done in house using the procedure described below. Blood typing can be done using commercial test kits or by sending samples away to outside laboratories. There is little risk of a reaction at the first transfusion although the life of the erythrocytes may be shortened by the formation of antibodies. If there is a second transfusion, life-threatening signs may develop within hours.

1. **Action:** Collect a small sample of donor blood in an EDTA tube and spin down at 3000 r.p.m. for 10 minutes.

   Rationale: EDTA will prevent clotting. The centrifugal force ensures that blood cells fall to the bottom of the tube.

2. **Action:** Draw off and discard the supernatant fluid.

   Rationale: The supernatant contains the plasma and the buffy coat, which are not needed.

3. **Action:** Resuspend the red blood cells in a little saline at 38°C.

   Rationale: This washes the red cells, which must be kept at blood temperature to ensure survival.

4. **Action:** Spin the sample again and remove the saline supernatant.

   Rationale: This leaves the washed red cells.

5. **Action:** Resuspend the red cells in a measured volume of warm saline to produce a 3–5% solution.

   Rationale: This produces a solution that is easier to work with.

6. **Action:** Collect a small sample of recipient blood in a heparinized tube and spin down in a centrifuge.

   Rationale: This is used to obtain plasma from the recipient.

7. **Action:** Place 1–2 ml of recipient plasma in a test tube, well plate or on a clean slide and add 1–2 drops of donor red cell suspension.

   Rationale: It is here that the reaction will be noted. The use of a slide produces a less reliable result.

8. **Action:** Gently mix by swirling the two liquids together and examine for evidence of haemolysis or agglutination.

   Rationale: Haemolysis is seen as reddening of the solution that does not separate out; agglutination is seen as irregular clumping within the solution, which forms a smooth button in the bottom of the tube.

9. **Action:** Compatibility is demonstrated by the absence of haemolysis or agglutination.

   Rationale: If the two blood samples are compatible there is no reaction.

Procedure: Collection of blood for transfusion

1. **Action:** Select equipment required for blood collection.

   Rationale: Blood collection bag containing anticoagulant such as citrate phosphate dextrose, citrate phosphate dextrose adenine or acid citrate dextrose; cats require a specific feline collection bag. Local anaesthetic cream, syringes and needles of appropriate size, extension tubing, surgical gloves, swabs, skin scrub, clippers, electronic scales. In addition, cats require an i.v. catheter and a 500 ml bag of crystalloid i.v. fluid.

2. **Action:** Select a suitable donor.

    Rationale: See Table 7.3 for selection criteria in dogs and cats.

3. **Action:** If necessary, check for compatibility.

    Rationale: This is important if this is a second or subsequent transfusion or if further transfusions are anticipated as the risk of a transfusion reaction is increased.

4. **Action:** If necessary, sedate the animal. Cats may be given a general anaesthetic.

    Rationale: Most dogs will tolerate the procedure, but cats usually require some form of sedation or anaesthesia.

5. **Action:** Ask your assistant to firmly restrain the animal in a position allowing clear access to the jugular vein, on a stable examination table.

    Rationale: If the animal feels secure and comfortable it will be less likely to try and escape.

6. **Action:** Position the dog in lateral recumbency or in a sitting position. Cats are more comfortable in sternal recumbency with the forelimbs over the edge of the table and the head raised.

    Rationale: The position must be comfortable for the animal and must allow the jugular vein to be raised ready for venepuncture (see Ch. 1).

7. **Action:** Clip and prepare the site over the jugular vein within the jugular groove aseptically.

    Rationale: It is vital to prevent the entry of infection into the blood stream.

8. **Action:** Infiltrate local anaesthetic into the area around the vein and massage gently. Local anaesthetic cream may be used instead.

    Rationale: To desensitize the area making the procedure less painful.

9. **Action:** Ask your assistant to raise the vein.

    Rationale: See Chapter 1.

10. **Action:** Wearing surgical gloves, introduce the needle bevel-side uppermost into the vein and draw back on the syringe.

    Rationale: Blood should flow into the syringe as you draw back. If no blood appears check on the needle's position.

11. **Action:** Detach the needle from the syringe and attach the needle to the tubing leading to the collection bag.

    Rationale: Blood will now begin to flow into the collection bag. Some collection bags have their own needle attached to the system.

12. **Action:** Position the bag lower than the animal and set it on some electronic scales.

    Rationale: Gravity will help the blood flow into the bag. The use of the scales allows you to monitor the weight of blood that has been collected. One ml of blood weighs approximately 1.053 g.

13. **Action:** Periodically invert the collecting bag.

    Rationale: To mix the blood with the anticoagulant in the bag.

14. **Action:** When the bag is full, clamp the tubing with a pair of artery forceps and remove the needle from the vein in the correct manner (see Ch. 1), applying pressure with a sterile swab for about 5 minutes.

    Rationale: One full bag (400 ml) is described as 1 unit of blood. Pressure will prevent the development of a haematoma.

15. **Action:** Apply a light neck bandage to the animal for several hours.

    Rationale: This will prevent haematoma formation and keep the site clean, preventing the entry of infection.

16. **Action:** If the blood is not to be administered immediately the tubing must be tightly clamped or heat sealed and labelled clearly with the species and date of collection. Blood can be stored at 4–8°C for a maximum of 3 weeks.

    Rationale: It is vital that infection does not enter the bag or that the blood does not deteriorate.

17. **Action:** Provide the donor with food and water and place in a warm, quiet kennel under observation for a few hours.

Rationale: To make sure that the donor does not suffer from hypovolaemic shock.

NB In cats a smaller volume will be collected and syringes containing anticoagulant may be used instead of collection bags. Following donation, cats should be given i.v. crystalloid fluid via an i.v. catheter placed in the cephalic vein, at the rate of 30 ml/kg over a period of 3 hours. If the cat has been given a general anaesthetic or sedation, it must be closely monitored during recovery. Once it is awake it should be given food and water and put into a warm quiet kennel.

BLOOD ADMINISTRATION

Procedure: Blood transfusion

1. **Action:** Select and prepare the equipment.

    Rationale: Bag(s) of blood, blood giving set, adhesive tape, bandage, patient (recipient) with large diameter i.v. catheter in place – this avoids red cell haemolysis.

2. **Action:** Make sure that the bag of blood is warmed to body temperature, particularly if it has been removed from storage.

    Rationale: To prevent cold shock and potential hypothermia.

3. **Action:** Hang the blood bag on a drip stand and set up the infusion set as described for fluid therapy. Insert the infusion spike into the correct port on the blood bag, taking care not to puncture the bag.

    Rationale: Puncturing the bag will cause leakage and may introduce infection.

4. **Action:** Squeeze both chambers of the infusion set to fill with blood to one-third in each of them (Fig. 7.1B).

    Rationale: The extra chamber within a blood infusion set provides a fibrin filter to collect any clots and prevent them from entering the circulation.

5. **Action:** Remove the cap from the infusion line and hold it over a bowl, making sure that you do not contaminate the tip.

    Rationale: It is essential to maintain sterility.

6. **Action:** Turn on the flow control to allow blood to flow through into the end of the line and out into the bowl. This must be done slowly to remove any bubbles and keep blood wastage to a minimum.

    Rationale: Bubbles must not enter the circulation as they may form an air embolism.

7. **Action:** Replace the cap on the end of the line and hang it over the drip stand ready for use.

    Rationale: Ensure that the equipment remains aseptic.

8. **Action:** Ask an assistant to restrain the patient within a warm comfortable kennel. The patient should be conscious or sedated and should be fitted with an intravenous catheter placed in the cephalic vein. Smaller exotics or neonates may be fitted with an intraosseus catheter (see Ch. 1).

    Rationale: Administration of a blood transfusion may take several hours and the patient must be warm and comfortable.

9. **Action:** Flush through the catheter with a small amount of heparinized saline in a syringe.

    Rationale: It is essential to check the patency of the catheter before attachment to the blood bag to avoid wastage of blood or unnecessary contamination.

10. **Action:** Remove the cap on the end of the fluid line and attach to the i.v. catheter. Switch on the flow control to allow the blood to flow into the patient.

    Rationale: If the blood is not flowing freely, check the catheter and reflush with heparin.

11. **Action:** When flowing freely, adjust the flow control to achieve the correct flow rate to deliver the required volume (Boxes 7.5 and 7.6).

    Rationale: Rapid transfusion should be avoided to prevent circulatory overload or reaction.

12. **Action:** Attach the line securely to the patient by means of tapes and bandages.

    Rationale: The line must be secure to avoid leakage or interference by the patient.

Box 7.5 To calculate the volume of donor blood required by the recipient

2 ml of blood/kg bodyweight raises the PCV by 1%.
For dogs:

$$volume\ of\ blood\ required = recipient\ bodyweight\ (kg)$$
$$\times 85 \times \frac{desired\ PCV - recipient's\ PCV}{PCV\ of\ donated\ blood}$$

For cats:

$$volume\ of\ blood\ required = recipient\ bodyweight\ (kg)$$
$$\times 60 \times \frac{desired\ PCV - recipient's\ PCV}{PCV\ of\ donated\ blood}$$

Box 7.6 Rate of administration of a blood transfusion

Rate of blood administration depends on the recipient's cardiovascular condition:
- For the first 20–30 minutes the rate should not exceed 0.25–1.0 ml/kg bodyweight/h.
- If well tolerated, increase the rate to deliver the remaining volume within 4–6 hours.
- In patients with a risk of volume overload (e.g. due to cardiovascular compromise or renal impairment) maintain the later rate at no more than 3–4 ml/kg bodyweight/h.

13. **Action:** Monitor the patient constantly for any signs of reaction. Record everything on the hospital chart.

    Rationale: Transfusion reactions require immediate attention and the patient must not be left for long periods on its own.

    The patient should be monitored every 15–30 minutes during the transfusion. Afterwards it should be checked within 1 hour, 12 hours and 24 hours.

14. **Action:** You should check for the following parameters:
    - Demeanour
    - Rectal temperature
    - Pulse rate and quality
    - Respiratory rate and character
    - Colour of mucous membrane
    - Capillary refill time
    - Plasma and urine colour
    - PCV and total proteins should be measured as the transfusion is completed and at 12 hours and 24 hours after completion.

    Rationale: Any abnormalities in these parameters may indicate a transfusion reaction.

TRANSFUSION REACTIONS

Assess the baseline parameters as listed above and take immediate action if any of the following are noticed:

- Pyrexia
- Salivation
- Dyspnoea
- Vomiting
- Diarrhoea
- Tachycardia
- Muscle tremors
- Facial oedema.

1. Acute haemolytic reaction with intravascular haemolysis:

   Clinical signs – include pyrexia, muscle tremors, tachycardia, dyspnoea, vomiting, weakness, collapse, haemoglobinaemia and haemoglobinuria. If left untreated the patient may progress to disseminated intravascular coagulation, renal damage and death.

   Treatment – immediately discontinue the blood transfusion and treat for the clinical signs of shock.

   This is most likely to be seen in blood type B cats receiving blood type A blood or in DEA 1.1 negative dogs sensitized to DEA 1.1 positive after repeated transfusions.

2. Non-haemolytic immune reactions:

   Clinical signs – include vomiting, dyspnoea secondary to pulmonary oedema, urticaria, pruritus, erythema and oedema.

   Treatment – immediately discontinue the blood transfusion. Assess the patient for signs of haemolysis and shock. Steroids and antihistamines may be used.

This type of reaction is an acute type 1 hypersensitivity reaction.

PLACEMENT OF FEEDING TUBES

In the majority of cases when an animal is ill it is important to provide some form of nutritional support, which will shorten recovery time, reduce time spent in the hospital and increase survival rates. A sick animal suffering from prolonged anorexia is likely to develop complications as a result of hypermetabolic stress. Whenever possible, nutrition should be supplied via the gastrointestinal tract (i.e. the enteral route rather than the parenteral route) – if the gut is functioning, then use it! If the gastrointestinal tract is deprived of nutrition the mucosa may develop stress ulcers leading to further complications and bacterial translocation through the gut wall into the blood stream may result in septicaemia, organ failure and death.

In providing enteral nutrition it may not always be possible or advisable to use the entire normal anatomical route; for example, if a cat has a fractured jaw then the rate of healing may be increased by bypassing the oral cavity with the use of an oesophagostomy tube. There are several types of feeding tube designed to deliver nutrition when normal ingestion is impossible. The choice of tube depends on the injury or disease process and the expected duration of the assisted feeding process. Table 7.4 lists the types of tube.

Procedure: Placement of a naso–oesophageal or nasogastric feeding tube

This procedure does not require anaesthesia or sedation and can be used for dogs, cats and rabbits.

Table 7.4 Types of feeding tubes

Type of tube/location	Indications	Contraindications
Naso-oesophageal – distal oesophagus via the nose	Short term nutrition where the upper GI tract is functioning normally	Long term nutritional support; comatose or recumbent patients; trauma to head, neck, nasal cavity, oesophagus; abnormal gag reflex; vomiting; functional or mechanical GI obstruction
Nasogastric – via the nose; lies in the distal oesophagus but more caudal than the naso-oesophageal tube to reduce the risk of gastric reflux	Can be left in place for 3–7 days; well tolerated; makes use of the majority of the GI tract	May be irritating to the eyes and nose
Oesophagostomy – distal oesophagus via surgical implacement through the skin over the cranial oesophagus	Facial trauma, injury or disease involving the mouth and pharynx; can be tolerated for a long time (months)	Oesophageal disorders; vomiting; comatose or recumbent patients; following oesophageal surgery
Gastrostomy – stomach via surgical laparotomy or endoscopically through the ventrolateral abdominal wall (PEG tube)	Injuries or surgery to oral cavity, larynx, pharynx or oesophagus	Ulceration or neoplasia of the stomach; intractable vomiting; peritonitis; lateral recumbency
Enterostomy (duodenostomy or jejunostomy) – small intestine via surgical laparotomy or endoscopically via a gastric tube and through the pylorus	When stomach or duodenum must be bypassed; pancreatic disease or surgery; disease of the biliary system	Patients must be stable enough to survive anaesthesia and surgery; dysfunction of the small intestine

GI = gastrointestinal; PEG tube = percutaneous endoscopically placed gastrostomy tube.

1. **Action:** Ask an assistant to restrain the animal in a sitting or standing position on a stable table covered in rubber mat.

   Rationale: The animal must feel comfortable and secure so that it does not feel the urge to move or to try and escape.

2. **Action:** Select a suitable naso-oesophageal or nasogastric tube.

   Rationale: These tubes are usually made of rubber or silicone and are available in a variety of bore size and length. The bore size will determine the type of liquid food given to the patient.

3. **Action:** On the outside of the animal (Fig. 7.2), run the tube from the tip of the nose to the appropriate rib space:

   - Naso-oesophageal tube – 7 / 8th rib space (cats) or 8 / 9th rib space (dogs)
   - Nasogastric tube – 9th rib space (cats) or 10th rib space (dogs).

   Rationale: The nasogastric tube is placed further down the oesophagus than the naso-oesophageal tube to reduce the risk of gastric reflux.

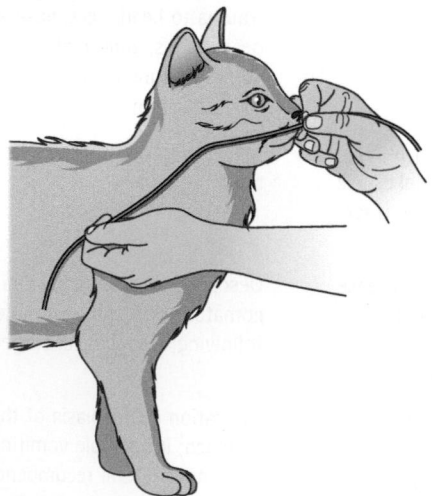

Figure 7.2 Naso-oesophageal tube placement. Before inserting the tube, determine the correct tubing length by measuring and marking the tube distance from the cat's mouth to the 7th or 8th rib space (8th or 9th rib space for dogs).

4. **Action:** Using a biro, mark the point on the tube close to the tip of the nose (Fig. 7.2).

   Rationale: This will be used to estimate the final position of the tube once it is placed within the oesophagus.

5. **Action:** Spray local anaesthetic around the entrance to the external nares.

   Rationale: To desensitize the nasal mucosa and reduce discomfort as the tube passes through the nasal cavity.

6. **Action:** Ask your assistant to restrain the animal firmly in a sitting or standing position with the head slightly raised but not overextended or flexed.

   Rationale: This allows you easy access to the external nares. If the animal is restrained it should not be able to move too much.

7. **Action:** Lubricate the tip of the tube with water soluble lubricant or anaesthetic gel. Do not use petroleum based jelly on silicone tubes.

   Rationale: Lubrication enables the tube to pass smoothly through the nasal cavity. Petroleum based jelly will react with silicone.

8. **Action:** Gently introduce the tube into the external nares, aiming it ventro-medially (towards the opposite ear) and slowly advance it into the pharynx and down into the oesophagus.

   Rationale: Aiming ventro-medially means that the tube will pass into the ventral meatus of the nasal cavity. This must be done slowly to avoid causing damage or discomfort to the patient.

9. **Action:** When the biro mark reaches the tip of the animal's nose stop advancing the tube.

   Rationale: The mark indicates that the end of the tube is in the desired location.

10. **Action:** Gently, using a syringe, introduce about 5 ml of water down the tube and observe the animal's response. Using a stethoscope, listen for borborygmi within the stomach.

    Rationale: If the tube is correctly placed in the oesophagus the animal should not respond, but you may hear borborygmi in the stomach. If the tube is in the larynx or trachea the animal will cough.

11. **Action:** A lateral radiograph may be taken.

    Rationale: To ensure that the tube is correctly placed within the distal third of the oesophagus and not kinked or twisted. The tube must be radio-opaque.

12. **Action:** Once the tube is correctly in place, occlude the end with a suitable bung.

    Rationale: The tube should be occluded at all times except when it is in use to prevent excessive swallowing of air.

13. **Action:** Secure the exterior part of the tube with the aid of tissue glue or sutures over the nose and between the eyes.

    Rationale: The tube must be held firmly in place to prevent it becoming dislodged.

14. **Action:** In some patients it may be necessary to use an Elizabethan collar.

    Rationale: To prevent displacement of the tube.

15. **Action:** The correct volume of prewarmed liquid food may now be syringed down the tube (Fig. 7.3).

    Rationale: The food must supply the correct calorific and nutritional requirements.

16. **Action:** Before removing the tube, free it from the sutures or tissue glue, seal the end with your thumb and pull it out gently.

    Rationale: This prevents the passage of air down into the oesophagus as it is removed.

NB Care of feeding tubes and correct methods of feeding are shown in Box 7.7.

Pharyngostomy tubes – this technique is no longer recommended as it has been associated with a high incidence of epiglottic entrapment and damage to the larynx and to the surrounding nerves.

Procedure: Placement of an oesophagostomy feeding tube

This tube is placed lower down the oesophagus, which reduces the risk of damaging nerves and blood vessels.

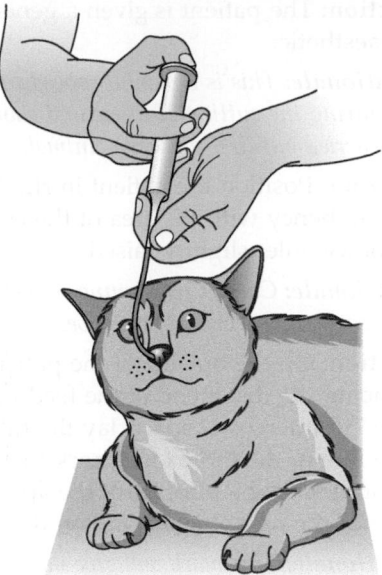

Figure 7.3 Naso-oesophageal tube feeding. Attach a syringe and instil 3 ml of water. Slowly administer food. After administration, flush with water to prevent blockage. Cap or cover tube opening.

Box 7.7 Care of feeding tubes

- Each time before feeding, flush the tube with a small volume of lukewarm water to make sure that the tube is still in place. If the animal coughs it may have become dislodged.
- Introducing a small volume of water into the tube also ensures that the tube is not blocked – small amounts of carbonated drinks may also be used as the bubbles help to clear blockage by debris.
- Only use warmed liquid food – cold food may induce vomiting.
- Total calorific requirement for the day should be administered in four separate feeds.
- Administer the food slowly by syringe.
- Observe the animal's reaction – licking the lips may indicate that the animal is feeling nauseous.
- After feeding, flush the tube with 5–10 ml of warm water to clear the tube – dried food may block it up.
- Never leave the end of feeding tube open as it will encourage excessive swallowing of air.
- Clean the area surrounding the open end (e.g. external nares or the skin wound) at least twice a day to aid respiration or to prevent wound infection and breakdown.

1. **Action:** The patient is given a general anaesthetic.

   Rationale: This is a painful procedure requiring the cutting of tissue and should never be carried out in a conscious animal.

2. **Action:** Position the patient in right lateral recumbency with the area of the cranial thoracic inlet slightly raised.

   Rationale: Correct positioning is essential in the correct placement of the tube.

3. **Action:** On the outside of the patient, placing the distal end of the feeding tube at the 7th intercostal space, lay the tube along the line of the thorax and neck towards the mouth. Using a biro, mark the approximate site of the oesophagostomy on the tube.

   Rationale: This mark will give you an indication of the correct placement of the tube when the procedure is complete.

4. **Action:** Ask your assistant to clip an area of the neck running from the angle of the jaw to the shoulder and prepare the site aseptically.

   Rationale: It is essential to maintain asepsis for the surgical procedure.

5. **Action:** Open the patient's mouth and carefully insert a long pair of curved artery forceps down the pharynx and into the oesophagus to the mid-cervical region (Fig. 7.4).

   Rationale: These will be used to grasp the tubing through the incision in the oesophagus.

6. **Action:** Turn the closed tips of the artery forceps to point laterally from the lumen of the oesophagus towards the superficial tissues.

   Rationale: From the outside you will be able to see the forceps pushing the tissues upwards.

7. **Action:** As you push the forceps up, using a scalpel, make a small 5–10 mm incision through the skin onto the point of the forceps. Bluntly dissect through the tissues until you can see the tips of the artery forceps in the oesophagus and then make an incision into the oesophagus.

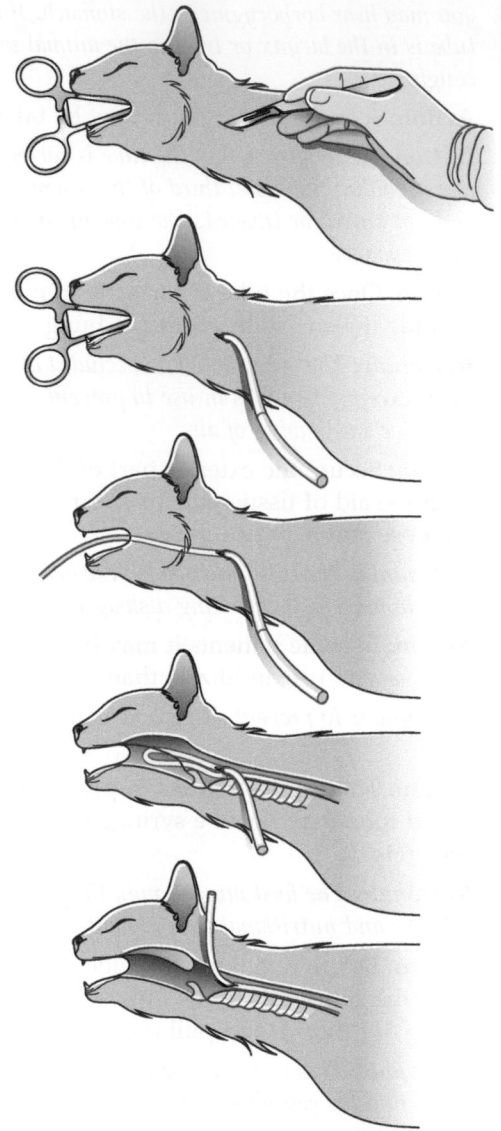

Figure 7.4 Placement of an oesophagostomy feeding tube. (Reproduced with permission from Nick Bexfield and Karla Lee: BSAVA Guide to Procedures in Small Animal Practice 2010, originally illustrated by Samantha J Elmhurst.)

   Rationale: Blunt dissection should prevent you from damaging any of the vessels or nerves that run in this area.

8. **Action:** As the points of the forceps come through the skin incision, open them and grasp the end of the tubing (Fig. 7.4).

   Rationale: You are now ready to pull the tube into the oesophagus.

9. **Action:** Holding the end of the tubing in the artery forceps, gently pull the tubing through the incision into the lumen of the oesophagus and then rostrally into the pharynx and then the mouth.

   Rationale: The other end will still be out of the oesophageal incision.

10. **Action:** Open the jaws of the artery forceps to release the tubing and then curl the end of the tube back into the mouth and ease it back down into the oesophagus.

    Rationale: This end of the tube will eventually lie in the distal oesophagus.

11. **Action:** Gently push the end down the oesophagus past the area of the incision and down into the distal oesophagus. You can use an endotracheal tube to help push the tube into the oesophagus.

    Rationale: The biro mark will now lie at the skin incision and will show you that the end of the tube has reached the correct site corresponding to the 7th intercostal space.

12. **Action:** The tube now lies between the distal oesophagus and skin incision. Slide it back and forth gently.

    Rationale: To make sure that it is free in the lumen and has not twisted or formed knot.

13. **Action:** Take a lateral thoracic radiograph.

    Rationale: To check that the tube remains in the oesophagus not in the stomach. The tube must be radio-opaque.

14. **Action:** Secure the end of the tube with a Chinese finger-trap suture (see Ch. 10). Close the end of the tube with a bung and cover the site with a sterile dressing and loose, soft padded neck bandage.

    Rationale: To keep the area clean, but you must still be able to access the opening of the tube to feed the patient.

Gastrostomy and enterostomy tubes – these are used to provide nutrition directly into the stomach or small intestine respectively. The placement of these tubes is a complicated surgical procedure and is not within the brief of this book. Their use

and care postoperatively is the same as for other tubes and is detailed in Box 7.7.

URINARY PROCEDURES

URINARY CATHETERIZATION

As the anatomy of patients varies, so too do catheterization techniques according to the species and sex of the patient. There are a range of urinary catheters (Fig. 7.5) and their details are summarized in Table 7.5.

The uses of catheterization include:

- Collection of a sterile urine sample for bacteriological culture and sensitivity testing
- Removal of blockages by hydropropulsion
- Emptying the bladder prior to surgery
- Placement of indwelling catheter to prevent urine scalding in recumbent animals
- Introduction of contrast material for cystography.

Procedure: Catheterization of the dog

1. **Action:** Ask an assistant to restrain the dog on a suitable examination table, in a standing position.

   Rationale: The dog should feel comfortable and secure.

2. **Action:** Wearing a disposable apron and gloves, wash the end of the prepuce and penis with a little dilute antiseptic.

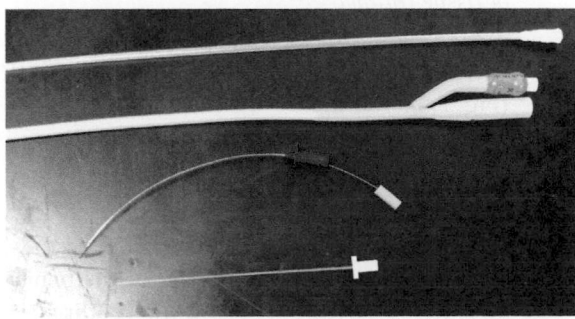

Figure 7.5 Examples of urinary catheter. From top to bottom: canine catheter, Foley catheter, tomcat catheter with stylet, 'slippery Sam' tomcat catheter.

Table 7.5 Types of urinary catheter

Type of catheter	Description and use
Jackson's cat catheter	Designed for use in tomcats but can be used in queens. Fine metal stylet provides stiffening during placement and is removed once in place. Reduced length enables the whole catheter to be placed in the urethra, which allows the plastic flange behind the Luer fitting to be sutured to the prepuce converting it to an indwelling catheter.
Plastic dog catheter	Rounded tip with two drainage holes in the tip. Designed for single use and can be used as an indwelling catheter. Range of gauges – choose as large a gauge as possible. Long enough to pass along the length of the dog urethra.
Foley catheter	Available in silicone (autoclavable) and latex (non-autoclavable so not reusable). Latex catheters are more flexible and placement is aided by a metal stylet. Inflatable balloon just behind the drainage holes at the tip – remember to deflate before removal. Inflation after placement makes it an indwelling catheter. Latex catheters must not be lubricated with petroleum based lubricants. Expensive.
Tieman's bitch catheter	Moulded curved tip makes it easier to place in the urethral orifice. Rest of the length is soft, flexible and difficult to control.

Rationale: To minimize the risk of entry of infection into the urethra. Protective clothing will prevent the spread of zoonotic disease.

3. **Action:** Remove the catheter from its outer packaging and then cut the end from the inner packaging, which is used as a feeder sleeve.

   Rationale: The use of a feeder sleeve allows the sterile catheter to be fed into the urethra without having to touch it.

4. **Action:** Lubricate the tip of the catheter.

   Rationale: This eases the passage of the catheter along the urethra and reduces the risk of tissue trauma.

5. **Action:** Standing on one side of the dog, extrude the end of the penis with one hand (Fig. 7.6).

   Rationale: This enables you to see the opening of the urethra and frees it from the overlying hair of the prepuce.

6. **Action:** With the other hand introduce the tip of the catheter into the end of the penis and gently advance it along the urethra using gentle pressure. Once the catheter is well within the urethra you can allow the prepuce to return to its normal position.

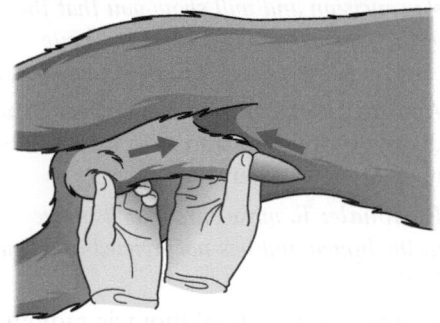

Figure 7.6 Extruding the penis.

Rationale: There may be slight resistance as the catheter passes over the ischial arch or through an enlarged prostate. If resistance is too great you may have to select a different gauge of catheter.

7. **Action:** Urine will start to flow when the catheter enters the bladder; collect it in a clean bowl (Fig. 7.7).

   Rationale: As the urethra passes through the bladder sphincter, urine is able to flow out.

8. **Action:** If you want to collect a sterile sample, attach a large sterile syringe to the Luer fitting on the end of the catheter and withdraw the required volume.

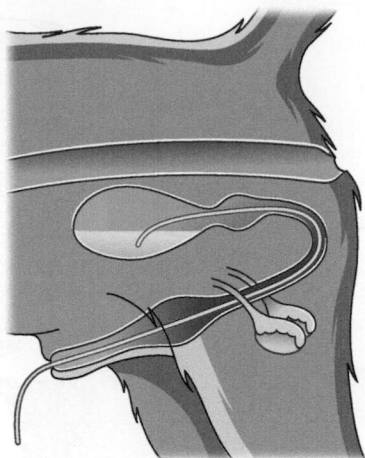

Figure 7.7 Passing a urethral catheter into the bladder.

Rationale: Urine withdrawn from the bladder will become contaminated only by organisms in the urethra or in the outside environment.

9. **Action:** If you wish to leave the catheter in the urethra (i.e. an indwelling catheter), apply a piece of zinc oxide tape around the Luer end.

   Rationale: There is no plastic flange on a standard dog catheter.

10. **Action:** Slide the prepuce back into a normal position and place 1–2 stitches between the tape and the edge of the prepuce.

    Rationale: This will prevent the catheter sliding out of the urethra.

11. **Action:** To remove the catheter, gently pull it out of the urethra.

    Rationale: Slow removal prevents tissue damage and urine splashes, which may spread zoonotic infection.

12. **Action:** Dispose of the catheter in the clinical waste bin.

    Rationale: To comply with legislation and prevent the spread of infection.

Procedure: Catherization of the bitch

1. **Action:** Some bitches may need to be sedated or given a general anaesthetic.

Rationale: This is not normally a painful procedure, unless there is an underlying problem such as a fractured pelvis, but some bitches may object.

2. **Action:** Ask an assistant to restrain the bitch in lateral or dorsal recumbency on a stable examination table. The bitch may also be placed in sternal recumbency with her hindlimbs hanging over the edge of the table.

   Rationale: The urethral orifice lies on the floor of the vestibule and the chosen position must provide as easy access as possible.

3. **Action:** Wearing a disposable apron and gloves, clean the vulva and its surroundings.

   Rationale: To prevent the entry of infection into the vestibule or vagina and the spread of zoonotic disease.

4. **Action:** If using a bitch catheter, remove it from its outer wrappings and cut the end off the inner wrapping to expose only the tip. If using a Foley catheter, remove it completely from its packaging, handle with sterile gloves and insert the stylet into the lumen.

   Rationale: Maintain sterility when handling either type of catheter to prevent the entry of infection.

5. **Action:** Standing at the tail end of the bitch, insert a speculum into the vestibule, taking care not to enter the ventral clitoral fossa, and position the slit of the speculum ventrally.

   Rationale: This position allows the slightly raised urethral papilla, which 'guards' the orifice, to be seen – it is often paler in colour than the surrounding vestibular mucosa.

6. **Action:** If necessary ask your assistant to pull the ventral vulval lips caudally to make visualization easier.

   Rationale: This action helps to straighten the vestibule.

7. **Action:** When you can see the urethral papilla / orifice, lubricate the tip of the catheter and insert it.

Rationale: Do not use petroleum-based lubricants on a latex Foley catheter as they may damage the material.

8. **Action:** Gently advance the catheter into the bladder.

    Rationale: Avoid causing damage to the urethral mucosa.

9. **Action:** If you want to use the Foley catheter as an indwelling catheter, advance it all the way into the bladder, remove the stylet and inflate the balloon using sterile water or saline.

    Rationale: The inflated balloon prevents the catheter slipping through the bladder sphincter.

10. **Action:** Once urine begins to flow then collect it in a clean bowl.

    Rationale: Urine will flow once the catheter has passed through the bladder sphincter.

11. **Action:** If you wish to collect a sterile sample, attach a sterile syringe to the Luer fitting of the bitch catheter and withdraw. There is no Luer fitting on a Foley catheter.

    Rationale: A Foley catheter can be attached to a urine collection bag with the appropriate fittings.

12. **Action:** When you have completed the procedure, slowly remove the catheter. If using a Foley catheter, remember to deflate the balloon first.

    Rationale: Slow removal and deflation of the balloon prevent tissue damage to the urethral mucosa.

NB It is possible to introduce a catheter blindly by digitally palpating the urethral orifice. Wearing sterile gloves, place a well-lubricated finger into the vestibule. Apply gentle pressure to the floor of the vestibule while moving your finger cranially. The urethral papilla will be palpable as a bulge of mucosa and the catheter can be then be guided into the orifice under your finger (Fig. 7.8).

Procedure: Catherization of the tomcat

1. **Action:** The cat must be anaesthetized for this procedure.

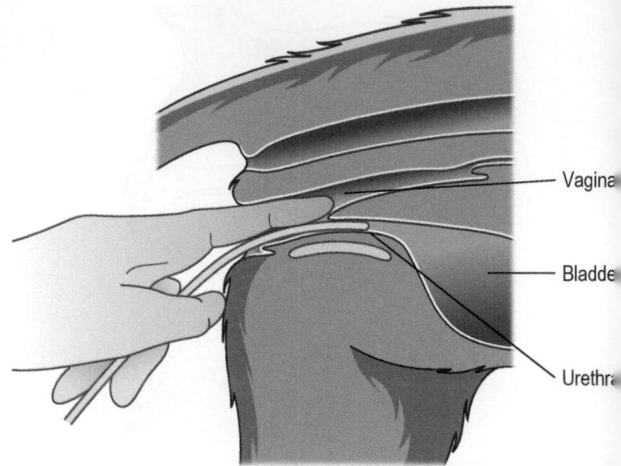

Figure 7.8 Using the blind approach to urinary catheterization.

Rationale: Catherization may be painful and struggling may lead to urethral rupture.

2. **Action:** Position the cat in dorsal or lateral recumbency with the tail out of the way and lying on a suitable examination or operating table.

    Rationale: You must be comfortable as this procedure can sometimes take time. You must have the best possible access to the hindquarters of the cat.

3. **Action:** Wearing disposable gloves and apron, clean the prepuce and the surrounding perineum.

    Rationale: To prevent the entry of infection into the urethra and the spread of zoonotic disease.

4. **Action:** Remove the cat catheter from its outer covering and cut the end off the inner wrapping, which will act as a feeder sleeve.

    Rationale: The use of a feeder sleeve allows the catheter to be fed into the urethra without touching it.

5. **Action:** Lubricate the end of the catheter.

    Rationale: This will aid the progress of the catheter along the urethra.

6. **Action:** Extrude the penis by applying gentle pressure on either side of the

prepuce and introduce the catheter into the urethra.

Rationale: If the cat is blocked with struvite crystals it is often difficult to introduce the catheter or to advance it further.

7. **Action:** Advance the catheter along the urethra and into the bladder until urine starts to flow.

   Rationale: Urine starts to flow when the catheter passes through the bladder sphincter.

8. **Action:** If a sterile sample is required then attach a sterile syringe to the end of the catheter and withdraw.

   Rationale: Urine withdrawn from the bladder will become contaminated only by organisms in the urethra or in the outside environment.

9. If the catheter is to be left in place, suture the plastic flange at the end to the prepuce.

   Rationale: This may be necessary in a blocked cat once the blockage has been relieved.

10. When the procedure is complete then slowly withdraw the catheter.

    Rationale: Slow withdrawal prevents damage to the urethral mucosa.

NB If the urethra of the tomcat is blocked with struvite crystals then it may be impossible to introduce the catheter more than a few millimeters, and it may be necessary to break up the plug by hydropropulsion using saline or water introduced via the catheter. This may take time, but must be continued until you can advance the catheter into the bladder. If the blockage is intransigent you can try using an ophthalmic irrigating cannula, which is narrower, then using the cat catheter after the blockage is removed.

CYSTOCENTESIS

Cystocentesis is the process by which urine is removed from the bladder by means of a sterile needle and syringe. The bladder must contain a reasonable volume of urine in order to palpate and stabilize it.

Indications for cystocentesis include:

- Collection of a sterile urine sample for bacteriological culture and sensitivity testing.

- Decompression of a distended bladder (e.g. where a blockage cannot be relieved or where neural damage interferes with normal emptying).

Procedure: Cystocentesis

1. **Action:** This procedure can usually be performed in a conscious but well-restrained patient or one that has been lightly sedated.

   Rationale: The procedure causes slight discomfort, but is completed quite quickly.

2. **Action:** Ask an assistant to place the patient in left lateral recumbency or in a standing position.

   Rationale: The patient should be restrained so that there is easy access to the bladder.

3. **Action:** Clip an area of about 5 cm^2 on the midline of the caudal abdomen and prepare it aseptically. In cats use an area on the flank.

   Rationale: To reduce the risk of infection.

4. **Action:** With one hand, palpate and immobilize the bladder by pushing it against the abdominal wall.

   Rationale: If the bladder cannot be palpated (e.g. in an obese animal) it may be identified by using ultrasonography.

5. **Action:** Using a 21G needle with a 5 ml or 10 ml syringe attached, insert it into the bladder at an angle of 45° to the bladder wall. The ideal site is just cranial to the neck of the bladder.

   Rationale: Try to cause as little trauma to the tissues as possible.

6. **Action:** Draw back on the syringe and, with the needle still in situ, pause and examine the contents.

   Rationale: To check that the contents are urine and not gut contents or blood.

7. **Action:** If urine is present in the syringe, continue to draw back until the bladder is almost empty or, if collecting a sterile sample, you have enough volume – normally about 2 ml.

   Rationale: For details of urinalysis see Chapter 5.

8. **Action:** As you remove the needle, apply gentle pressure to the site.

   Rationale: This encourages natural tissue recoil around the pierced area and prevents leakage.

9. **Action:** Urine should be disposed of in clinical waste.

   Rationale: To protect staff and other patients from contamination.

NB If the animal is in a standing position, gently push the bladder from the left side towards the opposite abdominal wall. Collect the sample from the right side, which should avoid penetration of the descending colon.

ENEMAS

An enema is a liquid substance administered per rectum in order to relieve an impaction or to empty the rectum prior to the administration of a contrast medium, such as barium, used in radiographical studies of the colon and rectum.

Materials commonly used as enemas are liquid paraffin or warm saline. Soapy water should be avoided as it is an irritant; phosphate enemas and glycerine, used in humans, should be avoided in cats as they are toxic. There are commercial mini-enemas designed for cats that are given orally.

The equipment designed for the administration of an enema is known as a Higginson's syringe (Fig. 7.9). This is made of rubber tubing with a nozzle at one end and a large bulb halfway along (Fig. 7.9B), which is designed to squirt the material into the rectum. The open end is used to suck up the liquid enema. The procedure is inevitably rather messy and should be carried out close to the prep room sink or on a tub table.

Procedure: Administration of an enema

1. **Action:** The patient should be fully anaesthetized or sedated.

   Rationale: This procedure is uncomfortable and it is preferable to have a relaxed anal sphincter.

2. **Action:** Check that there is no physical blockage such as a foreign body or

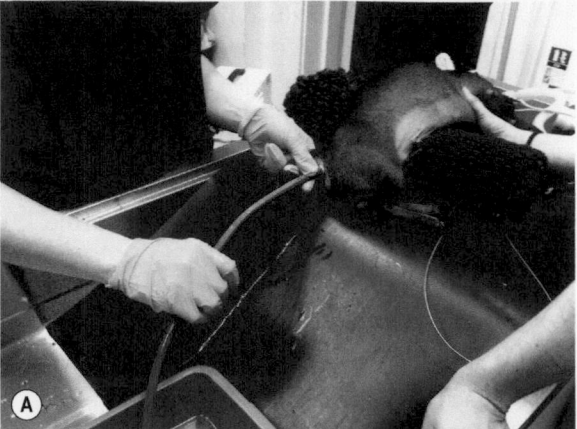

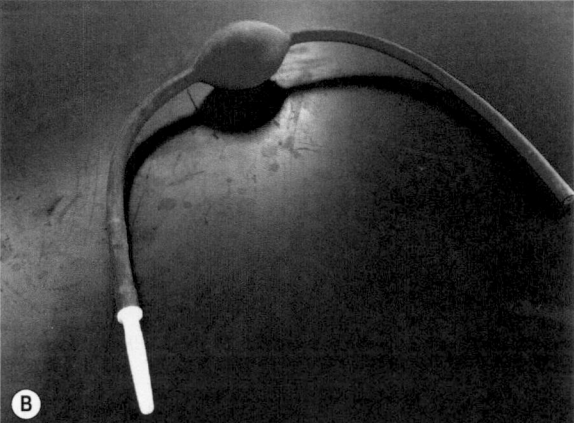

Figure 7.9 (A, B) Use of Higginson's syringe to perform an enema on a dog.

enlarged prostate before starting the procedure.

Rationale: If these are present then other methods of treatment should be adopted.

3. **Action:** Place the animal in lateral recumbency on the draining board of the sink with its anus towards the sink, or on the grill of a tub table.

   Rationale: Both of these sites will enable the faecal material to be disposed of easily.

4. **Action:** Wear gloves and a disposable apron. Sometimes boots are also necessary.

   Rationale: This is a messy procedure! Wearing protective clothing will protect you from faecal contamination and the potential spread of infection.

5. **Action:** Lubricate the nozzle end of the Higginson's syringe (Fig. 7.9). Lift the animal's tail and insert the nozzle into the rectum by gently twisting it.

    Rationale: This enables the tube to be inserted into the rectum more easily.

6. **Action:** Place the other end of the tube in the warmed enema solution and squeeze the bulb.

    Rationale: This pumps the liquid in one direction only – into the rectum. The enema solution must be warmed to prevent cold shock.

7. **Action:** Continue until the broken-down faecal mass begins to come out of the rectum. Sometimes gentle manipulation of the rectum and colon through the abdominal wall may help to break up the faecal mass.

    Rationale: The liquid enema hydrates and breaks up the faecal contents.

8. **Action:** Remove the Higginson's syringe and allow time for the faecal material to pour out. When it has stopped, repeat the process.

    Rationale: You may have to repeat the process several times depending on the amount of faeces in the rectum.

9. **Action:** When nothing more seems to come away, clean and dry the animal and place it in a warm kennel to recover from the anaesthetic.

    Rationale: You must take steps to prevent hypothermia.

10. **Action:** Check the animal at intervals and, when it is ready to go home, make sure it is clean and dry.

    Rationale: It is important to discharge the patient looking well cared for.

11. **Action:** Warn the owner that it may produce liquid faeces for a few hours.

    Rationale: The owner should understand the procedure and when they should be worried.

NB This can be done in a conscious animal and is performed in a standing position. After the enema has been administered, the animal must be given access to an outside run so that it can defaecate. Cats must have access to a litter tray.

FUNCTION TESTS FOR HORMONAL DISEASES

There are several hormonal conditions in dogs and cats that can be diagnosed and the progress of treatment monitored by function tests carried out within the practice. These tests measure the product of a hormonal pathway and assess how much it has deviated from normal within the affected patient.

Procedure: Water deprivation test

This test is used to diagnose cases of central or nephrogenic diabetes insipidus, caused by a lack of antidiuretic hormone (ADH), and primary or psychogenic polydipsia. It must not be carried out until all other possible causes of polydipsia and polyuria have been investigated and ruled out.

Depriving an animal of water is potentially dangerous and the test must be carried out with extreme care. It is always carried out within the practice and starting it early in the day means that it should be over and the animal ready to return home by the end of the normal working day.

Hormonal pathway – antidiuretic hormone (ADH), secreted by the posterior pituitary gland, changes the permeability of the collecting ducts of the renal nephrons to water, thus altering the concentration (specific gravity) of the resulting urine.

There are two types of diabetes insipidus:

- **Central** – affects the pituitary gland, which secretes little or no ADH.
- **Nephrogenic** – the pituitary gland secretes ADH, but the renal nephrons fail to respond.

In either case the clinical signs are of polydipsia, polyuria and production of urine with a low specific gravity (1.000–1.007).

(Normal specific gravity: 1.015–1.045 in dogs; 1.020–1.040 in cats.)

1. **Action:** Ensure that the animal is well hydrated and has normal blood urea levels.

   Rationale: To check that kidney and liver function are normal (i.e. there is no other concurrent condition).

2. **Action:** Empty the bladder by catheterization and measure the specific gravity (SG) of the urine using a refractometer.

   Rationale: It is important to have an accurate value for the SG as this will be the central criterion for assessing hormonal function.

3. **Action:** Weigh the animal accurately and calculate 5% of the bodyweight.

   Rationale: The animal must lose no more than 5% of its bodyweight in the test – this will be lost as fluid.

4. **Action:** Place the animal in a kennel with no access to food or water.

   Rationale: In a normal animal, ADH would start to act on the collecting ducts and conserve water by increasing the concentration of the urine.

5. **Action:** After 1 hour, empty the bladder, measure the SG of the urine and weigh the animal.

   Rationale: There should be a small decrease in weight.

6. **Action:** Record your findings.

   Rationale: So that you have results to refer back to.

7. **Action:** Return the animal to its kennel for another hour.

   Rationale: It should have no access to food or water.

8. **Action:** Repeat the process every hour until either there is a 5% loss in bodyweight or the SG of the urine has risen to above 1.030 (dogs) or 1.035 (cats).

   Rationale: If the SG has risen to within normal limits the animal does not have diabetes insipidus. If 5% of bodyweight has been lost and SG remains the same, the animal has diabetes insipidus.

9. **Action:** As soon as a diagnosis has been reached the animal must be given a drink of water.

   Rationale: If the animal is left without water any longer than is necessary for the test it may become fatally dehydrated as the kidneys cannot conserve water without the aid of ADH. Dehydration may lead to renal failure and CNS signs.

10. **Action:** If the animal fails to reach the 5% loss in bodyweight within the working day the test should carry on overnight, but monitoring urine, bodyweight and general demeanour of the animal must carry on and the animal must not be left unattended.

    Rationale: The test should stop immediately if the animal shows any signs of CNS depression.

11. **Action:** If overnight monitoring is not possible then the animal should be sent home and may be given maintenance amounts of water (2.5–3.0 ml/kg/h). The test should be continued the following morning.

    Rationale: This volume of water should prevent dehydration without threatening the life of the animal. The owner should be given strict instructions as to what to do and when to worry about the animal's condition.

Procedure: ACTH stimulation test

This test is used to diagnose Cushing's disease (hyperadrenocorticism), to aid in the diagnosis of Addison's disease (hypoadrenocorticism) and to assess the response to treatment with mitotane or trilostane.

Hormonal pathway – adrenocorticotrophic hormone (ACTH) secreted by the anterior pituitary gland controls the secretion of glucocorticoids and mineralocorticoids from the cortex of the adrenal glands. Levels of these hormones in the blood exert negative feedback on the anterior pituitary gland and 'switch off' secretion of ACTH. The most easily measurable glucocorticoid is cortisol.

There are two types of Cushing's disease:

- Caused by a pituitary tumour that oversecretes ACTH, resulting in overstimulation and thus oversecretion from the adrenal cortex.
- Caused by a tumour of the adrenal gland itself – this is the most common type.

In either case clinical signs include polyphagia, polydipsia, polyuria, bilateral symmetrical alopecia, potbellied appearance, calcinosis cutis and muscle wasting.

1. **Action:** Ask an assistant to restrain the patient for intravenous blood sampling using the jugular vein.

   Rationale: This vein provides an easy method of collecting a suitable volume of blood (see Ch. 1).

2. **Action:** Collect approximately 2 ml of blood and place it in a heparin or plain blood tube.

   Rationale: To enable the measurement of the basal levels of cortisol.

3. **Action:** Separate the plasma or serum before sending the sample to the laboratory (see Ch. 5).

   Rationale: Hormones are carried and can be measured within the plasma. The cellular fraction is not needed for the test.

4. **Action:** Make sure that the tubes are labelled correctly.

   Rationale: To ensure that the results relate to the correct patient and that the correct test is performed.

5. **Action:** Ask your assistant to restrain the patient for the administration of an intravenous injection using the cephalic vein and place an intravenous catheter (see Ch. 1).

   Rationale: Small amounts of drug are better given via an intravenous catheter. Placing a catheter in the cephalic vein is more comfortable for the patient.

6. **Action:** Inject 0.25 mg of synthetic ACTH into the vein.

   Rationale: For dogs of less than 5 kg and cats use only 0.125 mg of synthetic ACTH.

7. **Action:** After 30–60 minutes, ask your assistant to restrain the patient ready for blood sampling from the jugular vein.

Rationale: In this procedure it is best to sample from the jugular vein so that there is no chance of contaminating the sample with synthetic ACTH.

8. **Action:** Collect approximately 2 ml of blood and place it in a fresh heparin or plain blood tube. Label appropriately.

   Rationale: This will be used to measure the change in cortisol levels in response to the administration of ACTH.

9. **Action:** Separate the plasma or serum before sending the sample to the laboratory.

   Rationale: Hormones are carried and can be measured within the plasma. The cellular fraction is not needed for the test.

NB For a detailed interpretation of the results, please read a dedicated endocrinology textbook.

Excessively high levels of cortisol will indicate the presence of Cushing's disease.

Procedure: Dexamethasone suppression test – low dose test

This test is used to aid the diagnosis of Cushing's disease (hyperadrenocorticism).

Hormonal pathway – adrenocorticotrophic hormone (ACTH) secreted by the anterior pituitary gland controls the secretion of glucocorticoids and mineralocorticoids (corticosteroids) from the cortex of the adrenal glands. Levels of these hormones in the blood exert negative feedback on the anterior pituitary gland and 'switch off' secretion of ACTH. The most easily measurable glucocorticoid is cortisol. Dexamethasone is a synthetic corticosteroid.

1. **Action:** Ask an assistant to restrain the patient for intravenous blood sampling using the jugular vein.

   Rationale: This vein provides an easy method of collecting a suitable volume of blood (see Ch. 1).

2. **Action:** Collect approximately 2 ml of blood and place it in a heparin or plain blood tube.

   Rationale: To enable the measurement of the basal levels of cortisol.

3. **Action:** Separate the plasma or serum before sending the sample to the laboratory (see Ch. 5).

   Rationale: Hormones are carried and can be measured within the plasma. The cellular fraction is not needed for the test.

4. **Action:** Make sure that the tubes are labelled correctly.

   Rationale: To ensure that the results relate to the correct patient and that the correct lab test is performed.

5. **Action:** Ask your assistant to restrain the patient for the administration of an intravenous injection using the cephalic vein and place an intravenous catheter (see Ch. 1).

   Rationale: Small amounts of drug are better given via an intravenous catheter. Placing a catheter in the cephalic vein is more comfortable for the patient.

6. **Action:** Inject 0.01 mg/kg of dexamethasone into the cephalic vein.

   Rationale: The use of the intravenous catheter will ensure the entire dose is administered.

7. **Action:** Place the patient in a quiet kennel until required for the next part of the test.

   Rationale: Allowing the patient to relax in a quiet kennel will ensure that it is not stressed, which could affect cortisol levels.

8. **Action:** After 3 hours ask an assistant to restrain the patient while you collect a 2 ml blood sample from the jugular vein. Place it in a heparin or plain blood tube.

   Rationale: This will be used to measure the change in cortisol levels. It is collected from the jugular vein to reduce the risk of contamination of the blood sample by dexamethasone.

9. **Action:** Separate the plasma or serum and make sure that the tube is clearly labelled '+3 hours'.

   Rationale: This will distinguish it from the original sample.

10. **Action:** Return the patient to the kennel.

    Rationale: To allow it to relax thus reducing stress levels.

11. **Action:** After 8 hours repeat the sampling process and make sure that the sample is clearly labelled '+8 hours'.

    Rationale: To distinguish it from the other two samples.

NB A low dose of dexamethasone will suppress cortisol levels in a normal dog, but will cause incomplete suppression in a dog with Cushing's disease.

A high dose test can be used – using 0.1 mg/kg – but this is no longer considered a reliable means of diagnosing canine Cushing's disease and is rarely used. However, it may be used to distinguish between adrenal and pituitary dependent Cushing's disease. The technique is the same.

For a detailed interpretation of the results, please refer to a dedicated endocrinology textbook.

ELECTROCARDIOGRAPHY

This technique measures the electrical impulses within the heart that immediately precede contractions. It is used as a diagnostic or monitoring tool for a variety of cardiac conditions:

- Monitoring during anaesthesia or in critical care
- Evaluation of arrhythmias, pericardial and pleural diseases
- Evaluation of anatomical changes
- Evaluation of the efficacy of treatment for a range of cardiac conditions
- Investigation of clinical signs that may indicate a cardiac condition (e.g. dyspnoea, coughing, weakness, exercise intolerance and collapse).

An example of an ECG trace from lead II is shown in Figure 7.10. The different parts that make up the normal sinus complex are as follows:

1. **P wave** – the sino-atrial node begins the depolarization process, which spreads across the right atrium followed by the left atrium. When the process is complete the electrical difference returns to the baseline.

2. **P-R interval** – the wave of repolarization is delayed in the atrioventricular node.

3. **QRS complex** – represents depolarization of the ventricles. The R wave is a positive

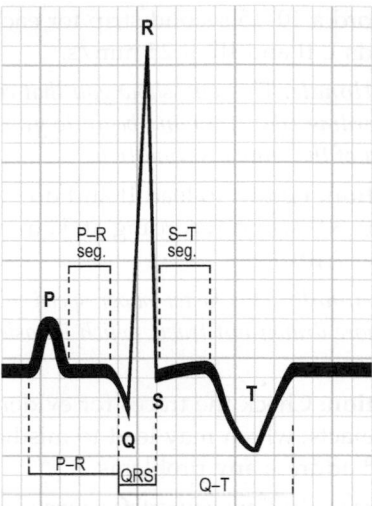

Figure 7.10 Example of a lead II ECG trace with the major deflections (waves) and intervals marked.

deviation representing depolarization through the bundle of His and the Purkinje fibres, whereas the Q and S waves are negative deviations representing depolarization of the ventricular septum and basal regions of the ventricles respectively.

4. **S-T interval** — depolarization of the ventricles is complete and the electrical difference returns to the baseline.

5. **T wave** – repolarization of the ventricles. The size and polarity of this part vary and it is of little diagnostic importance unless hyperkalaemia is a concern.

Procedure: Performing an electrocardiogram

1. **Action:** Perform the electrocardiogram (ECG) in a quiet room away from any noise or excitement.

   Rationale: Any stimulus such as a distant dog barking will be reflected on the ECG wave and a note should be made on the trace that this has occurred – failure to do so may lead to a misdiagnosis.

2. **Action:** The patient should be calm and relaxed and muscular activity, such as struggling, should be avoided as these may affect the heart rate and rhythm.

Rationale: Chemical sedation should be avoided as it may affect the heart rhythm. If it is used (e.g. acepromazine), a note should be made in the records.

3. **Action:** Place the patient in right lateral recumbency on a table covered in a rubber mat.

   Rationale: This is the conventional position, but if the patient is dyspnoeic or is uncomfortable in this position then allow it to adopt a neutral position. Cats may struggle in lateral recumbency and may be happier in sternal recumbency – purring may cause the baseline to tremble. The recognized normal ECG trace (Fig. 7.10) may vary in non-standard positions. A rubber mat electrically insulates the patient.

4. **Action:** Attach the ECG electrodes by means of crocodile clips, adhesive pads, plates or needles depending on the type of machine and the length of time they will be attached (e.g. crocodile clips for short periods; adhesive pads for long periods of recording).

   Rationale: Contact must be made directly with the skin by parting the fur and electrical conductivity is improved by cleaning the skin with spirit prior to attachment, or by the use of a coupling gel.

5. **Action:** Each electrode is attached to the machine by means of a colour-coded lead, which may be marked for human use. Attach to the limbs as follows:

   - Red – marked RA – right forelimb
   - Yellow – marked LA – left forelimb
   - Green – marked LL or F – left hindlimb
   - Black – marked RL or N (neutral) – right hindlimb.

   Rationale: Exact positioning is not critical but it is important that the electrodes are placed in a recognized way so that the resulting trace can be assessed against established criteria. Select relatively hairless areas. Placing the electrodes closer to the body reduces artefacts resulting from movement. Suggested sites are skin folds around the elbow, stifle or adjacent to the hock.

The neutral electrode may be placed anywhere, but is usually placed in front of the right stifle.

6. **Action:** Make sure that the leads are not tangled or touching each other as they lead away from the body. Do not place them over the trunk.

   Rationale: Tangled leads may cause artefacts on the trace. Placing them over the trunk may result in respiratory artefacts.

7. **Action:** Ensure that all non-essential electrical equipment is switched off (e.g. fluorescent lights, heat pads, diathermy).

   Rationale: The electrical fields generated by other equipment may interfere with the recording.

8. **Action:** Switch on the ECG machine and check the controls. There are four controls on most machines; these are the:

   • Paper speed
   • Calibration setting
   • Filter
   • Lead selector.

   Rationale:

   » Paper speed – controls the speed of the trace as the paper advances. Faster speed results in wider complexes, but fewer can be fitted on to the paper. Use 25 or 50 mm/s. Write the paper speed on the paper.
   » Calibration setting – allows the operator to control the number of centimetres that are equivalent to 1 mV. Typically a setting of 1 cm/mV is used, but if the complexes are too tall then decreasing the setting to 0.5 cm/mV will accommodate the trace. In cats you may increase it to 2 cm/mV to obtain a readable trace. Record the setting on the paper.
   » Filter – suppresses any artefacts, evening out the trace. May cause a decrease in the height of the QRS complex, which should be considered during interpretation. It is better to identify the cause of the artefact and eliminate it (e.g. electrical interference) than to use the filter control. Record its use on the paper.
   » Lead selector – this should allow manual selection of the three limb leads (I, II, III) and the three augmented leads (aVR, aVL, aVF) in turn.

9. **Action:** Once everything is set and the patient is calm, relaxed and is lying still,

record a 10–15 second strip for each of leads I, II and III at 25 mm/s.

   Rationale: This will show you that each lead is recording effectively and begin to give you an idea of the animal's condition.

10. **Action:** Return to lead II and do a 20–30 second recording at 50 mm/s (Fig. 7.10).

    Rationale: This faster paper speed will produce a more drawn-out trace, which is easier to interpret.

11. **Action:** Check the traces for evidence of artefacts, which may lead to misdiagnosis, and address any problems.

    Rationale: Common artefacts may be due to:

    » Movement – most common is respiration
    » Electrical interference from other equipment
    » Incorrect positioning of the leads
    » Poor skin contact
    » Tangled leads or leads that are touching.

12. **Action:** About 5 minutes of recording time is generally sufficient to identify intermittent arrhythmias.

    Rationale: Some arrhythmias, such as an AV block, may occur very intermittently and may require a form of 24-hour monitor.

NB Interpretation of an electrocardiogram can be complicated so you should refer to a specialist textbook; however, a simple interpretation can be carried out by asking the following questions:

• What is the heart rate?
• What is the rhythm?
• Is there a QRS complex for every P wave?
• Is there a P wave for every QRS complex?
• Are they consistently and reasonably related?
• What is the morphology of the QRS complex – is it narrow and upright or wide and bizarre?

FLUID COLLECTION FROM BODY CAVITIES

It may be necessary to collect fluid from either the abdominal or the thoracic cavity for diagnostic tests, or as a means of treatment.

Procedure: Abdominocentesis

This procedure may be used to collect a sample of peritoneal fluid for analysis or, when there is an excessive accumulation of fluid, it may be used to drain the fluid, thus relieving the pressure within the abdomen and making the patient more comfortable.

Abdominocentesis should not be performed in cases of:

- Noted distension of abdominal organs – identify by palpation, radiology or ultrasonography
- Coagulopathy.

Care must be taken to avoid penetration or laceration of distended organs.

1. **Action:** It may be necessary to sedate the patient.

   Rationale: Although not very painful, the patient may feel slight discomfort and be inclined to struggle.

2. **Action:** Restrain the patient in right lateral recumbency.

   Rationale: The ideal site is just caudal to the umbilicus on the midline.

3. **Action:** If necessary, empty the patient's bladder by urethral catheterization.

   Rationale: To prevent accidental penetration of the bladder.

4. **Action:** Clip an area in the ventral midline, centred on the umbilicus. This should be about 10 cm × 10 cm.

   Rationale: This should provide sufficient space for a single centesis or for several if necessary.

5. **Action:** Prepare the area aseptically and place a sterile, fenestrated drape with the umbilicus in the centre.

   Rationale: Aseptic preparation will prevent the entry of infection.

6. **Action:** Using a sterile hypodermic needle of suitable size and gauge – dog 21G, 1.5 inch (38 mm); cat 23G, ¾ inch (18 mm)– introduce the needle into the peritoneal cavity 1 cm right lateral of the midline and 2–3 cm caudal to the umbilicus. This is in the right cranial quadrant.

   Rationale: Inserting the needle without the syringe attached is more likely to result in fluid flow. Drawing back on the needle using a syringe may pull the omentum or viscera on to the point of the needle and block it.

7. **Action:** As you insert the needle twist it slightly.

   Rationale: This encourages fluid flow.

8. **Action:** Allow a few drops of fluid to flow into a sampling tube – EDTA is recommended for cytology.

   Rationale: See Chapter 4 for cytology and other analyses.

9. **Action:** Check the fluid in the sampling tube.

   Rationale: To check that the fluid is not blood, urine or gut contents that may have been collected by puncturing the relevant organ. If you are worried then use ultrasound-guided aspiration.

10. **Action:** If larger quantities of fluid are to be withdrawn, attach a 10–20 ml syringe and gently draw back allowing the syringe to fill slowly. Detach and empty the syringe as necessary and reattach to the needle.

    Rationale: Slight negative pressure when the syringe is drawn back will help the flow, but avoid too great a pressure. If the patient wishes to stand, gravity may speed up the flow.

11. **Action:** If fluid is difficult to obtain then repeat the process in other sites (e.g. right caudal quadrant, left cranial and left caudal).

    Rationale: If blood is aspirated, stop immediately. There is a risk of penetrating the spleen in the left cranial quadrant.

12. **Action:** When the process is complete, remove the syringe. The hole should seal itself, but if necessary apply gentle pressure for a few minutes with a sterile swab.

    Rationale: In some cases where a patient has a large abdominal effusion the centesis hole may continue to drain. This can be prevented by applying a pressure bandage – see Chapter 4.

Procedure: Thoracocentesis

Thoracocentesis may be used to collect samples of pleural fluid for analysis or, when there is accumulation of air or fluid in the pleural cavity, it may be used to relieve the clinical signs of dyspnoea and respiratory distress. In some cases this may be an emergency procedure.

The most important factor to remember is that in a normal animal the pleural cavity contains a vacuum. If during the procedure you let air into the cavity you risk causing extreme respiratory distress. It is therefore vital that you take steps to prevent this happening (e.g. by using a three-way tap).

1. **Action:** Minimal restraint is required in most cases. Sedation may be used if necessary.

    Rationale: Care should be taken with any dyspnoeic patient. Excessive struggling may also be detrimental.

2. **Action:** Place the patient in sternal recumbency, which allows efficient drainage, but a sitting or standing position or lateral recumbency may be used.

    Rationale: Allow the patient to adopt a position that is comfortable and allows it to breathe as easily as possible.

3. **Action:** Be prepared to administer oxygen by mask if necessary.

    Rationale: Some patients may become distressed and this could be life threatening.

4. **Action:** Clip the skin of the lateral thorax within a 15 cm radius of the proposed thoracocentesis site and prepare aseptically.

    Rationale: The site is usually the 7th or 8th intercostal space and depends on whether air or pleural fluid is present:

    » In the dorsal third of the thorax if air is present (Fig. 7.11A).
    » In the ventral third of the thorax if fluid is present (Fig. 7.11B).

5. **Action:** Instil local anaesthetic into the subcutaneous tissues and muscle at the site.

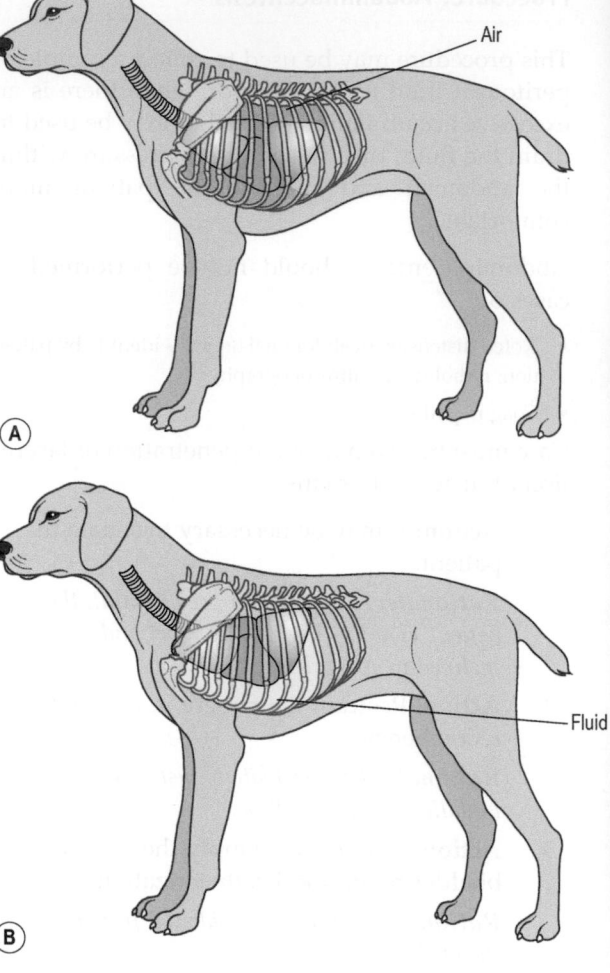

Figure 7.11 (A) Pleural air accumulates primarily in the dorsal and caudal thorax in the standing or sternal patient. (B) Pleural fluid accumulates centrally in the standing or sternal patient.

Rationale: This procedure is painful as the catheter passes through the superficial tissues.

6. **Action:** Attach a butterfly needle to a three-way tap and syringe, making sure that the tap is turned 'off' to the butterfly needle.

    Rationale: The tap must be closed at first to prevent an inrush of air into the pleural space.

7. **Action:** If a large amount of fluid is to be drained then use a large bore 'over-the-needle' intravenous catheter instead.

Rationale: A large bore catheter is blunt ended and is therefore less likely to lacerate the lung tissue. Cutting 2–3 small windows in the distal end of the catheter with a scalpel blade will reduce the risk of blockage while draining the fluid.

8. **Action:** Insert the butterfly needle (or catheter) into the selected intercostal space along the cranial border of the rib and advance it slowly, aiming slightly ventrally. The bevel of the needle should face the lung.

    Rationale: The intercostal nerves and blood vessels run on the caudal border of each rib.

9. **Action:** Once you feel the needle enter the pleural cavity, hold it steady. If using a catheter, slide the catheter over the needle into the pleural cavity and immediately attach the three-way tap.

    Rationale: There is a slightly increased risk of letting air into the cavity when using a catheter because there is a small time lag while you remove the needle and attach the three-way tap.

10. **Action:** Ask your assistant to turn the three-way tap to 'open' and apply gentle suction using no more than 2 ml of negative pressure.

    Rationale: Make sure that in doing this you do not dislodge the needle. The tubing between the needle and the syringe allows the syringe to be easily moved, which reduces the risk of lung laceration and the risk of pulling the needle out of the centesis site.

11. **Action:** When the syringe is full of air / fluid, turn the three-way tap to the position where the side port is 'open' to the syringe. Make sure that the needle port is blocked (i.e. you cannot push fluid / air back into the chest).

    Rationale: Air must not be able to enter the pleural cavity while you are emptying the syringe.

12. **Action:** Slowly push the plunger to expel the fluid or air into a collecting container.

    Rationale: The advantage of using a three-way tap is that you do not have to detach the syringe every time you want to empty it, which reduces the risk of displacing the needle or catheter and of letting air into the pleural cavity.

13. **Action:** When no further air or fluid can be withdrawn turn the tap to 'off' and withdraw the needle from the thorax.

    Rationale: The pleural cavity has now been drained of fluid or air.

14. **Action:** Repeat on the other side of the chest if necessary.

    Rationale: In many conditions both sides may be affected.

NB If using an 'over-the-needle' catheter, make a small nick in the skin with a scalpel blade about half an inch (12 mm) caudal to your chosen intercostal space. Push the nicked skin cranially over the intercostal space and then insert the catheter as described. This creates a skin 'valve' that prevents the escape of air into the chest when you remove the catheter.

Radiography should be carried out before the procedure to assess the state of the pleural cavity and after the procedure to monitor progress and to check for any iatrogenic injury (e.g. pneumothorax).

PRINCIPLES OF BARRIER NURSING

Barrier nursing, which may also be referred to as isolation nursing, is a method of creating a physical barrier between an infectious animal and a healthy / susceptible animal to prevent the spread of disease. In an ideal world, barrier nursing would be carried out within a dedicated isolation unit; however, the same principles relate to barrier nursing within a small veterinary practice or within an owner's home.

Most of the infectious diseases that we recognize in dogs, cats and rabbits are rarely seen nowadays, which is largely due to the fact that a proportion of the companion animal population is vaccinated. If the uptake of vaccinations were to fall, as it might do in a general economic downturn, then these diseases would be seen more frequently.

When a patient is diagnosed with an infectious disease it is the responsibility of the veterinary surgeon and the nurses within his / her employment to ensure that the infection does not spread to any other animal and, in the case of zoonotic diseases such as leptospirosis (Weil's disease), it is also vital that the disease does not spread to any human contacts. Even though the term 'barrier nursing' implies that this is the responsibility of the nurses in the team, it is important for the veterinary surgeon to understand the principles involved so that he / she can make sure that the regimen within the practice works effectively.

The first step in preventing the spread of infection is to understand the disease you are dealing with. Table 7.6 describes the most common infectious diseases, their clinical signs and methods of transmission. Box 7.8 lists some useful definitions of terms associated with the spread of disease.

Procedure: Factors to be considered in the design of an isolation unit

The aims of barrier nursing are to:

- Prevent the spread of an infectious disease
- Prevent neonates or susceptible young animals coming into contact with any disease
- Prevent immune-compromised animals coming into contact with any disease
- Prevent an animal that could be incubating a disease from spreading it to other animals – referred to as quarantine (Box 7.8).

1. **Action:** The isolation unit should be a self-contained room equipped with a range of kennels.

   Rationale: This provides physical separation from the rest of the practice. A range of kennels will satisfy the needs of a range of sizes of animal.

2. **Action:** The room should have a separate entrance and staff should access it via a footbath of disinfectant.

   Rationale: A separate entrance minimizes the risk of transferring infection into the practice. Disinfectant minimizes cross contamination.

3. **Action:** The room must have its own water supply and means of waste disposal.

Box 7.8 Common terminology associated with the spread of disease

- **Isolation** – physical separation of an animal that is known to have or is suspected of having an infectious disease
- **Quarantine** – physical separation of an animal that may have been exposed to an infectious disease and could be incubating it
- **Infectious disease** – a disease caused by a micro-organism that is capable of invading and growing within the tissues of the host animal
- **Pathogen** – a disease-causing organism
- **Direct contact** – method of spread when one animal touches another in some way
- **Indirect contact** – method of spread when there is no direct physical contact; the infectious agent will be spread by fomites or vectors
- **Fomites** – an inanimate object that can spread disease (e.g. litter tray, bowl, apron, shoes)
- **Vector** – an animate object that can spread disease (e.g. flea, fly, tick)
- **Carrier** – an animal that has previously been in contact with a disease and is not showing any clinical signs but can spread the pathogen; it may be a convalescent or a healthy carrier
- **Convalescent carrier** – an animal that is known to have had the disease and is now recovered but secretes the pathogen and is a source of infection to others (e.g. hepatitis, leptospirosis)
- **Healthy carrier** – an animal that has never had any overt signs of the disease (it may be immune) but secretes the pathogen and is a source of infection to others (e.g. ringworm in cats)
- **Incubation period** – time between the entry of the pathogen into the host animal and the appearance of clinical signs; an animal may be at its most infectious during the incubation period

Rationale: Water supply is used for cleaning and the preparation of food. Water, solids and consumables must not be taken into the practice for disposal.

4. **Action:** The ventilation system must be separate from the practice.

   Rationale: This must be in the form of extractor fans that vent directly to the outside not into the practice, to prevent cross contamination.

5. **Action:** There should be a separate kitchen area for the preparation of food.

Table 7.6 Infectious diseases of dogs, cats and rabbits

Disease	Infectious agent	Method of transmission	Incubation period	Clinical signs	Affected species	Zoonotic?
Distemper or hard pad	Morbillivirus	Inhalation and ingestion – virus is shed in nasal and oral discharges faeces and saliva	7–21 days	Pyrexia, anorexia, cough, nasal and ocular discharges; hyperkeratosis of nose and pads develops after a few weeks; recovered cases may be left with fits and chorea	Dogs and ferrets	No
Parvovirus	Canine parvovirus	Ingestion – virus is shed in faeces and vomit	4–7 days	Neonates may suffer with myocardial disease; severe haemorrhagic gastroenteritis, vomiting, anorexia, abdominal pain; death within 72 hours	Dogs	No
Infectious canine hepatitis	Canine adenovirus – CAV 1	Ingestion – virus is shed in vomit, faeces, saliva and urine; recovered cases may shed pathogen in urine	5–9 days	Acute – pyrexia and death within 24 hours; anorexia, vomiting and diarrhoea, conjunctivitis, photophobia	Dogs	No
Leptospirosis	Bacteria – *Leptospira canicola* and *L. icterohaemorrhagiae*	Ingestion – penetration through broken skin and mucous membranes; bacteria are shed in urine	Up to 7 days	*L. canicola* – affects the kidneys; polydipsia, polyuria, vomiting, renal failure *L. icterohaemorrhagiae* – affects the liver; sudden death; vomiting, jaundice, anterior abdominal pain	Dogs and rats	Yes – known as Weil disease
Infectious tracheobronchitis or kennel cough	*Bordetella bronchiseptica*, CAV2, parainfluenza virus, herpes virus, reovirus	Inhalation – pathogens are shed in nasal and oral secretions	5–7 days	Dry hacking cough; most cases remain well but some show pyrexia, nasal and ocular discharges, bronchopneumonia	Dogs	No

Table 7.6 *Continued*

Disease	Infectious agent	Method of transmission	Incubation period	Clinical signs	Affected species	Zoonotic?
Lyme disease	*Borrelia burgdorferi* – bacteria	Transmitted by ixodid ticks	Variable	Many are asymptomatic; pyrexia, anorexia, skin rash, enlarged lymph nodes, chronic arthritis	Dogs	Yes – results from tick bites
Feline infectious enteritis or feline panleucopaenia	Feline parvovirus	Ingestion – virus is excreted in saliva, vomit, faeces and urine	2–10 days	Lethargy, pyrexia, anorexia, vomiting, profuse dysentery; recovered cases may become carriers	Cats	No
Feline leukaemia	Retrovirus	Ingestion – virus is excreted in saliva; vertical transmission to kittens	Few weeks to several months	Wide variation including lymphosarcoma, anaemia, nephritis, polyarthritis, immunosuppression	Cats	No
Feline upper respiratory tract disease or cat 'flu syndrome	Feline herpesvirus, calicivirus, *Bordetella bronchiseptica*, *Chlamydia felis*	Inhalation pathogens are excreted in nasal and ocular discharges	2–10 days	Sneezing, conjunctivitis, oral ulcers, nasal and ocular discharge; secondary bacterial infection may lead to chronic infection; carrier state may develop in recovered cases	Cats	No
Feline immunodeficiency virus	Retrovirus	Ingestion – virus is secreted in saliva; neonates may become infected via the milk	Few weeks to a few months	Causes immunosuppression so clinical signs vary according to infection (e.g. respiratory tract disease, anorexia, loss of weight, gingivitis)	Cats	No

Feline infectious anaemia	*Mycoplasma haemofelis* (formerly *Haemabartonella felis*) – Rickettsia	Pathogen is found attached to the erythrocytes; presumed to be transmitted by blood-sucking insects (e.g. fleas)	Unknown	May be asymptomatic and occur when cat is stressed or has a concurrent disease; acute haemolytic anaemia, pyrexia, tachycardia, collapse	Cats	No
Feline infectious peritonitis	Coronavirus	Ingestion – virus is secreted in oral and nasal discharges	Variable	Signs depend on the immune status of the cat: If strong only the gut is affected – diarrhoea If moderate it may affect the CNS, liver, kidney and cause ataxia and convulsions If weak acute wet FIP develops – ascites, hydrothorax, pericardial effusion, diarrhoea and death	Cats	No
Myxomatosis	Poxvirus	Spread by insect vectors such as the rabbit flea and mosquitoes		Lethargy, depression and pyrexia, oedema of lips, ears, eyes, genitalia and anus; rapid death In the subacute form rabbits may recover	Rabbits	No
Viral haemorrhagic disease (VHD)	Calicivirus	Direct transmission via faeces during an outbreak; spread by fomites (e.g. feeding bowls, owner's clothing)	1–2 days	Death is often rapid with no apparent signs; lethargy, depression, pyrexia; rabbit may be found dead showing epistaxis and other signs of coagulopathy at post mortem	Rabbits	No

Rationale: Food provided to the patients in the unit should not have been in the practice or be taken back to the practice once the patient has left the unit, to prevent the risk of the spread of pathogens.

6. **Action:** Steps must be taken to prevent the entry of pests such as flies, cockroaches, mice or rats into the unit.

   Rationale: These creatures may act as vectors of disease from the unit to the practice or vice versa.

7. **Action:** There should be a separate treatment area that is well stocked with medicines.

   Rationale: Medicines should not be returned to the practice once the patient has left to prevent the risk of the spread of pathogens.

8. **Action:** All equipment (i.e. feeding, bedding, cleaning, bottles of disinfectant) should be used only within the unit. When the patient has recovered or died the equipment should be disposed of.

   Rationale: Select equipment that is cheap and/or disposable so that it can be thrown away or properly disinfected and used in the unit again. It must not be reused within the practice.

NB If a separate unit is not available then an infectious patient may be isolated in a room that is not normally used for animals (e.g. an office or storeroom). Always be aware of the dangers of zoonotic spread to people using those rooms.

Procedure: Designation of personnel to staff the unit

Access to the unit must be limited to the nursing team and the vet(s) in charge of the cases. No visitors are allowed in the unit. Lay staff must be made aware of the situation and warning notices should be displayed.

1. **Action:** A small team of two nurses should be allocated to the isolation unit and should not deal with any patients within the practice.

   Rationale: To reduce the spread of infection by the nurse's body. Having two nurses enables them to have a rota for being on and off duty.

2. **Action:** If specific nurses cannot be used, the care of the isolated patients should be done after nursing all other patients within the practice.

   Rationale: To prevent the spread of disease to patients whose immunity is reduced by surgery or other concurrent conditions.

3. **Action:** The same nurse should not be dealing both with infectious cases and with neonatal and immune-compromised cases.

   Rationale: Neonates and immune-compromised animals have lowered immunity to infectious diseases.

4. **Action:** All personnel entering or leaving the isolation unit must walk through a shallow foot bath containing a suitable disinfectant.

   Rationale: To prevent cross infection between the isolation unit and the practice. Not all disinfectants are active against all infectious diseases – always read the labels.

5. **Action:** Appropriate clothing must be worn when working in the unit. This should be left in the unit or disposed of before leaving the unit.

   Rationale: To prevent the spread of infection by fomites.

6. **Action:** A changing room should be provided. This is used only by the nurses and vets working in the unit. They must change before entering and before leaving the unit.

   Rationale: Clothes worn within the unit must remain there to prevent the spread of infection by fomites.

7. **Action:** Special footwear must be worn within the unit (e.g. disposable overshoes, clogs, wellington boots) and must not leave the unit.

   Rationale: To prevent the spread of infection by fomites.

8. **Action:** Disposable equipment such as gloves, masks, cap, aprons etc must be worn in the unit and must be disposed of before leaving the unit.

   Rationale: To prevent the spread of infection by fomites.

9. **Action:** Hair must be tied back and covered by a disposable cap.

    Rationale: Normal hygiene precautions to prevent the spread of infection by fomites.

10. **Action:** Personal hygiene must be observed and hand hygiene, using recommended alcohol rubs, must be carried out at regular intervals and between patients. Use disposable towels for drying.

    Rationale: To prevent the spread of infection by fomites to patients within and outside the unit.

NB Any inanimate object (e.g. pens, hospital charts) may act as a fomite (Box 7.8) in the spread of disease, so nothing must be taken out of the unit without prior, thorough disinfection.

Procedure: Isolation in a small practice or within an owner's home

1. **Action:** If a separate room is not available an infectious cat can be housed in the dog kennels and an infectious dog can be housed in the cat kennels.

    Rationale: Most dog diseases are not transmitted to cats and vice versa.

2. **Action:** Cages must be separated by solid walls and should be arranged in a straight line.

    Rationale: This prevents droplet infection by sneezing or coughing. The aerosol effect propels pathogens forwards in a straight line.

3. **Action:** If cages are arranged opposite each other then the gap must be greater than 1.2 metres.

    Rationale: Research has shown that this is the maximum distance a droplet can travel when sneezed out by a cat.

4. **Action:** If the patient cannot be put into a separate room then cover the cage with a towel or blanket.

    Rationale: This will prevent transmission by sneezed or coughed out droplets.

5. **Action:** Provide separate feeding bowls, litter trays, bedding and cleaning equipment. Do not use them for any other

animals and, after the animal has died or gone home, make sure they are disposed of or sterilized thoroughly.

    Rationale: To prevent the spread of infection by fomites.

6. **Action:** Wear protective clothing when dealing with the patient.

    Rationale: To prevent the spread of infection by fomites.

7. **Action:** Always wash your hands after dealing with the patient.

    Rationale: To prevent the spread of infection.

8. **Action:** Deal with the infectious patient after you have dealt with all other patients.

    Rationale: To prevent the spread of infection from one patient to another.

9. **Action:** If there are any other susceptible animals in the household they should be given booster vaccinations.

    Rationale: To boost their levels of immunity – remember that this may take time and may not necessarily provide total biosecurity, so instigate some form of barrier nursing in the household.

10. **Action:** Education, education, education – the owner must be told the methods of disease spread, the incubation period and the clinical signs of the disease in question (Table 7.6).

    Rationale: So that the owner can take appropriate measures and understands what to look out for in any in-contact animals. The earlier treatment is instigated the more likely it is to be successful.

DENTISTRY

Veterinary dentistry may be considered to consist of oral hygiene and the diagnosis and treatment of dental disease. The treatment of dental disease is a complicated and developing subject and it is recommended that you should refer to one of the many dedicated books written on the subject. The aim of this section is to provide you with sufficient information to deal with the more common and more minor problems.

If oral examination is to provide detailed diagnostic information it must be done under a general anaesthetic. Scaling and polishing of the teeth and / or removal of any diseased teeth can be a lengthy and possibly painful procedure and it would be an extremely placid patient that would satisfactorily tolerate the process without closing its mouth or, at the worst, biting you. To complete the job properly, records should be kept of any abnormalities detected so that you can monitor the animal's response to treatment.

ANAESTHESIA FOR DENTAL PROCEDURES

While the patient is anaesthetized (see Ch. 8) the following points should be considered:

1. **Airway security** – steps must be taken to prevent aspiration pneumonia as a result of inhalation of fluid, debris and blood, which may be by-products of the procedure. To prevent this:

   a. Always use an endotracheal tube and inflate the cuff.

   b. Always tie the tube using a light bandage around the adaptor and then around the back of the patient's head. In this way the bandage does not interfere with your examination.

   c. Always pack the pharynx for greater airway protection. It is simplest to use damp gauze swabs or a damp gauze bandage. Make sure you count the swabs to ensure that they are all removed at the end of the procedure or, if using a bandage, leave the end protruding from the mouth for easy removal. There is a risk that the swabs or bandage will become saturated during the process and may no longer provide protection – replace them at regular intervals. Do not pack the pharynx too tightly as venous return may be impeded.

2. **Eye protection** – the eyes should be protected using a lubricant ointment. Tear production is reduced when an animal is anaesthetized.

3. **Mouth gags** – should be used with care. They should be released and the jaws closed every 10–15 minutes. Keeping the jaws wide open for prolonged periods may cause neuropraxia and the inability to close the jaws. Recovery may take several weeks.

4. **Hypothermia** – this is a complication of prolonged anaesthesia and in addition the patient may become wet. Check the body temperature every 20–30 minutes, carry out the procedure on a tub table or put the patient's head over some form of a wire grid so that the water drains away and wrap the patient in bubble wrap, towels or blankets to minimize heat loss.

Procedure: Scaling/polishing the teeth and general oral examination

This procedure is recommended for any animal with halitosis, gingivitis, problems with eating or any evidence of tooth pain (e.g. excessive salivation).

1. **Action:** The patient is anaesthetized, intubated and the pharynx is packed with damp swabs or a damp gauze bandage. The eyes are lubricated with an eye lubricant.

   Rationale: See comments above.

2. **Action:** Position the patient in lateral recumbency on a tub table with the head slightly lower than the rest of the body. This can be achieved by tilting the table or placing a rolled up towel under the shoulders (Fig. 7.12).

   Rationale: This position will encourage fluids to run out of the mouth rather than down into the pharynx. A tub table consists of a wire grid over a large sink, which collects water from the ultrasonic scaler, leaving the patient reasonably dry.

3. **Action:** Put on a facemask, goggles and gloves.

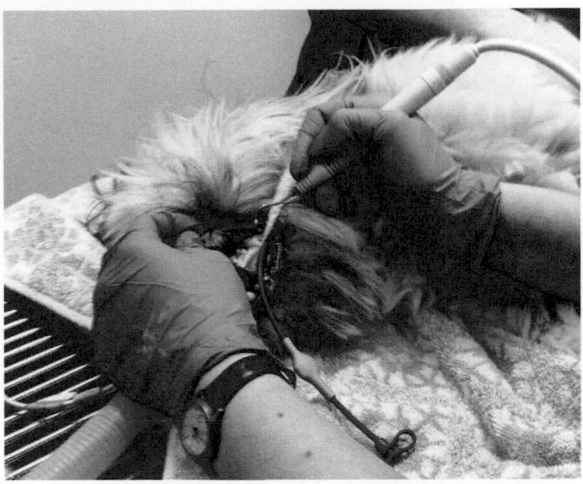

Figure 7.12 Canine patient undergoing a dental scale and polish

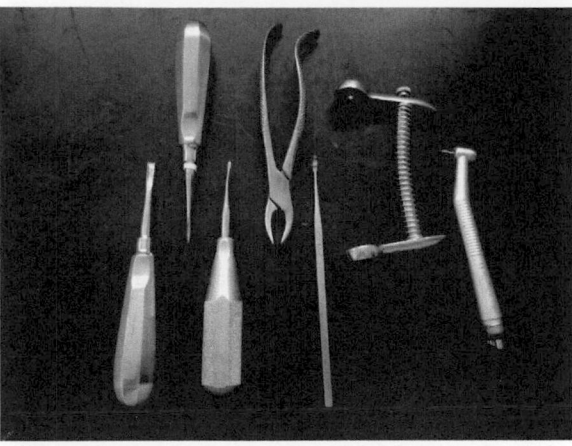

Figure 7.13 Dental instruments from left to right; three dental elevators in different sizes, extraction forceps, a hand scaler, a mouth gag, dental drill with burr attached (this is attached to the dental machine).

Rationale: This protective equipment will prevent you from inhaling any bacterial debris or getting chips of calculus in your eyes.

4. **Action:** Select a mouth gag of an appropriate size and insert it between the upper and lower canines.

   Rationale: To hold the mouth open facilitating examination and cleaning, but take note of the comments above.

5. **Action:** Make a detailed examination of each tooth on the uppermost side of the jaw looking for evidence of periodontal disease (Table 7. 7).

   Rationale: Make sure you record this so that you do not forget to instigate some form of treatment.

6. **Action:** Using an ultrasonic scaler, scale the teeth on the uppermost side of the jaw. Never leave the scaler on a tooth for more than 10 seconds.

   Rationale: The vibrating action of the scaler may generate heat, which may cause iatrogenic damage to the tooth if used for longer than 10 seconds. Make sure there is a plentiful supply of water to cool the tooth. You can return to the tooth later if it is still not clean.

7. **Action:** With the aid of appropriate instruments (Fig. 7.13, Table 7.8), check that all calculus (tartar) has been removed. Remember to check on the lingual side of each tooth.

   Rationale: Calculus is the hard brown deposit that forms as a result of bacterial action on plaque. Large accumulations may lead to gingivitis and should always be removed.

8. **Action:** Mop up any debris and excess fluid with gauze swabs or cottonwool.

   Rationale: It is important to clean up as you work. This prevents the patient becoming unnecessarily wet and cold and leaves less clearing up at the end of the procedure.

9. **Action:** Repeat your examination of the teeth.

   Rationale: Removing plaque and calculus may have revealed evidence of further disease.

10. **Action:** Remove any diseased teeth as necessary.

    Rationale: Some teeth may dislodge very easily whereas others will require a more complicated procedure – see below.

Table 7.7 Signs of periodontal disease*

Condition	Description	Treatment
Plaque	A soft layer composed of bacteria in an organic matrix that forms on the surface of a tooth	Brushing pet's teeth at home; change diet if necessary
Calculus	A calcified deposit that forms on the surface of the teeth as a result of bacterial action on plaque	Scaling and polishing
Gingivitis	Inflammation of the gums, which become swollen and bleed easily; caused by plaque at the base of the teeth	Removal of plaque and calculus by scaling and polishing; short term antibiotics to erase the infection
Periodontitis	Resulting from untreated gingivitis, the gum line recedes away from the base of the tooth	Extraction of the tooth; treatment for gingivitis
Caries	Decay and crumbling of the tooth due to acid produced by bacteria	Extraction or filling
Fracture of the crown	Caused by trauma to the tooth	Extraction or filling
Retained deciduous teeth	Teeth are not shed before permanent ones erupt. May cause misplacement of new teeth	Extraction

*After Aspinall 2003a, p 185, with permission of Elsevier Butterworth-Heineman.

Table 7.8 Dental instruments*

Name	Description	Use
Periodontal probe	A long, thin instrument with a 90° bend in the head; it has graduations on the probe; it is blunt ended	Used to examine and measure the subgingival margin, tooth mobility, inflammation and lesions
Dental probe	A long thin instrument with a rounded head; it has a sharp end	Used to examine caries, fractures and lesions
Dental mirror	A long handle with a small round mirror at the end	Used to visualize the inner and back surfaces of the teeth
Scaler	A long handle with a thin, bent head; it has a sharp, pointed tip	Used to remove supragingival calculus; if used subgingivally it will damage the tissue with its sharp tip
Curette	A long handle with a thin, bent head; it has a rounded tip	Used to remove supragingival and subgingival calculus
Luxator/elevator	A thick handle with a rounded and/or curved tip; various sizes available depending on the requirements of the patient	Used to break down the periodontal ligament, which holds the tooth in place
Periosteal elevator	A long thin handle with rounded or straight, and/or curved tips; various sizes are available depending on the requirements of the patient	Used when a periosteal flap is opened to facilitate the removal of a tooth
Extraction forceps	Various sizes available depending on the shape and size of the tooth	Used to lift a tooth out after being loosened by elevation; do not use to remove 'set in' teeth as the tooth can snap off leaving the root in place

*(See also Fig 7.1.)

11. **Action:** Turn the patient over, making sure that you do not dislodge the endotracheal tube or twist the anaesthetic circuit. If possible turn the body so that the legs pass under the body rather than over the top, which would be easier.

    Rationale: These are common problems associated with moving the patient. In some cases it may be easier to disconnect the circuit while you turn the animal over and then reconnect. Turning the body over in this manner reduces the chances of aspirating fluid.

12. **Action:** Repeat the examination and scaling process on this side. Remove any diseased teeth as before.

    Rationale: To complete treatment of the whole mouth.

13. **Action:** When you have completed the process, insert the polishing handpiece into the holder of the scaler and polish the teeth using prophylactic paste.

    Rationale: Polishing the teeth leaves them smooth; this reduces the ability of the oral bacteria to stick to the tooth and form pellicle, which becomes plaque. It also leaves the teeth looking clean and white, which will be appreciated by the patient's owner.

14. **Action:** Remove swabs or bandage from the pharynx before allowing the patient to return to consciousness.

    Rationale: To prevent the patient inhaling them or choking on them.

NB It is not a good idea to scale the teeth at the same time as a surgical procedure is taking place. There is a risk that pathogenic bacteria may be released into the blood stream, which may contaminate surgical wounds.

EXTRACTIONS – GENERAL GUIDELINES

Some badly diseased teeth will simply fall out of their sockets, but others may be more firmly attached and require the use of dental instruments (Table 7.8, Fig. 7.13).

Removal is done as follows:

1. Loosen the periodontal ligament all round the tooth using an elevator. This ligament holds the tooth in place and must be severed before the tooth becomes loose.

2. Gently rock the tooth in its sockets, being careful not to break the jaw. This might be a problem when removing the deep-rooted canine teeth, particularly those in the lower jaw.

3. As the tooth loosens, pull up vertically from the jaw using extraction forceps. It is important to try to remove the tooth with its roots intact. If the roots break off then they must be removed from the gum if they are not to become a focus for infection.

4. Teeth with multiple roots – that is, premolars, molars and the carnassials (1st lower molar and last upper premolar on each side) – may have to be sectioned using a drill or dental saw before they can be removed.

5. In some cases it may be necessary to open a periosteal flap over the tooth to facilitate removal. This must then be sutured to encourage healing.

COMPLICATIONS

Following tooth extraction, complications may include:

- Incomplete removal of the tooth – leading to a persistent infection and even osteomyelitis in the jaw
- Fracture of the mandible or maxilla
- Persistent haemorrhage from the tooth sockets – may occur in cases of Von Willebrand disease
- Creation of an oronasal fistula – may occur after removal of the upper canines.

MAINTENANCE OF ORAL HYGIENE

The effects of dental scaling and polishing are relatively short lived and if the owner does not instigate a regimen of dental home care the plaque will rapidly reform. Research shows that periodontal disease will be as bad again within 3 months if nothing is done to prevent it.

The key to maintaining oral hygiene is keeping plaque accumulation to as low a level as possible and the best way of doing this is tooth brushing. This depends on both patient cooperation and the owner's motivation and ability to handle the animal. It is easier to brush an animal's teeth if it has been trained from a young age, but it is never too late to start – in general kittens accept tooth brushing more readily than puppies.

There is a wide range of toothbrushes and toothpastes designed for use in animals, and client education and compliance accompanied by continuous monitoring and reinforcement will help to raise the levels of oral hygiene in your practice.

CHAPTER 8
Administration of anaesthesia

Anaesthesia may be defined as the production of a reversible state of insensitivity to pain. Pain is the conscious perception of a noxious stimulus.

Veterinary anaesthesia may be used for two main reasons:

- To obliterate the pain felt during a surgical procedure or other potentially painful procedure.
- To restrain the patient during a procedure required for diagnosis or treatment.

As such it is one of the most common daily procedures carried out in a small animal practice.

In anaesthetizing a patient the anaesthetist must not endanger the patient or the personnel involved in the administration of the anaesthetic. The correct choice of drugs and taking care during their administration will minimize the risks to both patient and personnel, and correct management of the anaesthetic process will significantly increase the chances of the animal's survival.

The types of anaesthesia may be divided into:

- **Sedation** – use of drugs to calm the animal. It is widely used to reduce the anaesthetic dose, and improve the induction and recovery stages of a general anaesthetic. It is usually given by injection – for a description of the techniques see Chapter 1.

- **Local** – infiltration with local anaesthetic (e.g. lidocaine) to desensitize a restricted area. This is not widely used in small animals, but may be used to stitch up small superficial wounds while the animal remains conscious. They may be used in cases where cardiovascular or metabolic problems make general anaesthesia dangerous. The anaesthetic may be administered by injection (see Ch.1) or in some cases by using creams or ointments designed to be absorbed through the skin.

- **Regional** – involves desensitization of a specified area by blocking the sensory nerves supplying that area. Requires accurate knowledge of the nerve's pathway and is widely used in large animal diagnosis and treatment (e.g. equine lameness, suturing wounds, caesarean section in cattle), but not used in small animals.

- **General anaesthesia** – the patient is rendered unconscious and, depending on the choice of drugs, will be insensitive to pain. A general anaesthetic can be considered to take place in two stages:
  - **Induction** – the administration of a drug to render the animal unconscious. In small animal practice these are usually injectable agents given intravenously or intramuscularly, although some exotic species may be induced using volatile agents in an induction chamber.
  - **Maintenance** – the process by which the patient is kept in a state of unconsciousness until such time as it is allowed to recover. This may be achieved by using injectable drugs or gases or volatile agents given via an anaesthetic machine and the appropriate circuit.

The use of injectable agents requires very little specific equipment and the administration techniques are no different from those of any other injection (see Ch. 1). The use of inhalational agents (i.e. gases or volatile liquids) requires the use of complicated and expensive anaesthetic machines and monitoring equipment and it is vital for the veterinary surgeon, who bears ultimate responsibility for the survival and recovery of the patient, to understand how the system works and is maintained.

It is not the responsibility of this book to describe the range and pharmacology of the anaesthetic agents used in practice; the reader is recommended to consult a dedicated textbook on anaesthesia.

PREPARATION FOR ANAESTHESIA

Procedure: Patient preparation for anaesthesia

Patients admitted for anaesthesia may fall into one of four groups:

- Normal healthy animals for elective routine procedures (e.g. neutering).
- Apparently normal animals to undergo diagnostic procedures.
- Sick animals for treatment – may present an increased anaesthetic risk.
- Emergency cases – pre-anaesthetic care and assessment may be minimal as they will be admitted quickly, but support and monitoring are vital.

1. **Action:** The patient should be starved for 12 hours prior to surgery and owners should be advised of this when they book their appointment.

   Rationale: Animals that are not fasted may vomit as a result of the anaesthetic drugs and may inhale their vomit. During anaesthesia the swallow reflex is lost and the airway is thus unprotected.

   NB This does not apply to rabbits as they are unable to vomit and if starved may suffer a fatal hypoglycaemia. Encouraging them to eat to within an hour of the anaesthetic may prevent postoperative anorexia, which may lead to gut stasis.

2. **Action:** If possible all patients booked in for elective procedures should be encouraged to urinate and defaecate before being brought to the surgery. Owners should be asked to do this.

   Rationale: This is not easy but is more pleasant for everyone involved in looking after the animal during the day.

3. **Action:** Weigh the patient – should be done for all patients.

   Rationale: This is essential for the accurate administration of premedicant and induction drugs.

4. **Action:** Take the client and patient into a consulting room and explain to the client exactly what will happen to their animal

during the surgical procedure. You should also give an estimate of cost and this should be written down on the case records.

Rationale: You may have already discussed cost and the details of the procedure, in which case it may be part of the practice's protocol for a veterinary nurse to admit the animal. Recording your estimate may prevent disputes later on.

5. **Action:** Ask the client to sign a consent form.

   Rationale: This may be done by a veterinary nurse. The client, or an agent of the client, must read, understand and sign the consent form – and must be over 18 years of age.

6. **Action:** At some time you should have taken a full history and carried out a detailed clinical examination (see Ch. 2).

   Rationale: If the patient is booked in to undergo a routine procedure (e.g. spaying) you may not have seen the animal for some time. It is important to check that the animal is healthy before proceeding. If the animal is sick you will have carried out a detailed clinical examination prior to deciding to admit the animal.

7. **Action:** Collect a blood sample for a pre-anaesthetic blood test.

   Rationale: This should be a routine procedure in any practice, but many practices will not do the test in young animals having routine operations such as neutering. The test is used to assess whether there are any underlying problems that may increase the anaesthetic risk. Parameters making up the pre-anaesthetic blood test are shown in Table 8.1.

8. **Action:** Administer your chosen premedicant drugs. The aim of the drugs is to calm the animal, enabling easy handling, and to allow for a smooth induction using a small dose of induction agent.

   Rationale: Choice of drugs depends on practice protocols and the condition of the patient. Routine predication may be administered by your veterinary nurse.

9. **Action:** The patient should then be placed in a warm, stress free kennel to await the procedure.

   Rationale: A calm, happy patient is less of an anaesthetic risk than a nervous, worried one.

THE ANAESTHETIC MACHINE

There are many designs of anaesthetic machine from simple small ones to large cumbersome pieces of equipment that are very often older or bought from hospitals. Whatever their shape and size, they are all designed to deliver accurate volumes of carrier gas and vaporized volatile liquids to the patient to produce anaesthesia. Figure 8.1 shows a generic form of a machine. Nowadays many practices have done away with oxygen cylinders attached to the machine and use piped oxygen from large cylinders kept outside the building. These are more convenient and more economical, although there may still be a small cylinder attached to the machine in case of emergency. There are also machines that extract oxygen from room air. Table 8.2 describes the parts and functions of the anaesthetic machine.

Procedure: Checking the anaesthetic machine before use

NB This may usually be done by a veterinary nurse, but the veterinary surgeon should also know how to do this.

1. **Action:** Turn on the spare oxygen cylinder and check that it is full. The pressure gauge should read 137 bar.

   Rationale: Oxygen is supplied in a black cylinder with a white collar and must be used at a minimum of 33% of the inspired gas mixture during anaesthesia. The contents of the spare cylinder ensure that there is a constant supply of oxygen throughout the anaesthetic if the cylinder in use becomes empty.

2. **Action:** Turn the cylinder off and label it as 'full'.

   Rationale: If the current cylinder and the spare cylinder are both on they will empty at the same rate.

3. **Action:** Turn on the in-use cylinder; check the contents by reading the pressure gauge and label it as 'in use'.

   Rationale: If the pressure reading is in the red area of the scale, indicating that it is almost empty, the cylinder should be changed.

Table 8.1 Biochemical and blood parameters that may be measured prior to anaesthesia

Pre-anaesthetic profile (PA6)	General profile (GP12) + electrolytes	Haematology
Alanine amino transferase (ALt) – raised values indicate acute liver damage	Alanine amino transferase (ALt) – raised values indicate acute liver damage	Haematocrit (HCT) – alternative to PCV – raised in cases of dehydration and lowered in cases of anaemia – see Table 5.3
Alkaline phosphatase (ALKP) – raised values indicate biliary stasis, but may also indicate intestinal or bone disease or raised steroid levels	Alkaline phosphatase (ALKP) – raised values indicate biliary stasis, but may also indicate intestinal or bone disease or raised steroid levels	Haemoglobin (HGB) – lowered in cases of anaemia – see Table 5.3
Blood urea nitrogen (BUN) – raised in cases of renal disease, dehydration, high protein meals or intestinal haemorrhage	Blood urea nitrogen (BUN) – raised in cases of renal disease, dehydration, high protein meals or intestinal haemorrhage	Mean corpuscular haemoglobin content (MCHC) – see Table 5.3
Creatinine – raised in cases of severe renal disease or dehydration	Creatinine – raised in cases of severe renal disease or dehydration	White blood cell count (WBC) – raised in cases of inflammation and infection – see Table 5.2
Glucose – raised in diabetes mellitus and in stressed cats. Reduced in insulinomas, some liver tumours and starved neonates	Glucose – raised in diabetes mellitus and in stressed cats. Reduced in insulinomas, some liver tumours and starved neonates	Granulocyte – numbers (Grans) – see Table 5.2
Total protein – raised values may be due to dehydration or high globulin levels. Low values in protein-losing diseases and severe liver disease	Total protein – raised values may be due to dehydration or high globulin levels. Low values in protein losing diseases and severe liver disease	% granulocytes (% Grans) – see Table 5.2.
	Albumin – gives a more specific guide to levels of one of the total proteins	Lymphocytes/monocytes – numbers (L/M) – see Table 5.2
	Globulin - gives a more specific guide to levels of one of the total proteins	% lymphocytes/monocytes (%L/M)) – see Table 5.2
	Amylase – non-specific but may indicate pancreatic disease	Platelets (PLT) – see Table 5.2
	Cholesterol – raised values may indicate liver disease	
	Calcium – raised values may indicate 1° hyperparathyroidism and is seen in some malignancies	
	Phosphate – raised values may indicate renal disease	
	Sodium	
	Potassium – high resting potassium could indicate hypoadrenocorticism (Addison disease). Poor storage of the blood sample will raise potassium levels	
	Chloride	

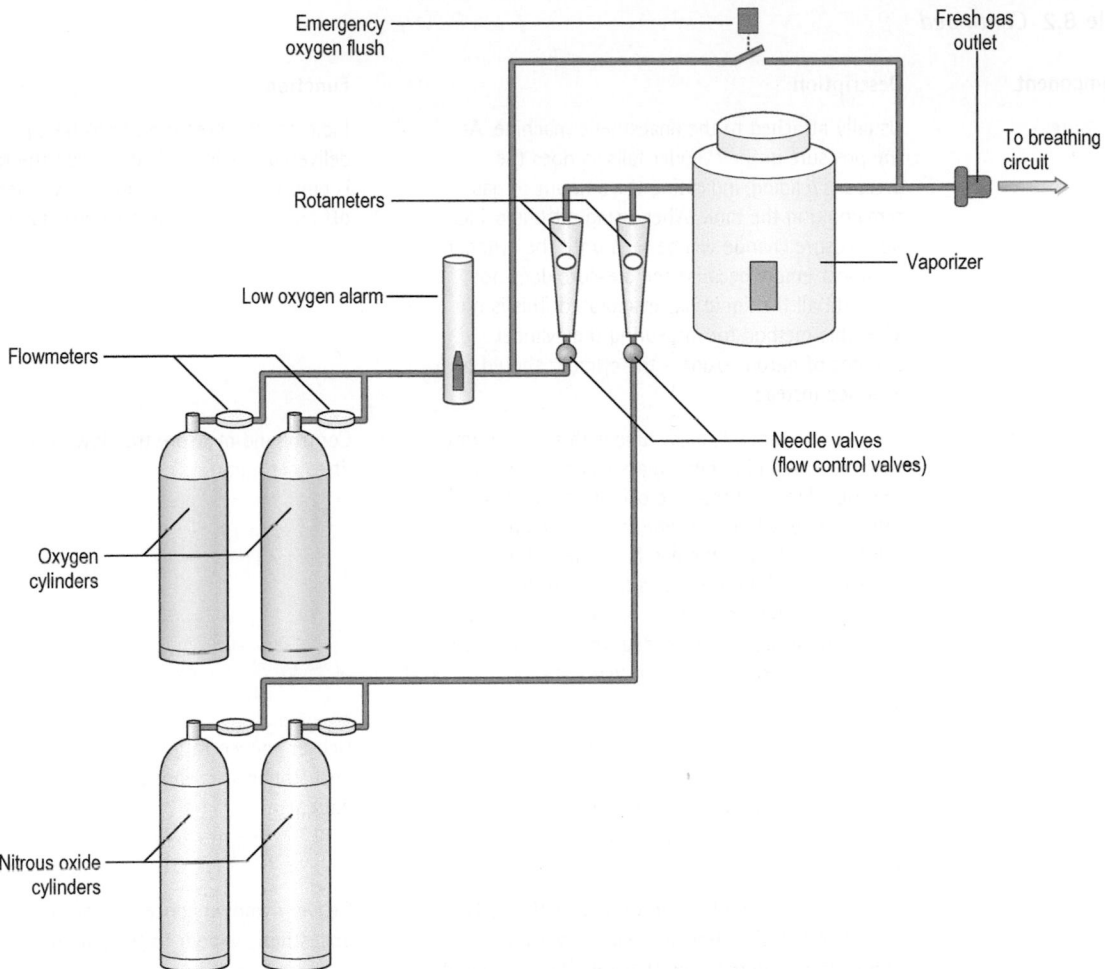

Figure 8.1 Diagram to represent a generic form of anaesthetic machine. (With permission from E. Mullineaux, M. Jones, BSAVA Manual of Practical Veterinary Nursing (2007).)

Table 8.2 Parts of the anaesthetic machine

Component	Description	Function
Gas supply	Oxygen cylinders are black with a white collar. Nitrous oxide cylinders are blue. Smaller cylinders, such as E and F, can be incorporated into the anaesthetic machine. Larger cylinders, J and G, may be kept separate and gas supply to the anaesthetic machine is through pipes in the wall	Supplies fresh oxygen and nitrous oxide to the patient. An E-sized cylinder contains enough oxygen to supply a 20 kg dog for 3 hours
Pressure-reducing valve or regulator	Usually incorporated into the yoke and is therefore impossible to identify	Reduces the pressure of the gas leaving the cylinder to ensure a constant flow to the anaesthetic machine regardless of the pressure changes within the cylinder. It provides a safe operating pressure for the machine

Table 8.2 *Continued*

Component	Description	Function
Pressure gauge	Usually attached to the anaesthetic machine. As the pressure in the cylinder falls so does the pressure reading, indicating the amount of gas remaining in the tank. When using nitrous oxide, no pressure change will be seen until the cylinder is almost empty because the pressure does not fall until all the liquid has evaporated. This is not a reliable method for measuring the cylinder content of nitrous oxide – the cylinder should be weighed instead	Indicates the pressure of gas being delivered. It will read zero when the tank is empty or when the tank is switched off and the gas in the pipe evacuated
Flowmeters or rotameters	Consist of a tapered, glass tube with the flow rate written on it and either a glass ball or bobbin in the tube. Provided that the ball or bobbin can rotate freely within the tube, it will give an accurate reading of the gas flow rate. A bobbin must be read from the top, a ball from the middle. Flowmeters are gas specific and control knobs are usually colour coded: they should never be overtightened as the valve seat is easily damaged	Control and measure the flow of gas in litres per minute
Vaporizers: uncalibrated	The Boyle's bottle (sometimes seen on very old machines) is an example of an uncalibrated vaporizer: whilst output can be varied, it fluctuates with temperature and gas flow changes	Deliver concentrations of volatile anaesthetic, in a vapour form, to the patient
Vaporizers: calibrated	The Tec, Penlon and Plenum vaporizers (Fig. 8.1) are calibrated. They remain accurate despite temperature and gas flow changes. They are agent specific. High and low flow rates may cause problems with accuracy	Deliver a known concentration of anaesthetic vapour to the patient
Back bar	Flowmeters and vaporizers can be attached to the back bar in series. This allows more than one volatile agent to be available. The 'Selectatec' manifold allows swift attachment or removal of Tec 3 and 4 vaporizers	Supports the flowmeters and vaporizers
Common gas outlet	Location varies between anaesthetic machines	Connects anaesthetic circuits, ventilators or oxygen supply devices to the machine
Oxygen flush valve	Oxygen reaches this valve swiftly, bypassing the vaporizer. High flow rates are produced. The valve may be locked open in some cases, by rotating it 90°	Provides oxygen in emergency situations and purges anaesthetic from the circuit before disconnection to minimize pollution
Low oxygen alarm	An alarm sounds or, in some cases, a light flashes when oxygen levels become dangerously low	Warns the anaesthetist of low oxygen levels

4. **Action:** Repeat the process for the nitrous oxide cylinder. The spare full cylinder should read 44 bar.

    Rationale: Nitrous oxide is supplied in blue cylinders. The pressure gauge will read full until the cylinder is almost empty. It has marked analgesic properties and will reduce the amount of volatile agent needed.

5. **Action:** Check for leaking gas as you turn the cylinders on.

    Rationale: A faulty Bodock seal can lead to gas leakage.

6. **Action:** Open and close the flowmeter valves.

    Rationale: To ensure that the ball or bobbin can move and rotate freely in its cylinder.

7. **Action:** Check the low oxygen alarm by turning the oxygen cylinder off and pressing the oxygen flush valve. Turn the oxygen back on.

    Rationale: The alarm is designed to sound as the oxygen pressure falls to a dangerously low level. This also confirms the flow of fresh gas through the oxygen flush valve.

8. **Action:** Check that the correct type of vaporizer is fitted to the back bar and that it is full. If more than one vaporizer is fitted, check that only one of them is switched on.

    Rationale: Each type of vaporizer is calibrated to take a different volatile agent and it is important to select the correct one. In reality most practices stick to one type. The control valve on the vaporizer should move freely. The level of liquid inside can be checked through the viewing port (Fig. 8.2).

9. **Action:** Select the correct anaesthetic circuit and check it for faults.

    Rationale: This prevents blockage by artefacts in the tubing or leakage at joints or from cracks in the tubing. Check particularly detachment of coaxial tubing or holes in reservoir bags.

10. **Action:** Connect the scavenging system and if appropriate switch it on. Anaesthetic machines must not be used without some form of scavenging to protect personnel in the area.

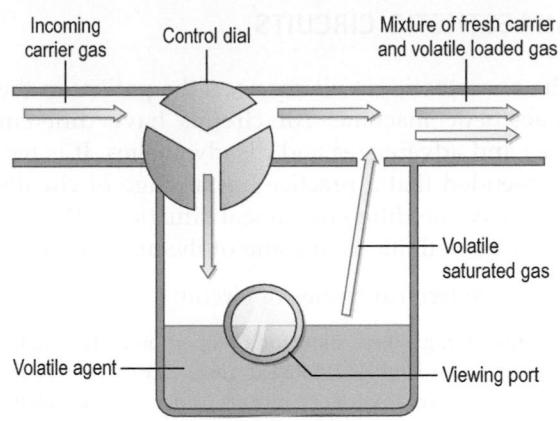

Figure 8.2 A plenum vaporizer.

Rationale: Scavenging systems may be active, in which case the waste gases are sucked out of the building, or passive, in which case the waste gases pass into a canister containing activated charcoal – these do not remove nitrous oxide.

Procedure: Shutting down the anaesthetic machine

1. **Action:** Check the contents of the gas cylinders and remove any empty ones. Replace them with full cylinders.

    Rationale: To ensure that the machine is ready for the next use.

2. **Action:** Open the oxygen flowmeter and allow a flow of 2 litres/min. Close the nitrous oxide cylinder and turn on the nitrous oxide flowmeter until the reading has fallen to 0. Close the flowmeter control.

    Rationale: This will flush all nitrous oxide out of the pipes. Any gas in the pipes could register when the flowmeter is switched on, implying that the cylinder is open.

3. **Action:** Turn the oxygen cylinder off and press the oxygen flush valve until no pressure reads on the pressure gauge.

    Rationale: All oxygen must be flushed from the pipes, as in step 2.

4. **Action:** Wipe the anaesthetic machine with disinfectant.

    Rationale: This minimizes the risk of contamination.

ANAESTHETIC CIRCUITS

The anaesthetic circuit connects the patient to the anaesthetic machine. All circuits have different uses and advantages and disadvantages. It is recommended that a practice has a range of circuits to satisfy the different clinical situations. Box 8.1 provides definitions of some of the terms used.

There are two categories of circuit:

- **Rebreathing** – these allow for a proportion of the exhaled gases to be reinhaled. Inhaled gases consist of only the carrier gas (i.e. oxygen or nitrous oxide) and the volatile liquid anaesthetic, whereas the exhaled gas contains carrier gas, volatile gas, carbon dioxide, water vapour and heat. If these can be reinhaled, less carrier and volatile gas are required to achieve unconsciousness and heat and water vapour are retained. A build-up of carbon dioxide could be fatal so this must be removed from the exhaled gases using soda lime.

  Soda lime is used in a granular form contained in some form of canister through which the exhaled gases pass. The material is coloured and this changes as the soda lime reacts with the carbon dioxide. Different companies produce different colours and it is important to familiarize yourself with the colour that indicates fresh and exhausted soda lime in your practice. Soda lime is an irritant so care must be taken when handling it; wear gloves, goggles and a mask when filling a canister. It is also dangerous if inhaled by staff or patients and can cause bronchiolitis.

- **Non-rebreathing** – these rely on the flushing out of exhaled gases, including carbon dioxide, by the fresh gas inflow. They are therefore less economical and there is a loss of heat and moisture. As the exhaled gases pass out into the atmosphere, efficient scavenging is very important. These circuits are simple, relatively cheap and easily sterilized. They allow accurate control of inspired gases and soda lime is not required.

REBREATHING CIRCUITS

1. Circle system (Fig. 8.3)

This is suitable for patients over 15 kg. Flow rate = 10 ml × bodyweight per minute. There is no circuit factor and minute volume is not required.

Advantages

- Mechanical dead space remains unchanged during surgery
- Bronchiolitis is unlikely because the soda lime canister is some distance from the patient
- High gas efficiency
- Intermittent positive pressure ventilation (IPPV) can be carried out
- Less circuit inertia than with the 'to-and-fro' system (see below)

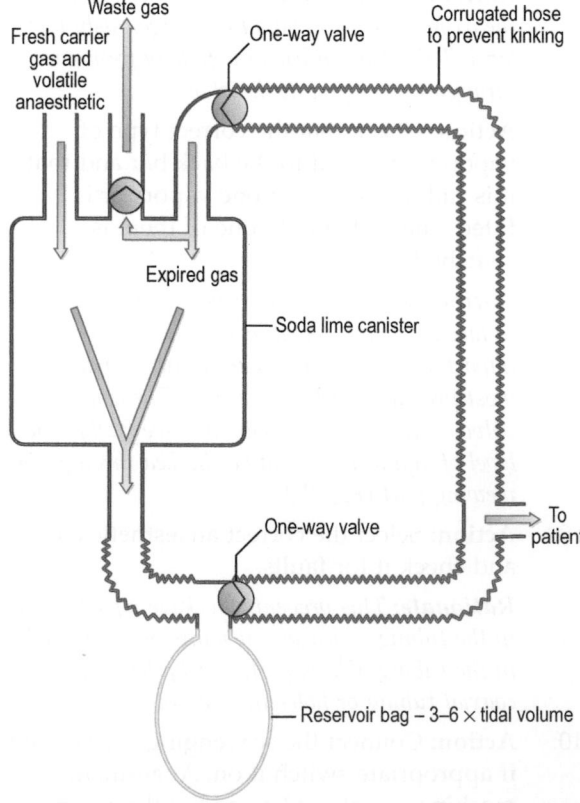

Figure 8.3 The circle system.

Box 8.1 Definitions of respiratory measurements

Tidal volume – volume of air inspired at each breath.
Respiratory rate – number of breaths per minute.
Minute volume – tidal volume × respiratory rate.
Dead space – area in which gaseous exchange does not take place. It may be the:
- **anatomical dead space**, i.e. trachea, bronchi and bronchioles
- **mechanical dead space**, i.e. endotracheal tube and exhausted area of soda lime.

Airway resistance – resistance to the flow of gas through the airway. It depends on the viscosity of the gas and the diameter and length of the circuit tubing.

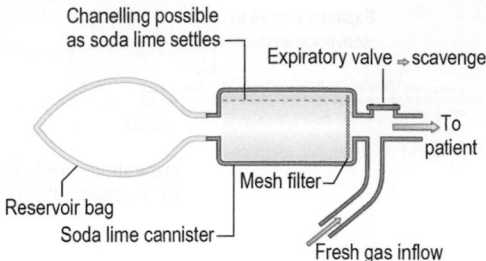

Figure 8.4 The to-and-fro system.

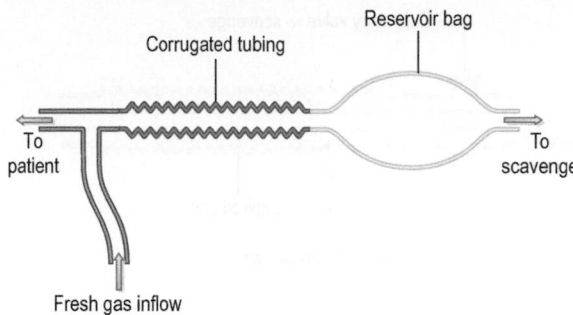

Figure 8.5 Jackson-Rees modified Ayre's T-piece.

Disadvantages

- Expensive and cumbersome
- High resistance
- Cannot use nitrous oxide
- Bulky and difficult to clean and sterilize

2. To-and-fro system (Fig. 8.4)

This is suitable for patients weighing over 15 kg. Flow rate = 10 ml × bodyweight per minute. There is no circuit factor and minute volume is not required.

Advantages

- Good heat conservation, although hyperthermia may be a problem with prolonged use
- Bi-directional flow improves the removal of carbon dioxide
- As circuit volume is low, denitrogenation (breathing out of all nitrogen in the blood) is achieved rapidly and gas concentrations can be altered quickly
- As the fresh gas inflow is close to the patient, the concentration of the volatile gas can be measured accurately
- High gas efficiency
- Less resistance
- Cheaper than a circle system

Disadvantages

- Channelling may occur in the canister if it is not completely filled with soda lime
- Mechanical dead space increases during surgery as the soda lime is exhausted
- Bronchiolitis may occur, but the risk can be minimized by placing a gauze filter at the patient end of the canister
- Sited close to the patient so may be a problem during head surgery

- Bulky and can cause a drag on the tubing
- Cannot use nitrous oxide in the circuit

NON-REBREATHING CIRCUITS

1. Jackson–Rees modified Ayre's T-piece (Fig. 8.5)

The Jackson-Rees modification includes an open-ended bag added to the expiratory tubing and is the circuit of choice for animals below 10 kg. The original Ayre's T-piece does not have a reservoir bag and is unlikely to be used in practice. Flow rate = 2.5–3 × minute volume.

Advantages

- IPPV can be carried out
- Bag movement acts as a convenient respiratory monitor
- Minimal apparatus and dead space resistance

Disadvantages

- High gas flow rates required
- The incorporation of an expiratory valve, placed just in front of the bag and using a closed bag, increases the resistance
- Scavenging is difficult if expired air is vented through an open-ended bag

2. Bain circuit (Fig. 8.6)

This is suitable for animals of 10–20 kg. Flow rate = 2.5–3.5 × minute volume.

Advantages

- Can be used for continuous IPPV
- The length of circuit between the patient and the bag improves access to the patient

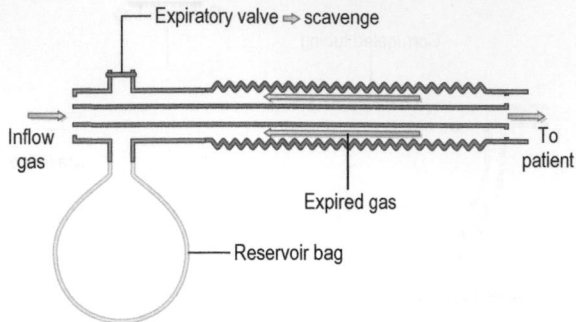

Figure 8.6 Bain circuit.

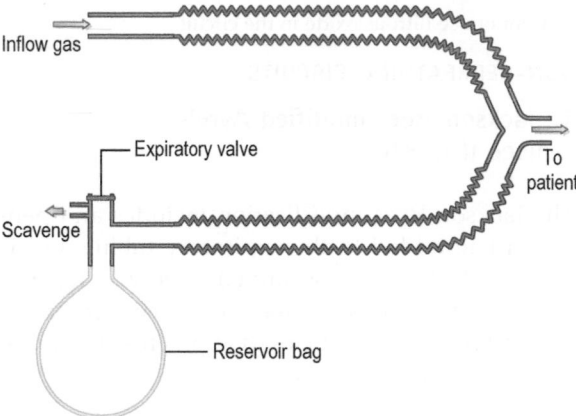

Figure 8.7 Modified Bain circuit.

- Expired air in the outer tube warms the inspired air in the inner tube of the coaxial tubing so conserving the patient's body temperature
- Low resistance and reduced mechanical dead space

Disadvantages

- The inner tube may become disconnected, which could cause rebreathing problems. Check by plugging the end with a syringe while the oxygen is flowing – the flowmeter indicator will fall if the tubing is connected
- High flow rates are required
- Higher resistance than a T-piece

NB Modified Bain (Fig. 8.7) does not use coaxial tubing so inspired air is not warmed but the expiratory tube is of a greater diameter so resistance is reduced.

3. Magill circuit (Fig. 8.8)

This is suitable for patients of over 8 kg. Flow rate = 1–1.5 × minute volume.

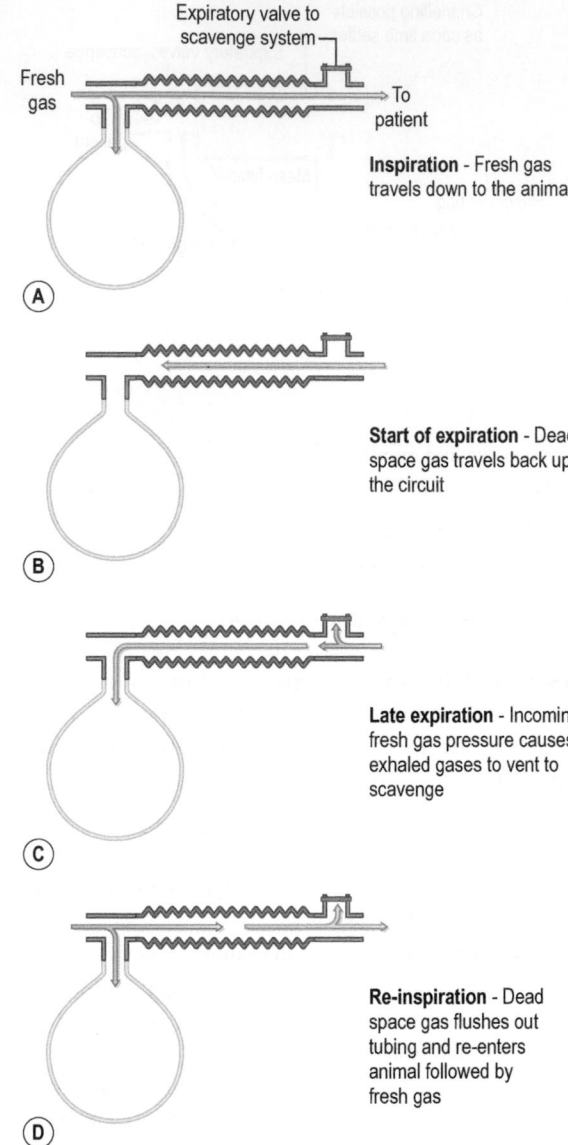

Inspiration - Fresh gas travels down to the animal

(A)

Start of expiration - Dead space gas travels back up the circuit

(B)

Late expiration - Incoming fresh gas pressure causes exhaled gases to vent to scavenge

(C)

Re-inspiration - Dead space gas flushes out tubing and re-enters animal followed by fresh gas

(D)

Figure 8.8 Movement of gas within the Magill circuit.

Advantages

- Efficient general purpose circuit
- Readily maintained and sterilized

Disadvantages

- Location of the expiratory / Heidbrink valve close to the patient is inconvenient for scavenging and surgery around the head area
- Should not be used for IPPV because rebreathing will occur and cause hypercapnia. If it is used for IPPV then

increase the flow rates to 1.5 × minute volume to flush out the carbon dioxide

- Offers considerable resistance and increased mechanical dead space

4. Lack circuit (Fig. 8.9A)

This is suitable for patients of 10–60 kg. Flow rate = 1–1.5 × minute volume.

Advantages

- The position of the expiratory valve allows improved access to the head and to the scavenging attachments
- The length of the circuit allows the anaesthetic machine to be positioned away from the patient
- Circuit is lightweight and exerts less drag than the Magill

Disadvantages

- Cannot be used properly for IPPV, but is easier than the Magill

- The coaxial tubing may become disconnected causing rebreathing

NB The **parallel Lack** circuit (Fig. 8.9B) does not use coaxial tubing, which makes maintenance easier and reduces the risk of a disconnected inner tube. The flow resistance is reduced and there is a paediatric version for animals of below 5 kg. Incoming air is not warmed. Flow rate is the same the Lack.

5. Humphrey ADE system (Fig. 8.10)

This is a relatively new system that can be used either as rebreathing or a non-rebreathing circuit because it has a soda lime canister that can be switched into or out of the circuit. It provides one system for all animals and is gaining in popularity.

Advantages

- Semi-closed mode can be used for animals under 10 kg
- Rebreathing mode is economical to use
- One system for all animals therefore saving on the expense of buying several circuit types

Disadvantages

- Expensive to buy
- Cannot be used with nitrous oxide

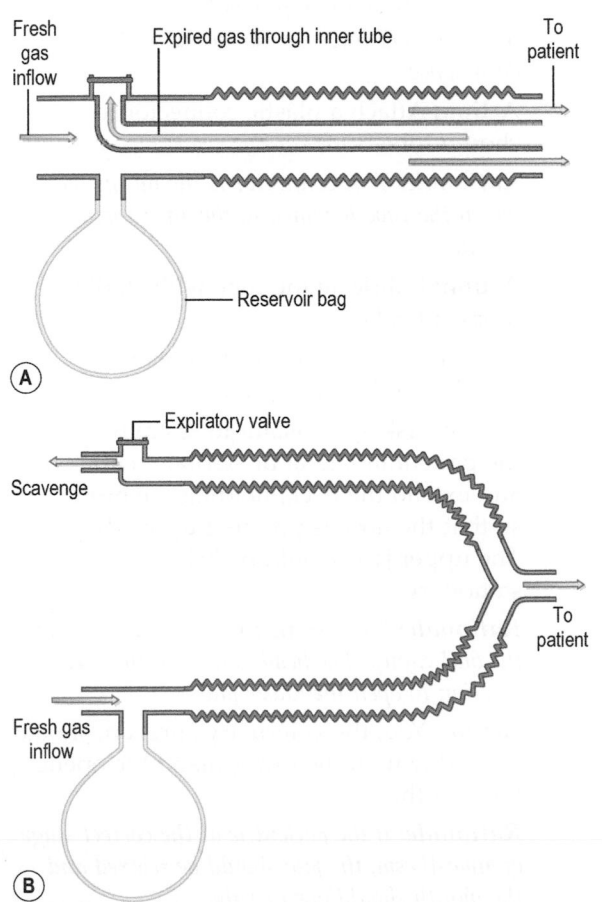

Figure 8.9 (A) The Lack circuit. (B) The parallel Lack circuit.

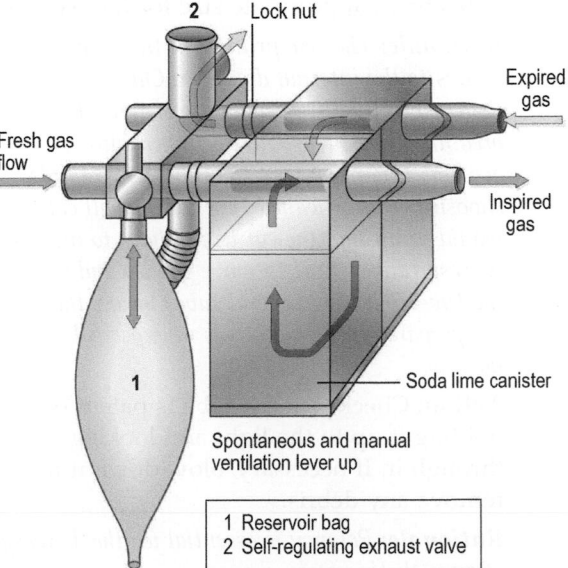

Figure 8.10 The set-up for the Humphrey ADE system.

- Difficult to clean
- Not very efficient in conserving anaesthetic gases – the Bain is 24% better

INTUBATION

This is carried out after the induction of anaesthesia and is the placing of an endotracheal tube into the patient's airway. The tube is connected to the anaesthetic circuit and is the means by which the anaesthetic gases are conducted from the machine into the patient's trachea and lungs. The typical Magill endotracheal tube is made of red rubber and has an inflatable cuff at the distal end. When inflated the cuff fills the gap between the tube and the tracheal mucosa, preventing the inhalation of debris and the animal breathing in anything but the anaesthetic mixture.

Intubation cannot be carried out until the patient is sufficiently anaesthetized. The indicative signs are:

- The jaw is relaxed
- The tongue is flaccid and can be held without resistance
- When the tube is introduced there is no gagging reflex.

Procedure: To intubate a canine or feline patient

1. **Action:** Select at least three endotracheal tubes of an appropriate size for the patient.

   Rationale: The size printed on the tubes relates to the internal diameter. Once inside the trachea the tube causes a resistance to breathing and this should be taken into account when selecting the tube; for example, choosing a thick-walled tube for a small cat would mean that the cat would have to increase its respiratory effort to move gas up and down the tube. Selecting several tubes means that you are prepared if the trachea is unexpectedly narrow.

2. **Action:** Check that the tube is patent by holding it up to the light and looking through it. If necessary, blow down it to remove any debris.

   Rationale: Patency is essential for the delivery of anaesthetic gases.

3. **Action:** Check that the tube is clean.

   Rationale: There should be no blood or debris remaining from the previous use. All cleaning fluids should have been rinsed off – these can damage the tracheal mucosa.

4. **Action:** Check that the cuff is functioning correctly by gently inflating it using a syringe.

   Rationale: If the cuff leaks it is better to throw the tube away. Leakage will enable the patient to breath fresh air around the tube thus diluting the effect of the anaesthetic mixture, and/or debris and fluid may be inhaled.

5. **Action:** Measure the length of the tube against the patient's head and neck.

   Rationale: The tube should be of sufficient length to reach to the level of the scapula. Excessive length (i.e. protruding beyond the nose) will increase the mechanical dead space.

6. **Action:** Attach a plastic connector to your chosen tube.

   Rationale: This connector is the means by which the tube is joined to the anaesthetic circuit.

7. **Action:** Lubricate the tube with sterile lubricant jelly.

   Rationale: To enable smooth atraumatic introduction into the trachea.

8. **Action:** Ask an assistant to restrain the patient in lateral or sternal recumbency and extend the neck, holding the head so that the nose is pointing upwards. The upper jaw should be held stationary.

   Rationale: This position gives good access to the oral cavity. The head is now in the correct position to open the lower jaw.

9. **Action:** You, the veterinary surgeon, should press down on the lower mandible opening the mouth.

   Rationale: If the patient is at the correct stage of anaesthesia, the jaw should be relaxed and the mouth should open easily.

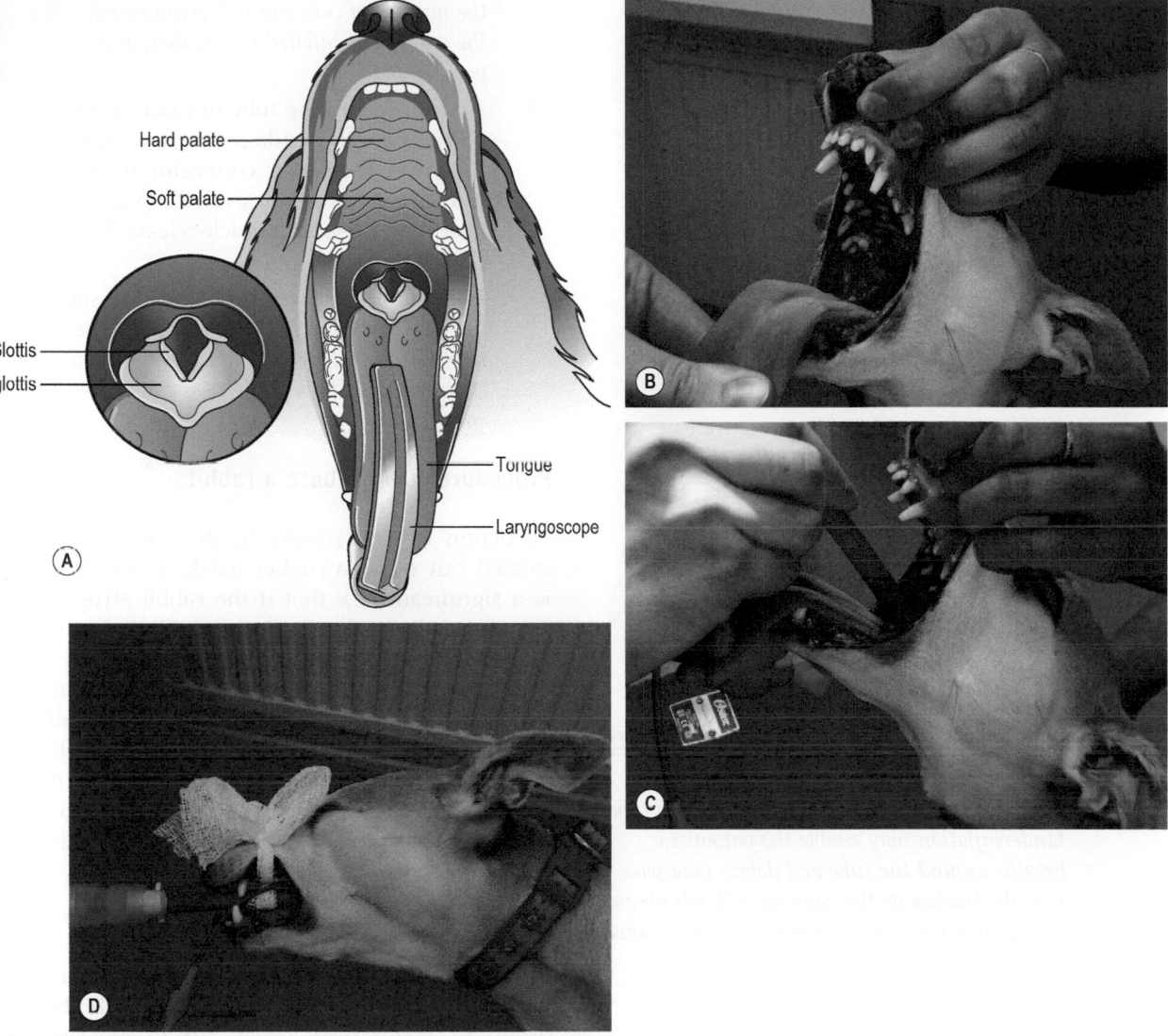

Figure 8.11 (A) Anatomy of the pharynx. Inset: When the epiglottis is depressed, the glottis is exposed. The endotracheal tube is advanced through the glottis. (B) Visualizing the pharynx and larynx prior to intubation. (C) Introducing the endotracheal tube into the larynx. (D) The cuff is inflated and the tube is secured by tying it to the upper jaw.

10. **Action:** Take hold of the tongue and pull it down until you can see the epiglottis (Fig. 8.11A, B).

    Rationale: Some people use a dry swab to hold the slippery tongue. In this position you can clearly see the anatomy of the pharynx.

11. **Action:** Using the bevelled end of the selected lubricated tube, push down the epiglottis and insert the tube between the vocal folds into the trachea (Fig. 8.11C). It may be necessary to push the soft palate dorsally.

    Rationale: The bevelled end makes insertion of the tube easier. The soft palate sometimes obscures the view of the epiglottis.

12. When intubating a cat, spray local anaesthetic onto the larynx. Introduce the tube at inhalation when the vocal folds will open.

Rationale: The feline larynx may go into spasm when it is touched. The use of local anaesthetic will prevent this.

13. **Action:** A laryngoscope may be useful when intubating cats and brachycephalic dogs.

   Rationale: The smooth blade of the handle enables the operator to move the epiglottis aside and the light illuminates the pharyngeal area.

14. **Action:** Once the tube is inserted, attach the tube to the anaesthetic circuit and ventilate the patient with 100% oxygen and apply pressure to the reservoir bag. Observe the chest movements.

   Rationale: The tube should lie within the trachea (Fig. 8.12). If the tube is pushed into one of the bronchi then only one lung will be inflated; if the tube is incorrectly placed in the oesophagus then the stomach will inflate and the animal will begin to come round.

15. **Action:** Inflate the cuff just enough to prevent oxygen escaping around the cuff.

   Rationale: Overinflation can damage the tracheal mucosa or cause occlusion of the tube. Underinflation may enable the patient to breathe around the tube and debris may pass into the trachea as the gagging reflex is absent at this depth of anaesthesia. It is easy to damage

the mucosa of cats and it is recommended that the cuff is not inflated unless there is a particular reason.

16. **Action:** Secure the tube in place using a piece of gauze bandage. Tie it around the tube over the plastic connector, then pass it over the maxilla or over the patient's head and tie with a quick-release bow (Fig. 8.11D).

   Rationale: The plastic connector will support the tube preventing it from being occluded if the tie is pulled tight. A quick-release bow enables the tie to be undone in case of an emergency.

Procedure: To intubate a rabbit

Induction of anaesthesia in the rabbit may be carried out using a rubber mask; however, there is a significant risk that if the rabbit struggles it may break its back or a limb so this technique is not recommended. An induction chamber, in which the rabbit quietly inhales the anaesthetic mixture, may be used but may be too small for some of the larger breeds. As rabbits are obligate nose breathers it is possible to obtain a small mask that fits over the nose. The rabbit will breathe through it leaving the mouth clear for dental procedures.

Rabbit intubation is a difficult technique because the glottis is small and is often covered by the long tongue, the oropharynx is narrow and the larynx is prone to spasm; however, rabbits are prone to respiratory arrest during anaesthesia and ventilation may be difficult to assist using a facemask so intubation is a useful technique to perfect. Rabbit endotracheal tubes are usually made of clear plastic and are uncuffed. There are two techniques:

1. Intubation using an otoscope

1. **Action:** Place the anaesthetized rabbit on its back on a stable operating table.

   Rationale: This position gives the optimal view into the oral cavity and the oropharynx.

2. **Action:** Administer 100% oxygen for 1–2 minutes.

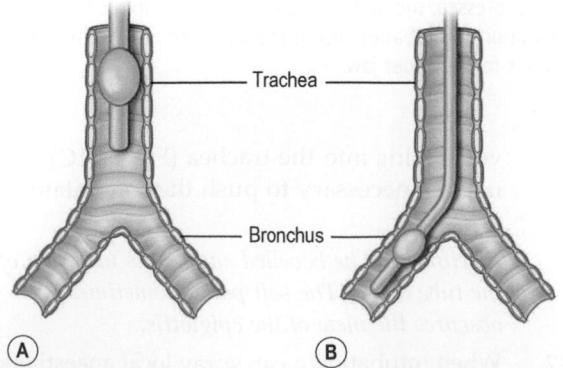

Figure 8.12 Placement of endotracheal tube in the trachea: (A) correct placement; (B) endobronchial intubation (incorrect).

Rationale: To prevent hypoxia and respiratory arrest.

3. **Action:** Standing at the head of the rabbit, bend your knees until you are approximately level with the head.

    Rationale: If necessary you can kneel on the floor, but make sure that you are comfortable and steady.

4. **Action:** Using an otoscope, advance it through the gap (diastema) between the incisor and cheek teeth until you can see the larynx.

    Rationale: For 2–4 kg rabbits use a medium speculum.

5. **Action:** If you can see the larynx, spray it with local anaesthetic spray.

    Rationale: To prevent laryngospasm.

6. **Action:** With the tip of the speculum, disengage the epiglottis from the soft palate.

    Rationale: If the tip of the epiglottis is positioned on the nasal aspect of the soft palate you may inadvertently enter the oesophagus.

7. **Action:** As you further advance the speculum you should see the larynx and should be able to pass an introducer through the speculum and into it.

    Rationale: Purpose-made introducers are available, but you can use a bitch or urinary catheter having first removed the Luer fitting as this will not pass through the tip of the speculum.

8. **Action:** When the introducer (or catheter) has been placed in the larynx, remove the otoscope by carefully sliding backwards over it.

    Rationale: Make sure that you do not shift the position of the introducer.

9. **Action:** Thread an endotracheal tube over the introducer and advance it into the trachea.

    Rationale: To ensure that the tube is positioned correctly. Uncuffed tubes of 2.5–5 mm are recommended as this allows a slightly larger internal diameter, which reduces the resistance of the circuit.

10. **Action:** Withdraw the introducer through the endotracheal tube.

    Rationale: This is no longer needed.

11. **Action:** Tie the endotracheal tube in place using a gauze bandage as described for the dog and cat.

    Rationale: To prevent the tube slipping out of the trachea.

NB Anaesthetic circuits for rabbits should have a low dead space – a T-piece or Bain is recommended. As the tidal volume is often only 5–10 ml/kg, low dead space connectors on the end of the endotracheal tube should be used.

2. Intubation using the 'blind technique'

1. **Action:** Place the anaesthetized rabbit in sternal recumbency on a stable operating table.

    Rationale: This makes it easier to insert the endotracheal tube.

2. **Action:** Administer 100% oxygen for 1–2 minutes.

    Rationale: To prevent hypoxia and respiratory arrest.

3. **Action:** Place one hand over the head of the rabbit and gently bend the neck so that the mouth is vertical.

    Rationale: This provides easy access to the oral cavity.

4. **Action:** Insert the endotracheal tube into the oral cavity through the diastema and advance it slowly down towards the larynx.

    Rationale: Placing the tube through the diastema protects it from damage by the incisor teeth.

5. **Action:** Monitor the breath sounds by putting your ear to the free end of the tube or by looking for signs of condensation within the clear tube.

    Rationale: This will show you that the end of the tube is approaching the larynx.

6. **Action:** Continue to advance the tube into the larynx. As it enters the larynx you may hear a small coughing sound.

Rationale: If you are in the larynx the breathing sounds and signs of condensation will continue; if you are in the oesophagus then they will no longer be apparent.

7. **Action:** If you have entered the oesophagus, withdraw the tube slightly, reposition the head by tilting it slightly forwards or backwards and advance the tube again.

   Rationale: Repositioning the head will slightly alter the position of the larynx, which may make the procedure a little easier.

8. **Action:** Sometimes the use of local anaesthetic spray helps intubation. This can be sprayed towards the back of the throat at maximum inspiration.

   Rationale: To prevent laryngospasm.

9. **Action:** When the tube is correctly in place, secure it using a gauze bandage tied around the tube and the back of the head. Tie with a quick release bow.

   Rationale: To prevent the tube slipping out of the trachea.

10. **Action:** Attach it to the anaesthetic circuit.

    Rationale: To ensure that anaesthesia is maintained.

NB 100% oxygen should be administered every 4 minutes while you attempt intubation to prevent the rabbit becoming hypoxic.

Procedure: Removal of the endotracheal tube – extubation

(This relates to all species.)

1. **Action:** Untie the gauze bandage holding the endotracheal tube in place when the procedure is finished.

   Rationale: This is usually done before the signs of recovery begin so that the tube can be quickly removed as the gag or swallowing reflex returns.

2. **Action:** Deflate the cuff.

   Rationale: Removing an inflated cuff may damage the tracheal mucosa. After oral surgery, the cuff may be left partially inflated to dislodge debris and blood clots in the larynx as the tube is removed.

3. **Action:** In dogs, the tube is left in place until the swallowing reflex returns. This may be deduced by curling of the tongue and slight movements of the jaw.

   Rationale: The swallowing reflex protects the airway from aspirating solid matter in the event of vomiting. If the tube is left in too long the dog may bite it in half and part of the tube may pass further down the trachea.

4. **Action:** In cats, the tube should be removed just before the swallowing reflex returns. This may be deduced by limb, head and tail movements or an active palpebral reflex.

   Rationale: Delayed extubation may result in laryngospasm.

MONITORING ANAESTHESIA

Drugs used to achieve anaesthesia do so by depression of the central nervous system (CNS) resulting in a state of unconsciousness and a varying reduction in the awareness of pain, depending on the type of drug. The particular signs of anaesthesia described for many years were related to certain anatomical levels or 'planes', which could be used to assess the progress of the 'journey' through the anaesthetic until the patient reached the correct depth. This method, originally used to help inexperienced human anaesthetists during World War I who were mainly working with diethyl ether, is now largely discounted. Nowadays we use a large range of drug types (e.g. analgesics, sedative, gaseous and volatile anaesthetics, muscle relaxants, etc.) and they have varying effects, depending on their pharmacology, their combination with others, the species of the patient, the dosage, etc., so it is impossible to produce a 'one size fits all' system of assessment. The term 'depth of anaesthesia', although now rendered obsolete, is still in common usage and must be assessed by regular and careful monitoring of the patient.

Monitoring should begin once the premedication has been given and should cease only when the animal is returned to its owner. A variety of critical parameters are used in monitoring and they are listed below – you should know what these are and how they are changed by the drug(s) that you are using. It is important to know their normal values so that you can detect and interpret any variations and alter the anaesthetic appropriately and rapidly.

It is important to be aware that the responses of rabbits to anaesthesia are different to those of the dog and the cat:

- Rabbits are never as relaxed as dogs and cats.
- The most reliable method of assessing the depth of anaesthesia is by monitoring the rate and depth of respiration. Laboured breathing and pauses between breaths indicate deep anaesthesia.
- The absence of a head shake when you pinch the ear of a rabbit indicates an acceptable level of anaesthesia.
- The pedal reflex remains for longer than in the dog and cat. The response in the forelimbs goes before that in the hindlimbs and when this is lost the rabbit is too deeply anaesthetized.
- The corneal and palpebral reflexes are similar to those in the dog and cat.

The required depth of anaesthesia in any species depends on the type of procedure being undertaken; for example, a dog undergoing radiography merely needs to be restrained, a dog undergoing a minor lumpectomy requires deeper anaesthesia, and a dog undergoing fracture fixation requires a still deeper level as well as muscle relaxation and analgesia. It is down to the skill and experience of the veterinary surgeon to achieve this by the correct selection of the drugs and management of the whole process.

MONITORING PARAMETERS

The following parameters should be routinely monitored during anaesthesia:

- Cranial nerve reflexes
- Body temperature
- Cardiovascular function
- Respiration.

Normal values are shown in Table 8.3.

Table 8.3 Normal clinical parameters used to monitor anaesthesia

Clinical parameter	Dog	Cat	Rabbit
Body temperature (°C)	38.3–38.7	38.0–38.5	38.5–40.0
Pulse or heart rate (b.p.m.)	70–120	120–180	180–300
Respiratory rate (b.p.m.)	10–20	20–30	30–60
Capillary refill time (s)	1–2	1–2	1–2
Mean arterial blood pressure (mmHg)	60–120	60–120	–
Normal pH of blood	7.31–7.41	7.24–7.40	–
Oxygen saturation (%)	99	99	–
P_aO_2 – room air (mmHg); – 100% O_2 (mmHg)	85–105 500	100–115 500	–
P_aCO_2 (mmHg)	29–42	29–42	–

Procedure: Monitoring the depth of anaesthesia using cranial nerve reflexes

1. **Action:** Palpebral reflex – lightly touch the medial canthus of the eye to stimulate a blink.

   Rationale: Present in light anaesthesia, but may become sluggish if repeated too frequently. Should be very slow or absent to indicate an adequate depth for surgical procedures.

2. **Action:** Corneal reflex – gently touch the cornea with a moistened cotton bud to stimulate a blink.

   Rationale: Not very useful as it may be present even in deep anaesthesia. Best used to ascertain brain death.

3. **Action:** Eye position – as the depth increases the eye moves to a ventromedial position and then returns to the centre.

Rationale: May be confusing as the eye is in a central position when the animal is both light and deep, but when the animal is deeply anaesthetized there is no palpebral reflex. In ketamine anaesthesia the eye remains in a central position.

4. **Action:** Pupil diameter – pupil dilates as the depth of anaesthesia increases, but it should remain responsive to light.

   Rationale: This reflex may be influenced by drugs such as atropine and ketamine.

5. **Action:** Jaw tone – during light anaesthesia the jaw tone is strong, but this decreases as the depth increases.

   Rationale: During light anaesthesia the animal may move its jaws.

6. **Action:** Tongue curl – during light anaesthesia the tongue may curl when the jaw is opened.

   Rationale: This is a useful indicator when preparing to intubate. If the tongue curls when the mouth is opened then the depth of anaesthesia should be increased.

7. **Action:** Lacrimation – present during light anaesthesia, but absent in deeper planes.

   Rationale: The cornea should be protected by the use of ocular lubricants. This is particularly important in rabbits as they have more protuberant eyes.

8. **Action:** Salivation – may be profuse in light planes of anaesthesia.

   Rationale: The use of ketamine will increase salivation.

NB Although the pedal reflex is not a cranial nerve reflex it is widely used to assess the depth of anaesthesia. Absence of withdrawal when the web between the toes is pinched indicates that a surgical plane of anaesthesia has been reached.

Procedure: Monitoring the body temperature during anaesthesia

Anaesthesia disrupts the body's ability to maintain its temperature within normal limits. It depresses the CNS response to temperature change, such as shivering or muscular movement, and core temperature may fall drastically. Hypothermia is more common during anaesthesia than hyperthermia and patients that are most prone to it are those with a thin or a wet coat, those that are metabolically compromised and those that have a small volume to surface area ratio (i.e. small exotic species such as guinea pigs and hamsters).

The following steps must be taken to minimize heat loss during anaesthesia:

- Clip as small an area as possible around the surgical site, but it must still be aseptic.
- Wrap the body in bubble wrap or space blankets.
- Use heat pads, hot water bottles, etc., taking care to avoid burning the patient, as it is unable to move away from the heat source.
- Increase the ambient temperature – operating lights also help.
- Avoid the use of spirit-based surgical scrubs in small exotic species.
- Check the body temperature every 15 minutes during surgery and continue until the patient regains consciousness.
- Remember that heat is lost from rebreathing circuits (e.g. T-piece, Magill, etc.).

  1. **Action:** Feel the patient's extremities at regular intervals.

     Rationale: This will give you an estimate of the body temperature, but tells you little about the core temperature.

  2. **Action:** Measure temperature using a rectal thermometer.

     Rationale: Provides a measurement of peripheral temperature.

  3. **Action:** Measure core temperature using an oesophageal thermometer.

     Rationale: Core temperature is the most significant parameter as shocked animals may have a low peripheral temperature but an adequate core temperature.

The effects of hypothermia are:

- Increases the depth of anaesthesia by depressing CNS activity
- Reduces cardiac output
- Increases blood viscosity
- Increases the risk of cardiac arrhythmias
- Increases the recovery time.

Procedure: Monitoring cardiovascular function during anaesthesia

Increasing the depth of anaesthesia by increasing the amount of anaesthetic drug may have a deleterious effect on the heart and the lungs, resulting in tissue hypoxia and even death, and this is likely to be a limiting factor to the anaesthetic regimen as a whole. Nowadays there are many technological aids to monitor the cardiovascular system, but there is nothing to beat regular accurate observation of the clinical signs and the correct use of a stethoscope.

1. **Heart rate and rhythm** – Use a stethoscope as follows.
   - **Action:** Palpate the apex beat.
     Rationale: Used when the peripheral pulse is difficult to detect.
   - **Action:** Precordial auscultation.
     Rationale: Useful, but positioning and draping of the operation site may make it difficult.
   - **Action:** Oesophageal auscultation using an oesophageal stethoscope.
     Rationale: Place stethoscope into the oesophagus so that the tip lies next to the heart – this is critical. It is good for non-oral surgery. The nurse can remain remote from the patient.

2. **Pulse rate and quality** – **Action:** Digital palpation of a peripheral artery should be carried out every 5 minutes. Use femoral, lingual, facial, digital and coccygeal arteries.
   Rationale: Peripheral arteries will be the first to indicate developing hypotension – the pulse will be absent or weak. Pulse rate should be the same as the heart rate.

3. **Mucous membrane colour** – **Action:** Check the colour of the gums at regular intervals. Pigmentation of the gums may obscure your observations, in which case use the conjunctiva or inside the vulval lips.
   Rationale: Used to assess tissue perfusion and oxygenation. The normal colour is pale salmon pink. Mucous membranes become pale in cases of anaemia, vasoconstriction and hypotension, blue

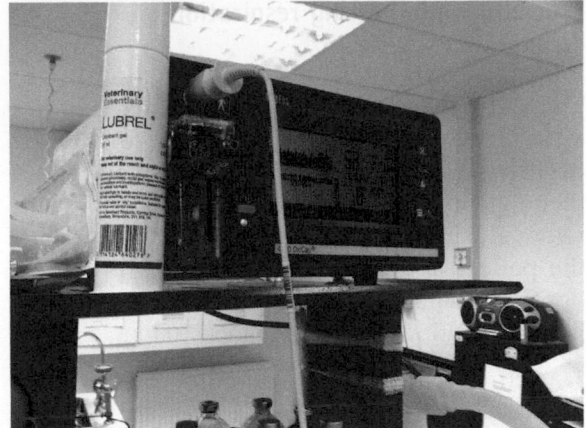

Figure 8.13 Pulsoximeter machine measuring pulse rate and percentage saturation of oxygen.

in cyanosis, brick red in hypercapnia, and yellow with jaundice.

4. **Capillary refill time** – **Action:** Press on the gum and then release. Time the return to normal colour. You can also pinch a non-pigmented claw.
   Rationale: Indicates tissue perfusion. Normal capillary refill time is 1–2 seconds.

NB Dead animals may still show refill for a time.

5. **Pulse rate and haemoglobin levels** – **Action:** A pulse oximeter (Fig. 8.13) is attached to the tongue, lip, vulval labia, prepuce or toe web.
   Rationale: Gives an audible 'beep' at every pulse. Also measures oxygen saturation of blood expressed as a percentage.

6. **Heart rate** – **Action:** Electrocardiography using a cardiac monitor records the electrical activity of the heart.
   Rationale: It may detect arrhythmias – although only some arrhythmias are important whereas others such as sinus arrhythmia, are not.

7. **Blood pressure** – **Action:** Indirect measurement using a cuff is the most common method, but results may be unreliable in small dogs and cats.
   Rationale: The cuff occludes arterial blood flow distal to the cuff; as it is deflated the pressure of the returning blood flow is detected.

Procedure: Monitoring respiration during anaesthesia

The body tissues must be well oxygenated during anaesthesia and this is achieved by providing an oxygen-enriched carrier gas for the volatile anaesthetic agent. However, respiration must also ensure removal of waste gases; if the respiratory rate of the patient is within normal parameters but the depth is shallow the waste gases may be accumulating, resulting in a rise in blood pH.

1. **Action:** Observe the effect of the chest movements on the reservoir bag.

   Rationale: The respiratory rate can be measured by counting the movements of the bag.

2. **Action:** Use of a respiratory monitor.

   Rationale: Detects the difference in temperature between the cool inspired air and the warmer expired air. Does not register depth of respiration.

3. **Action:** Use of a capnograph.

   Rationale: Measures the adequacy of respiration – probes are connected between the endotracheal tube and the anaesthetic circuit and measure the respiratory rate and levels of carbon dioxide in each breath, which provides information about the efficiency of gas exchange. High levels of carbon dioxide indicate hypercapnia and subsequent acidosis. More advanced monitors also measure inspired and expired oxygen content.

4. **Action:** Use of pulse oximeter.

   Rationale: Measures oxygen tension of patient's blood as a percentage and an audible beep highlights the pulse rate. Sensor is attached to tongue, interdigital web, lip, vulva or prepuce as appropriate.

5. **Action:** Apnoea alert monitors.

   Rationale: An alarm is triggered after a period of apnoea. The time interval can be set by the operator.

6. **Action:** Blood gas analysis.

   Rationale: Used in equine anaesthesia, but rarely in small animal practice. A blood sample is collected from a peripheral artery and analysed for levels of oxygen, carbon dioxide, bicarbonate and various electrolytes. This detects adequacy of ventilation, oxygen supply and respiratory and metabolic imbalances, enabling them to be corrected.

ANAESTHETIC EMERGENCIES

In most anaesthetic emergencies the final consequence is hypoxia of the tissues. This is particularly serious for the brain cells, which are easily damaged, and loss of oxygen for even a short time may result in a loss of intelligence and change in nature. Hypoxia of the myocardium reduces contractility and, if coupled with hypercapnia, may precipitate cardiac arrest. Lack of oxygen to the liver and kidneys may cause damage that may not be apparent until after recovery from the anaesthetic. To ensure that tissues are oxygenated the blood must carry an adequate supply of oxygen and the circulation must be in such as state as to be able to carry the blood to and from the tissues. Monitoring should ensure that this is occurring, while resuscitation is aimed at reinstating oxygen levels and the removal of waste from the tissues.

Most emergencies can be prevented by monitoring and avoiding becoming overconfident with a familiar anaesthetic regimen. Problems may arise suddenly and catastrophe can be averted by recognizing the cause and applying the appropriate remedy, but most serious emergencies are the result of a summation of smaller problems that have been ignored or not noticed. Most disasters can be avoided by accurate assessment of the patient preoperatively, thus identifying where a problem might occur, and by careful monitoring during the anaesthetic. The most frequent time for emergencies is during the recovery period, when hypotension, lack of a protected airway, shivering and relapse into unconsciousness are the most common.

A resuscitation regimen should follow a simple 'A for airway, B for breathing, C for circulation' routine. This is an oversimplification, but it provides a straightforward mantra on which to base both monitoring and resuscitation protocols. It is essential that, in any anaesthetic emergency, cerebral circulation is restored within 3 minutes to prevent irreversible brain damage.

Resuscitation must be performed rapidly and this is facilitated by having a well-stocked emergency kit. You may consider that the whole practice is one big emergency kit, but time is wasted by rushing around opening cupboards trying to find the correct equipment. Table 8.4 lists the contents of a kit and it is important to make sure that it is regularly checked and restocked with in-date drugs. Table 8.5 provides a list of potential anaesthetic emergencies and their treatment. Figure 8.14 provides an algorithm to follow in cases of any emergency.

Table 8.4 Suggested contents of an anaesthetic emergency kit

Contents	Action	Rationale
Epinephrine (adrenaline) (0.05–0.1 mg/kg)	Increases cardiac output by increasing heart rate and force	Cardiac arrest; unresponsive hypotension
Atropine (0.02–0.05 mg/kg)	Vagolytic	Bradycardia
Doxapram (5–10 mg/kg)	Respiratory and central nervous stimulant	Apnoea; respiratory arrest
Dobutamine (Dogs: 2.5–20 µg/kg/min; Cats: 1–5 µg/kg/min by constant i.v. infusion)	Increases the force of cardiac contractions	Hypotension
Lidocaine (Dogs: 1–6 mg/kg; Cats: 0.25–1.0 mg/kg)	Antidysrhythmic	Ventricular premature contractions and ventricular tachycardia
Naloxone (0.01–0.02 mg/kg)	Reverses the effect of opioid agonists	Reverse accidental overdose of pethidine, fentanyl, morphine, etorphine
Dexamethasone (1–2 mg/kg)	Anti-inflammatory	Treatment of shock
Atipamezole (Dogs 0.05–0.2 mg/kg; Cats 0.5 mg/kg)	Reverses the effects of alpha$_2$-agonists	Reverse accidental overdose of medetomidine, xylazine and detomidine
Sodium bicarbonate (1.0 mmol/kg)	Alkali	Reversal of metabolic acidosis
Propranolol (Dogs 0.02–0.08 mg/kg; Cats: 0.02–0.06 mg/kg i.v. slowly)	Non-selective beta blocker	Management of cardiac arrhythmias
Tracheostomy tube	To perform emergency tracheostomy	Laryngeal or oropharyngeal obstruction
Syringes and needles in a range of sizes	For the administration of drugs	—
Intravenous catheters, giving set and tape	To administer intravenous fluids	Hypovolaemic shock

Table 8.4 *Continued*

Contents	Action	Rationale
Swabs, emergency surgical kit and dressing materials	To perform cardiac massage via a thoracotomy incision	Cardiac arrest
A range of endotracheal tubes (these may be kept within the prep room for everyday use)	Maintains a clear airway and conducts oxygen into the lungs	Patients should be intubated in all emergencies if possible to keep the airway clear and allow attachment to an anaesthetic machine ensuring adequate oxygenation
Defibrillator and paddles	Shocks the heart from a chaotic non-pulse-producing rhythm to normal sinus rhythm – can be used externally or internally	Cardiac arrest caused by ventricular fibrillation or rapid ventricular tachycardia – rare causes of arrest in dogs and cats

Table 8.5 Anaesthetic emergencies

Emergency	Potential cause	Signs	Action
Premature awakening	Most likely to be due to machine/circuit problems or to choice of anaesthetic drug	Apnoea or transient hypoventilation; spontaneous movement; exaggerated breathing; tachycardia; awareness of pain	Check anaesthetic machine and circuit for leakage or other evidence of malfunction Check vaporizer controls for correct level of administration Check that the cuff of the ET tube is inflated and that the tube is in the correct position
Bradypnoea or apnoea	May be a normal symptom of induction or of an anaesthetic that acts as a respiratory depressant. May be serious if it occurs during the operative period	Slow or absence of breathing; spasmodic contractions of the diaphragm; dilated pupils; cyanosis; no movements of the reservoir bag	Administer 100% oxygen by IPPV Give respiratory stimulants (e.g. doxapram)
Tachypnoea	Associated with deeper planes of anaesthesia or is related to hypercapnia, hypoxia, hypotension and hyperthermia	Fast, shallow breathing	Check for any obvious cause and instigate appropriate treatment If tachypnoea interferes with the surgical procedure use IPPV to override the natural rhythm

Table 8.5 *Continued*

Emergency	Potential cause	Signs	Action
Hypercapnia	Caused by excessive carbon dioxide production by the tissues or by impaired elimination by the lungs, e.g. hypoventilation due to respiratory depression by anaesthetic, airway obstruction, restriction of the thoracic cavity, pleural space occupying disorders (e.g. pneumothorax), excessive circuit dead space, failure of soda lime absorption	Hypoventilation; cyanosis Low reading on capnograph	Observe reading on the capnograph for P_aCO_2 Identify the problem and treat appropriately if possible Administer 100% oxygen by IPPV
Hypoxia	May be due to low flow rate of inspired oxygen, low oxygen levels in the cylinder, excessive circuit dead space, hypoventilation, low cardiac output	Cyanosis; eventual cardiac arrest	Observe reading on the pulse oximeter P_aO_2 Check anaesthetic circuit and flow rates Identify the problem and treat appropriately if possible. Administer 100% oxygen by IPPV
Airway obstruction	If it occurs before intubation consider presence of a tumour or other mass, pharyngeal or laryngeal collapse, e.g. brachycephalic breeds If it occurs post intubation consider ET problems: blockage, e.g. dried debris or lubricant, kinking, bevelled end positioned against the tracheal wall	Non-productive respiratory effort; inspiratory snoring; cyanosis; eventual cardiac arrest	If this is expected pre-oxygenate for 5 minutes before induction – this delays the onset of hypoxia. Prepare to use a smaller ET tube. Be careful not to dislodge a mass into the trachea If obstruction is unexpected check the ET tube and its position If necessary, perform an emergency tracheostomy (see Ch. 3) Administer 100% oxygen by IPPV
Vasoconstriction	Increase in sympathetic tone, which may be caused by hypovolaemia, hypothermia or hypercapnia. May be common during the excitement stage of recovery. It impairs perfusion of the visceral tissue	Pale mucous membranes; prolonged capillary refill time; cool extremities; oliguria	Identify the underlying cause and treat appropriately. Do not administer vasodilator drugs
Hypotension	May be due to hypovolaemia, reduced cardiac output, e.g. due to anaesthetic drugs or some forms of heart disease or peripheral vasodilation caused by, e.g. sepsis, certain drugs such as propofol, surface rewarming of hypothermic patients	Prolonged capillary refill time; pale mucous membranes; weak thready pulse	Administer fluid therapy and epinephrine or dobutamine

Table 8.5 *Continued*

Emergency	Potential cause	Signs	Action
Hypothermia	May be due to excessive use of water, spirit-based surgical scrubs, cold uninsulated operating table, cold environment, exposed body cavity, removal of hair from a large area and size of patient (small animals lose more heat than larger ones)	Cold extremities; low body temperature; bradycardia; pale mucous membranes; prolonged recovery time; reduced anaesthetic requirement; cardiac arrest	Identify the problem and instigate appropriate measures (see monitoring during anaesthesia) Minimize surgical time Monitor body temperature every 5 minutes during recovery and then every 15 minutes until full recovery If patient is shivering, provide oxygen-enriched environment until full recovery
Bradycardia	May be due to deep anaesthesia, excessive vagal tone caused by pressure by stimulation of the pharynx, larynx or trachea by the ET tube, traction on the viscera, some drugs and hypothyroidism	Slow heart rate of less than 60 b.p.m. in dogs and 60–80 b.p.m. in cats; reduced cardiac output and tissue perfusion	Identify the cause and instigate appropriate measures Administer 100% oxygen by IPPV Give vagolytic drugs (e.g. atropine)
Tachycardia	Light level of anaesthesia, pain, hypovolaemia, hypotension, hypercapnia, sepsis, some drugs and organ failure	Fast heart rate of over 180–200 b.p.m. in dogs and 240 b.p.m. in cats	Identify the cause and instigate appropriate measures Use of beta blockers (e.g. propanol)

Procedure: Anaesthetic emergency protocol

1. Airway
   - **Action:** Ensure that the airway is patent by looking into the mouth, clear the pharynx with your fingers, extend the tongue, loosen the collar and extend the head.

     Rationale: The larynx may become blocked with blood or saliva. It must be clear to allow the passage of air/oxygen into the lungs.
   - **Action:** Intubate using the appropriate-sized tube.

     Rationale: To ensure a good supply of oxygen.
2. Breathing
   - **Action:** Attach the endotracheal tube to an appropriate circuit.

     Rationale: Use a non-rebreathing circuit appropriate to the size of the animal – a Bain is preferred.

   - **Action:** Supply 100% oxygen.

     Rationale: To ensure optimal oxygenation.
   - **Action:** Patient should be in right lateral recumbency. Compress the chest wall in an area immediately caudodorsal to the heart in medium / large dogs and directly over the heart in small dogs and cats. Begin chest compressions every 5 seconds (see Fig. 3.5).

     Rationale: To circulate oxygen around the body in the blood, expiration of carbon dioxide and to encourage a return to autonomous respiration.
   - **Action:** If the chest starts to move and the colour of the mucous membranes returns to normal, autonomous respiration has restarted.

     Rationale: Continue to monitor the patient for at least 10 minutes as respiration may stop again. Do not detach from the circuit until the swallowing reflex is clearly present.

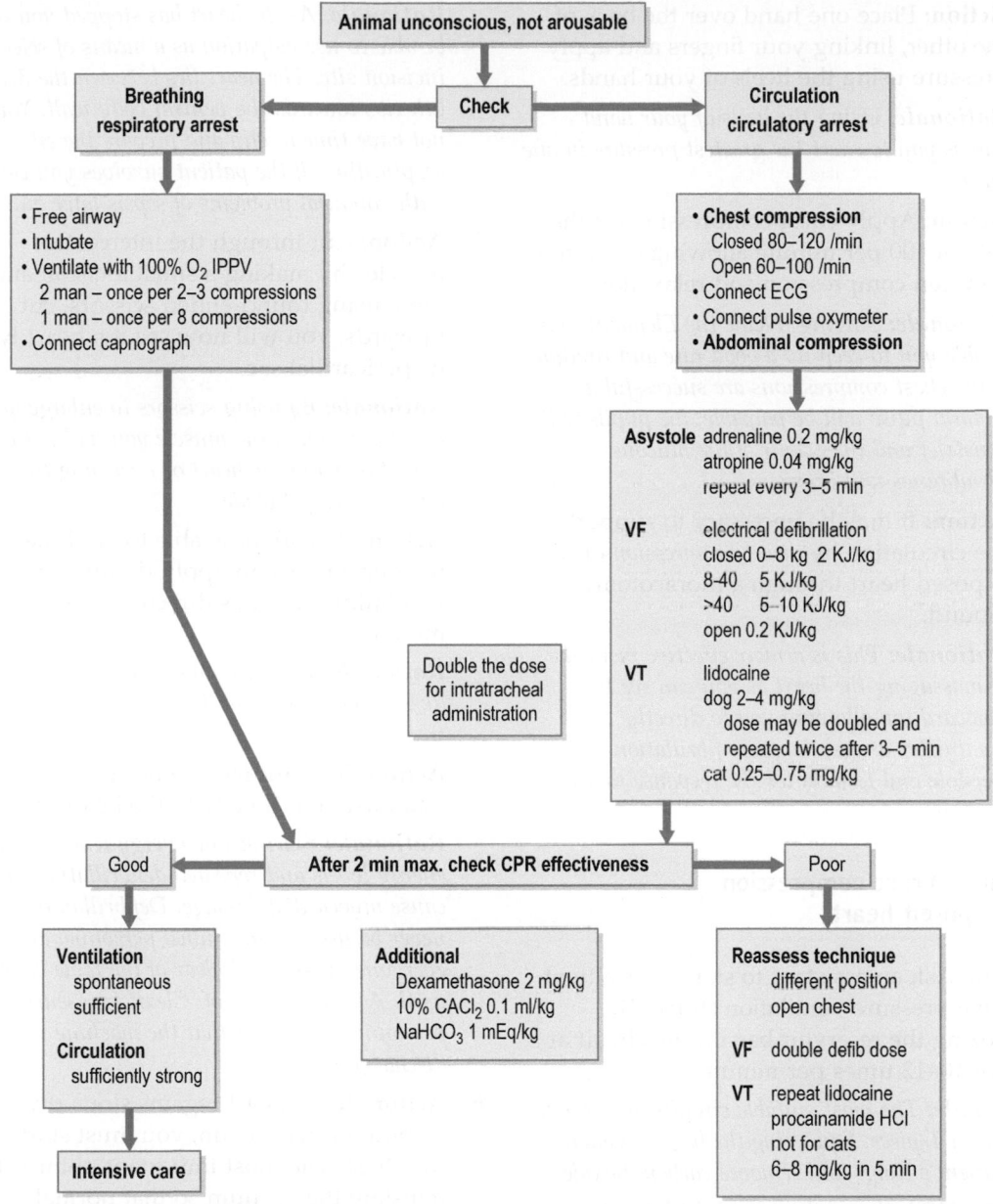

Figure 8.14 Life support algorithm. (Adapted with permission from How, K.L., Fleens, N., Stokhof, A.A., Hellebrekers, L.J., 2001. Current concepts in resuscitation of dogs and cats. EKCAP 11, 19–26, originally printed in 'het Tijdschrift voor Diergeneeskunde' (NL)).

3. Circulation

- **Action:** Support the circulation by *external thoracic massage*. Patient should be in right lateral recumbency. Compress the chest wall in an area immediately caudodorsal to the heart in

medium / large dogs and directly over the heart in small dogs and cats (see Fig. 3.5).

Rationale: This position ensures that the hands are as close as possible to the heart on the outside of the body.

- **Action:** Place one hand over the back of the other, linking your fingers and apply pressure using the heels of your hands.

  Rationale: Using the heels of your hand allows you to exert the greatest pressure in one place.

- **Action:** Apply chest compressions at the rate of 100 per minute allowing equal time between compression and relaxation.

  Rationale: Singing 'Nellie the Elephant' will enable you to keep up a good rate and rhythm. If the chest compressions are successful a femoral pulse will be palpable, the pupils will constrict and the colour of the mucous membranes will improve.

- **Action:** It may be necessary to support the circulation by *direct compression* of the exposed heart through a thoracotomy wound.

  Rationale: This is a more effective method of massaging the heart as you can see the myocardium allowing you to directly administer drugs, diagnose fibrillation or asystole and to monitor the response to direct pressure.

Procedure: Direct compression of the exposed heart

1. **Action:** Ask an assistant to start intermittent positive pressure ventilation (IPPV) by squeezing the reservoir bag on the circuit at a rate of 10–12 times per minute.

   Rationale: The most suitable circuits are a circle, Bain or a T-piece. Squeezing the bag oxygenates the patient's lungs and removes carbon dioxide.

2. **Action:** With the patient in right lateral recumbency, select an area immediately over the heart, part the fur and make an incision with a scalpel blade running from dorsal to ventral through the skin and superficial chest muscles.

   Rationale: As the heart has stopped you will not be able to use palpation as a means of selecting the incision site. The heart lies between the 3rd and 6th ribs towards the ventral body wall. You will not have time to clip and prepare the site aseptically – if the patient survives you can deal with potential problems of sepsis later on.

3. **Action:** Cut through the intercostals muscles by making a small incision and then, using round-ended scissors, cut upwards. You will now see the heart lying in its pericardial sac.

   Rationale: By using scissors to enlarge your incision through the muscle you will reduce the risk of incising the heart or overlying lung tissue with the scalpel blade.

4. **Action:** You are now able to hold the heart in your hands and apply rhythmic pressure or to administer drugs directly to the heart muscle.

   Rationale: This also allows you to monitor directly how the heart is responding to treatment.

5. **Action:** If necessary a defibrillator can be administered directly to the heart muscle.

   Rationale: Start at low energy levels as high energy levels and repeated defibrillation can cause myocardial damage. Defibrillators should never be used by untrained personnel and everyone must stand clear of the table before it is used. A warning cry of 'Clear' is essential to alert personnel to the fact that the machine is about to discharge.

6. **Action:** If the heart regains sinus rhythm and respiration has begun, you must start to close the chest. The most important point is to reinstate the vacuum so that normal respiration can take place.

   Rationale: Only a small percentage of patients survive this drastic procedure, but it is always worth trying to revive the animal.

   For suture techniques see Chapter 10.

CHAPTER 9
Theatre practice

CHAPTER CONTENTS

Before undertaking a surgical procedure, whether it is minor (e.g. blood sampling) or major (e.g. a bitch spay or an exploratory laparotomy), it is vital that you consider all the steps involved in aseptic preparation. Any technique that involves the breaching of the skin, which acts as the body's primary barrier against the outside environment, must be carried out under sterile conditions. Even a simple injection risks the introduction of pathogens into the body, and when opening up a body cavity the risk of infection is far greater.

To ensure asepsis within the operating theatre, each surgical procedure should be classified according to the degree of infection (Table 9.1) and this should be taken into account when organizing the day's operating list. To reduce the chances of breaking asepsis, always start with the clean procedures and progress through the operations, finishing with the dirty ones.

Every aspect of a surgical procedure must be prepared aseptically and this includes:

- Preparation of the surgical environment
- Sterilization of all instruments and drapes and anything that may come into contact with the surgical site
- Preparation of the surgical site
- The surgical scrub
- Donning suitable sterile surgical attire.

Although preparation of the surgical environment may be largely done by your nursing team, it is important that you, the veterinary surgeon, understand the principles behind this vital job. It takes very little disruption to any of the routine procedures to compromise asepsis, which may lead to wound breakdown, systemic infection, reduced surgical success rate and thus inevitably the reputation of the practice.

PREPARATION OF THE SURGICAL ENVIRONMENT

Surgical procedures are carried out within a dedicated operating theatre. The preparation of the

Table 9.1 Classification of surgical procedures

Classification	Types of procedure	Comment
Clean	Non-traumatic elective procedures; orthopaedic procedures with no connection to traumatic wounds; simple tumour removals	Gastrointestinal, respiratory and urinary tracts are not entered; asepsis maintained throughout; no acute inflammation
Clean-contaminated	Ovariohysterectomy and orchidectomy	Procedures in which the gastrointestinal, respiratory and urinary tracts are entered but there is no spread of contents; minor break in aseptic technique
Contaminated	Cystotomy, enterotomy, urethostomy, fresh traumatic wounds that are less than 4 hours old	There is no infection but if there is spillage of contents there is a risk of contamination; major break in aseptic technique
Dirty	Abscess, pyometra, traumatic wounds of more than 4 hours duration, perforated viscera with the presence of pus	Pus is present and area involved in surgical procedure is infected

patient and some dirty procedures (e.g. tooth cleaning) may be carried out in the preparation room. To ensure a high standard of asepsis, practice protocols should include a strict monthly, weekly and daily cleaning routine for the operating theatre and preparation room. This is almost always carried out by the nursing staff, but it is the job of the veterinary surgeon to make sure that the task is being carried out effectively.

It is not the brief of this book to describe cleaning protocols, but there are rules governing the use of the operating theatre that should be adhered to if asepsis is to be maintained:

1. The theatre should contain only the equipment that is strictly necessary for the surgical procedure and it should be removed afterwards.
2. Only personnel involved in the procedure should be present in the theatre and should remain within the sterile area to minimize the risk of cross contamination.
3. The surgeon should concentrate on the procedure and should not be talking excessively. The act of talking releases droplets full of bacteria.
4. Body movements should be restricted as much as possible to reduce air movement and the chance of contamination.
5. All personnel should understand that they are either sterile or non-sterile and there should be no cross contamination between the two.
6. Sterile and non-sterile equipment should be identified and grouped separately and kept a reasonable distance apart to reduce the risk of cross contamination.
7. Sterile tables are sterile only at table height; gowns are sterile only from mid-chest to waist; gloved hands are sterile only from the tips of the fingers to 2 inches (5 cm) above the elbow.
8. Always hold your sterile hands together above waist height and when passing another sterilized person you should pass back to back to avoid contamination.
9. All waste must be disposed of correctly and efficiently.

STERILIZATION OF SURGICAL EQUIPMENT

Sterilization may be defined as the destruction of all micro-organisms including bacterial spores. It is much more effective than disinfection, which destroys or removes micro-organisms but does not destroy bacterial spores.

Everything that comes into contact with the surgical site must be sterilized prior to use. This includes all instruments, drapes, swabs and all the equipment used for the procedure (e.g. orthopaedic screws, plates, fixators, drill bits, urinary catheters, feeding tubes, etc.). If sterilization is not carried out properly there is a risk of introducing infection into the body and/or the wound, which may result in wound breakdown and/or systemic infection.

Sterilization can be achieved by various methods:

1. **Irradiation** – the use of gamma irradiation can be carried out only in a controlled environment and is not done in practice. Prepackaged items such as needles and syringes are sterilized in this way.

2. **Heat** – micro-organisms are killed by high temperatures and the different methods aim to raise the temperature as high as possible.

   • **Boiling water** – this is the simplest form of sterilization, but it is not always the most reliable. Instruments may be sterilized in boiling water, but it must be kept at a rollicking boil for at least 10 minutes. It can be used when nothing else is available, but there is a risk of melting some plastic items and blunting others.

   • **Dry heat** – using a hot air oven. Micro-organisms are killed by oxidative destruction of their protoplasm, but they are more resistant to this if there is a dry atmosphere. To counteract this a hot air oven is designed to reach higher temperatures of 150–180°C. If the temperature is below 140°C then microbial spores will not be killed in less than 4–5 hours.

   These ovens are used to sterilize equipment such as orthopaedic drill bits, glass syringes and other glass equipment, cutting instruments and powder and oil that cannot be sterilized in the presence of moisture. Fabric, plastic and rubber will be damaged by the high temperatures.

The disadvantage of a hot air oven is that a long cooling period is needed before the instruments can be handled and the moment the door of the oven is opened there is a risk of contamination by airborne organisms. There is also a risk of burning yourself and for this reason they are not recommended by the Health and Safety Executive (HSE).

   • **Moist heat (steam) under pressure** – this is the most common method in a practice. Under normal circumstances water cannot reach temperatures higher than boiling point before producing steam but if pressure is applied, the boiling point is raised and the temperature of the steam is higher. The moisture in the steam increases the permeability of the packs of instruments and drapes to heat, which then kills the micro-organisms.

   a. **Pressure cooker** – simple form of an autoclave. Water is boiled in an enclosed space and the air vent in the lid is closed when all the air has been driven out. The pressure then builds up to 15 p.s.i. ($\approx$107 kPa). There is a risk of trapping a layer of air under the steam and this may not reach sufficient temperatures to sterilize effectively. The system is manually operated so there is room for human error.

   b. **Autoclave** – there are various designs the most efficient of which are vacuum assisted and incorporate a second cycle, which removes moisture and dries the load. Most are fully automatic with a choice of programmes and have fail-safe mechanisms.

   Effective sterilization relies on loading the packs of instruments, etc. correctly, making sure that there is adequate space for the free circulation of steam. Instruments must be free of grease and protein to enable the steam to penetrate and the autoclave must not be overloaded otherwise there is a risk of blocking the inlet and exhaust valves.

3. **Cold chemicals** – these are not always very effective and it usually takes at least 24 hours to ensure adequate sterility. Instruments and

other equipment are soaked in alcohol-based chemicals or glutaraldehyde. The method is sometimes used to sterilize needles and suture materials in a shallow dish ready for use in emergencies. Chlorhexidine may also be used, but it has poor activity against bacterial spores, fungi and viruses so this is really only a form of disinfection.

4. **Ethylene oxide** – this gas sterilizes by inactivating the pathogen's DNA thus preventing its replication. The sterilizer is in the form of a plastic container fitted with a ventilation system. Items to be sterilized are placed in a sealed polythene bag with a gas ampoule, which is then snapped from the outside to release the gas that permeates through the bag. Sterilization takes 12 hours, followed by 2 hours ventilation and a further 24 hours for the gas to dissipate. The process is usually done overnight and the sterilizer must be used only in a well-ventilated area away from the working environment.

Most equipment can be sterilized in this way, but the limiting factor is the size and shape of the sterilizer. It is usually used to sterilize things that may otherwise be damaged by heat (e.g. fibreoptic endoscopes, plastic catheters, anaesthetic tubing and optical equipment).

MONITORING STERILIZATION

It is essential that sterilization is carried out effectively and this must be constantly monitored. There are several different methods of monitoring and it is important to select a method that is appropriate to the type of sterilizer used within your practice. If you do not then false results may be obtained.

- **Chemical indicator strips** (TST strips) – placed in the centre of the pack and change colour when the correct temperature, pressure and time have been reached. It is important to select the correct strip for the autoclave cycle. They are also used to monitor ethylene oxide sterilizers.
- **Browne's tubes** – small glass tubes filled with orange liquid that turn green when the correct temperature is reached for the correct amount of time. Used in autoclaves and hot air ovens.
- **Bowie Dick tape** – beige-coloured tape impregnated with a chemical strip that turns brown when it reaches a temperature of 121°C. Used to seal packs of instruments or drapes, but is of limited value as it does not ensure that the temperature has been maintained for a set time. Used in autoclaves.
- **Spore tests** – strips of paper impregnated with bacterial spores (usually *Bacillus stearothermophilus*) are placed within the load. After sterilization, the paper strip is placed on a culture medium and incubated at room temperature for 72 hours. Lack of growth indicates effective sterilization. It is an accurate method, but delay in culture results is a disadvantage. Used in autoclaves, ethylene oxide and hot air ovens.
- **Thermocouples** – electrical leads with temperature sensitive tips. The tips are placed within the load and the leads are passed out of the autoclave door and attached to a recording device. The temperature is recorded at intervals during the autoclave cycle.
- **Ethylene oxide tape** – similar to Bowie-Dick tape, but the lines are green and change to red on exposure to the gas.

There are many types of packaging used for sterilizing surgical equipment and the choice depends on factors such as cost, method of sterilization and personal choice. All sterilized packs should be labelled with the contents (e.g. spay pack), the date and the name of the person responsible. It should not be assumed that once a pack is sterile it will remain so forever – if the pack has not been used within 3 months it should be resterilized.

PREPARATION OF THE SURGICAL SITE

The skin and hair of the patient are the greatest potential sources of wound contamination because it is never possible to remove all micro-organisms; however, careful preparation of the surgical site following established practice protocols will minimize the risk. Much of the preparation of the surgical site may be carried out by the nurse, but in small practices it may be done by the veterinary surgeon.

Procedure: Clipping the site

This should be carried out within the preparation room to minimize contamination of the operating theatre.

1. **Action:** The patient should be anaesthetized, and placed in the correct position for the surgical procedure.

Rationale: The patient will not move, thus making the task easier. If the patient is considered to be an anaesthetic risk, clipping prior to induction will reduce anaesthetic time.

2. **Action:** Ensure that the clippers are clean, sharp and in good working order.

   Rationale: Poorly maintained clippers are more likely to nick the skin and cause 'clipper rash'.

3. **Action:** Select the site for the surgical incision and clip with the grain of the hair first and then repeat against the grain.

   Rationale: Removal of long, thick hair is easier with the grain. Clipping against the grain achieves a closer clip.

4. **Action:** Clip at least 5–15 cm beyond the line of the incision.

   Rationale: This allows the surgeon to extend the incision if necessary. Do not clip unnecessarily as this may annoy the owner.

5. **Action:** Make sure that the finished edges are neat.

   Rationale: Owners are not impressed by untidy clipping.

6. **Action:** If clipping around an open wound or close to the eyes, apply an appropriate water soluble gel to the area before clipping. Wipe away the gel before cleaning the site.

   Rationale: This will trap tiny hairs, which may act as foreign bodies in an open wound or cause irritation in the eye.

Procedure: Cleaning the surgical site

This is carried out in the preparation room until step 8, when you should move to the operating theatre. This is done to minimize contamination of the operating theatre.

1. **Action:** Put on a pair of surgical gloves – they do not need to be sterile at this stage.

   Rationale: This will protect the patient's skin from your hands and will protect your hands from the antiseptic skin scrub.

2. **Action:** Use an appropriate skin scrub (e.g. chlorhexidine or povidone iodine) at the correct dilution.

Rationale: Always read the manufacturer's instructions. Both of these have disinfectant and detergent properties and are safe to use on skin (i.e. they are antiseptics).

3. **Action:** Use lint free swabs.

   Rationale: They will not contaminate the site with minute threads or particles.

4. **Action:** Select one hand to be your 'clean' hand and the other as your 'dirty' hand. If you are right-handed use your right hand as the 'dirty' hand as this hand does the majority of the action.

   Rationale: If you can remember to do this it minimizes contamination of fresh swabs and the cleaned area.

5. **Action:** With the 'clean' hand, pick up a fresh swab and pass it to the 'dirty' hand. Dip it in the bowl of skin scrub solution and, starting at the incision site and working with a circular motion, wipe the skin towards the edges of the clipped area.

   Rationale: By moving with a circular motion you should not miss any part of the site. Working from the centre towards the outside ensures that you do not bring dirt from the coat to the surgical site.

6. **Action:** Once the edge is reached then discard the dirty swab.

   Rationale: To avoid recontamination of the cleaner area.

7. **Action:** Select a fresh swab with your 'clean' hand, pass it to your 'dirty' hand and keep repeating the process until the used swab is not discoloured.

   Rationale: This indicates that all visible dirt has been removed. Take care not to return to the centre of the area once it is clean.

8. **Action:** Include the hair at the edges in your cleaning.

   Rationale: This removes debris and flattens the hair. Do not make the hair too wet as this may promote 'strike-through' (i.e. the passage of micro-organisms, suspended in water, through the cloth from inside to outside thus recontaminating sterile areas) or hypothermia.

9. **Action:** Transfer the patient to the operating theatre and position for surgery using appropriate restraints if necessary (e.g. ties).

   Rationale: The site will now have been recontaminated.

10. **Action:** Wearing sterile gloves and using sterile swabs and water, repeat the scrub procedure as described before.

    Rationale: Sterile equipment is used in the clean theatre to maintain an aseptic environment as much as possible.

11. **Action:** The final skin preparation is carried out by a member of the surgical team using sterile swabs held in Rampley sponge-holding forceps. An alcoholic solution of a skin disinfectant is applied and left to dry on the skin.

    Rationale: The alcohol solution will remove any remaining detergent and provide residual bactericidal activity. Do not apply to open wounds or mucous membranes. Do not use diathermy if alcohol solution has been applied.

DRAPING THE PATIENT

In order to maintain asepsis, draping is carried out by a member of the surgical team who is appropriately gowned and gloved. Correctly prepared drapes should be evenly sterilized and when handled should unfold easily.

Procedure: Draping the patient with four plain drapes

1. **Action:** Pick up the first drape and let it unfold away from the instrument trolley or table.

   Rationale: The drape is sterile and must not be allowed to become contaminated by touching anything non-sterile.

2. **Action:** Fold back the edge of the drape underneath itself.

   Rationale: This will line the edge of the incision forming a double layer, which will protect from strike-through.

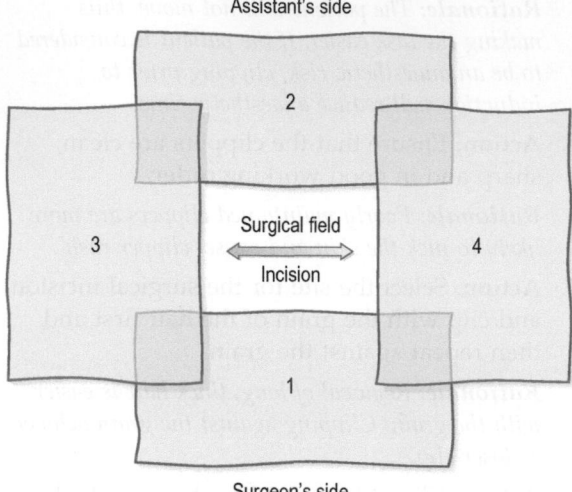

Figure 9.1 Draping with four plain drapes. (With permission from E. Mullineaux, M. Jones, BSAVA Manual of Practical Veterinary Nursing (2007).)

3. **Action:** Hold the drape along the folded edge with your hands inside the drape.

   Rationale: This prevents your hands from touching the patient when you place the drape.

4. **Action:** Apply the first drape on the surgeon's side (Fig. 9.1).

   Rationale: To prevent contamination of the surgeon when leaning over the patient to place the subsequent drapes.

5. **Action:** Place the second drape on the opposite side to the first (Fig. 9.1).

   Rationale: The surgeon may place this drape by leaning across the patient or an assistant may place it from his/her side.

6. **Action:** The third and fourth drapes are placed at either end of the surgical site (Fig. 9.1).

   Rationale: To complete the area all around the planned surgical incision.

7. **Action:** If necessary, apply further drapes to cover any remaining exposed parts of the patient or table.

   Rationale: It is important to cover the patient, the entire table and the area between the instrument trolley and the surgical site to prevent any risk of breaking asepsis.

8. **Action:** Place a towel clip diagonally across each corner with one tip on each drape. Secure by including a small fold of skin within the jaws.

   Rationale: Do not pierce the drape with the jaws of the clip as this will contaminate the clip.

9. **Action:** Cover each clip with the edge of the drape.

   Rationale: This will prevent the clips becoming accidentally caught and pulled.

Procedure: Draping a patient with a fenestrated cloth (e.g. cat spay cloth)

1. **Action:** Pick up the drape and allow it to unfold away from the instrument trolley or table.

   Rationale: Avoid touching anything that will break the sterility of the drape. If asepsis it broken, discard the cloth and use another one.

2. **Action:** Hold the drape along the edge with your hands inside the drape.

   Rationale: Your hands must not touch the patient's skin or coat.

3. **Action:** Looking through the fenestration, place the drape over the proposed surgical site.

   Rationale: If the fenestration is too large, place another smaller fenestrated drape over the top to make the hole smaller; if it is too small, discard the drape and start again with a fresh one.

4. **Action:** Secure the drape with a towel clip at each corner.

   Rationale: The clips cannot be concealed under the drape and are therefore more likely to be caught on instruments during surgery.

Procedure: Draping a limb

1. **Action:** Cover the distal part of the limb with a bandage and hold it upright (Fig. 9.2A). You may ask an assistant to hold it or tie it to a drip stand using a tape.

   Rationale: The lower part of the limb is a source of contamination. It has to be lifted out of the way to allow further drapes to be placed under it.

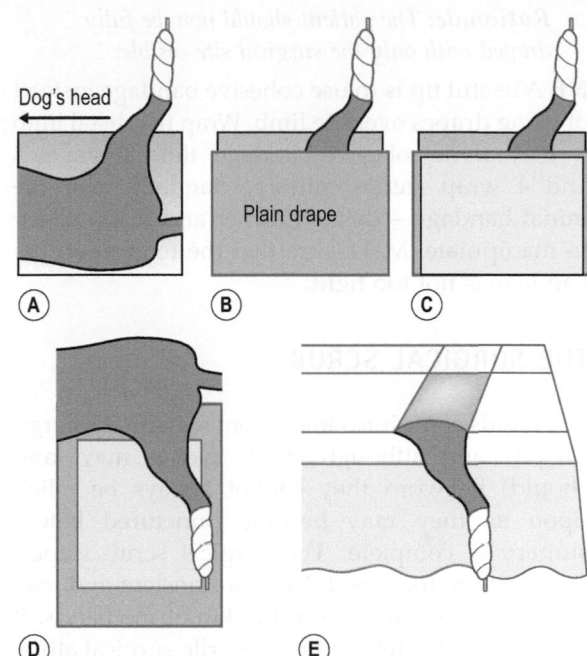

Figure 9.2 Draping a limb for surgery: (A) The lower limb is bandaged and attached by tape to a transfusion stand. (B) A plain drape is laid over the body and the opposite limb of the patient. (C) A smaller plain drape is laid on top of this. (D) The tape is then cut and the limb lowered onto the inner drape. (E) The drape is carefully wrapped around the limb and secured with a towel clip. Plain drapes or a fenestrated drape is then applied over the surgical site.

2. **Action:** Place a large plain drape or several smaller ones over the rest of the body and the opposite limb of the patient (Fig. 9.2B).

   Rationale: This reduces the risk of contamination from the rest of the body.

3. **Action:** Place a smaller drape on top of the initial drape and lower the limb (Fig. 9.2C, D).

   Rationale: The limb should be in contact only with this drape.

4. **Action:** Wrap this second drape firmly around the limb and secure with a towel clip (Fig. 9.2E).

   Rationale: The limb now has two layers wrapped around it to prevent it from contaminating the surgical site.

5. **Action:** Place further drapes around the surgical site.

Rationale: The patient should now be fully draped with only the surgical site visible.

NB A useful tip is to use cohesive bandage instead of using drapes over the limb. Wrap the distal limb in non-sterile cohesive bandage, then at stages 3 and 4 wrap sterile cohesive bandage over the initial bandage – this is quicker and much easier to manipulate. Make sure that the tension on the bandage is not too tight.

THE SURGICAL SCRUB

The hands come into closest contact with the surgical site and although sterile gloves may (and should) be worn they cannot always be relied upon as they may become punctured before surgery is complete. The surgical scrub is performed to reduce levels of both transient and resident micro-organisms on the skin of the hands. It is carried out before donning sterile surgical attire.

It is good practice to undertake a general hand wash at the beginning of the day, and with the increase in resistant organisms such as MRSA it is now becoming increasingly important that hands are cleaned using an alcohol-based scrub at regular intervals throughout the day (e.g. between patients). Personnel are encouraged to have small bottles of skin scrub in their pockets or pinned to their clothing. A full surgical scrub lasting 10 minutes should be performed before your first surgical procedure then a shorter scrub, usually lasting about 3 minutes, between subsequent procedures providing there has been no major contamination of the hands. Having a clock above the scrub sink will ensure that this important part of surgical preparation is carried out properly.

The choice of surgical scrub depends on the range of activity of the chemical against micro-organisms, length of activity, cost and personal choice. At the time of writing, new skin scrubs are coming onto the market that significantly shorten the time spent 'rubbing up' as they do not use water and take a much shorter time to become effective.

Before beginning any hand-washing procedure, all rings and watches must be removed, nails should be short and clean and free from nail varnish.

Procedure: General hand-washing routine

1. **Action:** Turn on the water and adjust to a warm temperature.
   Rationale: The use of taps with elbow, knee or foot controls reduces the risk of cross contamination.

2. **Action:** Allow the water to wash over your hands and drain from the wrists to the fingertips.
   Rationale: This will remove any gross contamination.

3. **Action:** Clean the fingernails with an orange stick or nail file.
   Rationale: Once this has been done each day it can be omitted from subsequent washings.

4. **Action:** Apply plain soap and massage into the hands from the wrists to the fingertips in a circular motion including the backs of the hands.
   Rationale: This will remove all traces of organic dirt, which may inactivate the antiseptic solution used in the surgical scrub.

5. **Action:** Rinse allowing the water to drain from the fingertips. Repeat step 4.
   Rationale: Repeating the action will ensure the removal of residual organic matter.

6. **Action:** Turn off the water.
   Rationale: Your hands should not touch the tap otherwise they may become recontaminated. You may have to ask an assistant to do this or use a paper towel to cover the taps – discard the paper towel afterwards.

7. **Action:** Dry your hands thoroughly using a paper towel.
   Rationale: Powered hand dryers are not recommended as they spread micro-organisms around the environment. Reusable towels are unsuitable as they harbour micro-organisms.

Procedure: Routine hand hygiene using an alcohol-based rub (based on the WHO guidelines)

This should be done as often as possible during the working day as it helps to reduce the risk of spreading micro-organisms between patients and around the hospital environment. Research shows that regular hand cleaning significantly reduces the risk of nosocomial infections (WHO 2009).

1. **Action:** Remove all rings and watches and roll up your sleeves.
   Rationale: *Dirt and micro-organisms may accumulate under rings or watch straps.*

2. **Action:** Apply 3–5 ml of alcohol rub to your right or left palm (Fig. 9.3).
   Rationale: *Sterilizing alcohol rub is widely available in many forms.*

3. **Action:** Rub the palms of your hands together using a minimum of three strokes.
   Rationale: *To ensure that the rub is spread well.*

Duration of entire procedure: 20-30 seconds

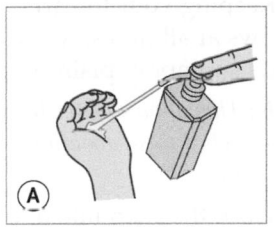
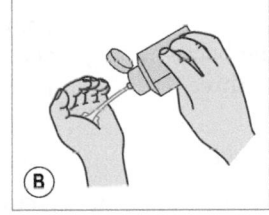
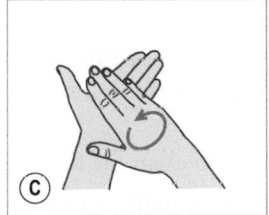

Apply a palmful of the product in a cupped hand, covering all surfaces

Rub hands palm to palm

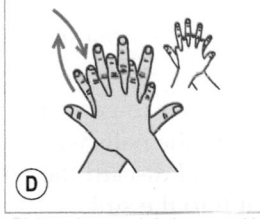
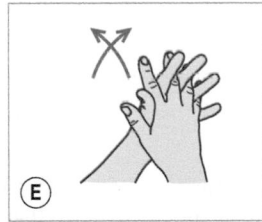
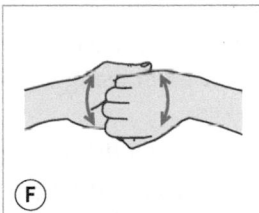

Right palm over left dorsum with interlaced fingers and vice versa

Palm to palm with fingers interlaced

backs of fingers to opposing palms with fingers interlocked

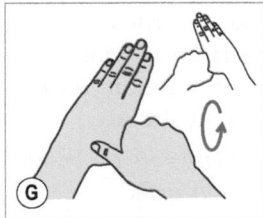
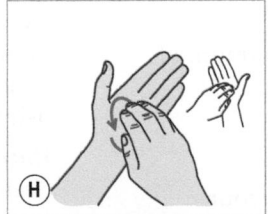
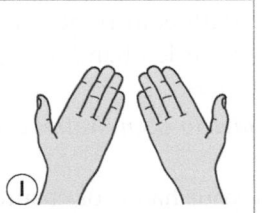

Rotational rubbing of left thumb clasped in right palm and vice versa

Rotational rubbing, backwards and forwards with clasped fingers of right hand in left palm and vice versa

Once dry, your hands are safe

Figure 9.3 Hand hygiene technique with alcohol-based formulations: (A, B) Apply a palmful of the product in a cupped hand, covering all surfaces. (C) Rub hands palm to palm. (D) Right palm over left dorsum with interlaced fingers and vice versa. (E) Palm to palm with fingers interlaced. (F) Backs of fingers to opposing palms, with fingers interlocked. (G) Rotational rubbing of left thumb clasped in right palm and vice versa. (H) Rotational rubbing, backwards and forwards with clasped fingers of right hand in left palm and vice versa. (I) Once dry, your hands are safe. (Reproduced with permission from WHO 2009 Guidelines on hand hygiene. WHO Press, Geneva.)

4. **Action:** Rub your right palm over the back of your left hand using a minimum of three strokes.

   Rationale: To clean the back of your left hand.

5. **Action:** Rub your left palm over the back of your right hand using a minimum of three strokes.

   Rationale: To clean the back of your right hand.

6. **Action:** Interlace your fingers and rub the palms together using a minimum of three strokes.

   Rationale: To clean the interdigital spaces and the palms.

7. **Action:** Clasp your fingers to rub the backs of your fingers using a minimum of three strokes.

   Rationale: To clean the backs of your fingers.

8. **Action:** Rotationally rub the left thumb with the right palm using a minimum of three strokes.

   Rationale: To clean the left thumb.

9. **Action:** Rotationally rub the right thumb with the left palm using a minimum of three strokes.

   Rationale: To clean the right thumb.

10. **Action:** With your left fingertips, rub the palm of your right hand using a minimum of three strokes.

    Rationale: To clean the tips of the left fingers.

11. **Action:** With your right fingertips, rub the palm of your left hand using a minimum of three strokes.

    Rationale: To clean the tips of the right fingers.

12. Air dry your hands or ensure that your hands are dried before continuing to do anything else.

    Rationale: To ensure that moist alcohol rub does not contaminate sensitive parts of the patient and that your hands are not sticky.

NB As the alcohol rub is designed to evaporate quickly you may need to use a bit more than recommended as it dries before you reach the end of the procedure.

Procedure: Surgical scrub

This is carried out before a surgical procedure and before you don surgical clothing.

1. **Action:** Turn on the tap to produce a gentle stream and adjust the temperature so that it is warm but not too hot.

   Rationale: A gentle stream will minimize splashing.

2. **Action:** Keeping your forearms higher than your elbows at all times, wet your arms and hands and apply plain soap.

   Rationale: This allows water to run away from the scrubbed area, avoiding recontamination.

3. **Action:** Work the soap into a lather and spread it over the hands and arms to about 5 cm above the elbow then rinse in the stream of water.

   Rationale: To remove any surface dirt or grease.

4. **Action:** With your fingers under the stream of water, clean the nails with a file or an orange stick and discard the file by dropping it into the sink.

   Rationale: If you place it back on a surface you risk possible recontamination.

5. **Action:** Take a sterile nail brush, moisten it under the stream of water and apply surgical scrub solution. Scrub your nails using a straight stroke.

   Rationale: Make sure the bristles of the brush clean under your nails.

6. **Action:** Starting with your little finger and using the brush, scrub each of the four planes of each finger in straight strokes (Fig. 9.4A).

   Rationale: Remember to include the interdigital spaces.

7. **Action:** With the brush, clean the palm and back of the hand using a circular movement.

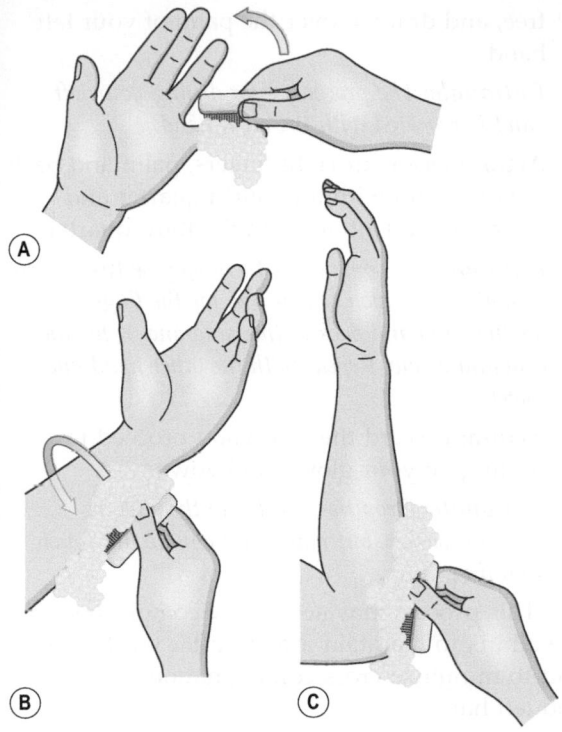

Figure 9.4 The surgical scrub sequence: (A) Starting with the little finger and working across to the thumb, scrub each surface of each digit. (B) Scrub the forearm, again scrubbing the entire circumference. (C) Scrub elbow area to 5 cm (2 inches) above the elbow, including all surfaces.

Rationale: Take care not to overscrub the back of the hand because the skin there is more delicate and therefore susceptible to trauma.

8. **Action:** Scrub the forearm up to 5 cm above the elbow using a circular movement (Fig. 9.4B, C).

   Rationale: Maintain the lather at all times, adding more water or scrub solution if necessary.

9. **Action:** Repeat the process for the other hand and forearm.

   Rationale: Use the same method making sure that no area of skin is missed.

10. **Action:** You can use another sterile brush – discard the first brush into the sink and take the second brush from the sterile pack with your scrubbed hand. If not, rinse the brush and add more scrub solution before transferring it to the other hand.

    Rationale: Once one hand is scrubbed it must not become recontaminated otherwise you will have to repeat the procedure.

11. **Action:** Keeping your hands above your elbows, rinse both hands thoroughly and allow the water to drain into the sink.

    Rationale: Avoid getting water on to your clothing because this may lead to strike-through.

12. **Action:** Wash the hands and arms again using the surgical scrub solution, but this time do not include your elbows.

    Rationale: This ensures that your hands do not come into contact with any area that has not been scrubbed.

13. **Action:** Rinse then dry your hands using a sterile towel (see next procedure).

    Rationale: To avoid recontamination.

14. **Action:** Hold your hands above your elbows with your palms facing your chest. Do not allow your hands to touch each other.

    Rationale: To avoid recontamination.

NB When you encounter another person who has scrubbed up you should pass back to back. The back of a person prepared for surgery is considered to be non-sterile. Passing back to back reduces the risk of recontamination.

Procedure: Drying your hands after the surgical scrub

1. **Action:** Your hands are now considered to be sterile and they are wet. Ask an assistant to open the pack containing a sterile towel.

   Rationale: Do not handle the outside of the pack as it is non-sterile, and do not encourage your assistant to remove the sterile towel as she will contaminate it.

2. **Action:** Pick up the corner of the towel in the pack with your right hand. Stand clear of any surfaces and take the towel out.

   Rationale: Avoid touching any surfaces with the sterile towel or your scrubbed hands.

3. **Action:** Allow the towel to unfold without shaking it. Imagine that the towel is divided into four quarters.

   Rationale: Shaking the towel increases the risk of it touching a non-sterile object and will also increase airborne movement of micro-organisms. You are going to use the imaginary quarters of the towel to dry different parts of your two hands.

4. **Action:** Let the towel fall over the palm of your right hand and use the first quarter to dry the fingers, palm and back of your left hand. Dry each finger separately and ensure that the interdigital spaces are included (Fig. 9.5).

   Rationale: The right hand supports the towel and dries the left hand, but it must not touch the top of the towel or directly touch the left hand so as to prevent cross contamination between hands.

5. **Action:** Using the second quarter of the towel, dry the left forearm and elbow.

   Rationale: Using a separate quarter for each hand and arm increases the degree of asepsis.

6. **Action:** With your dry left hand, pick up the towel by the fourth quarter, which is hanging free, and drape it over the palm of your left hand.

   Rationale: The procedure for drying your left hand is repeated with the right hand.

7. **Action:** Dry your right fingers, palm and back of your hand with the fourth quarter and your arm and elbow with the third quarter.

   Rationale: In some cases there may be two towels available, in which case use ⅓ for the fingers, ⅓ for the palm and back of the hand and ⅓ for the arm and elbow. Repeat with the other hand and towel.

8. **Action:** Discard the towel and proceed to putting on your gloves and gown.

   Rationale: Drop the towel into the sink or washing basket, but make sure you do not touch anything.

NB This process may seem very complicated, but the aim is to maintain asepsis after scrubbing up and to minimize cross contamination of the right and left hand.

DONNING THEATRE ATTIRE

To achieve and maintain asepsis within the operating theatre environment, normal outdoor clothes should be replaced by specific theatre scrub suits. These should be worn by the entire theatre team and should not be worn around the practice as they may become contaminated. Although these 'scrubs' are not sterile they act as a barrier to micro-organisms and they are covered by sterile attire just prior to the surgical procedure.

Clothing worn within the theatre includes:

- **Scrub suits** – a top and trousers. The top should be tucked in and the trousers should be tucked into surgical boots or have cuffed legs. Usually made of cotton, which is easy to wear and reduces static electricity. Must be changed daily and changed more often if soiled.

- **Footwear** – shoes, boots or clogs are designed to be non-slip, antistatic, comfortable and easily cleaned. They should not be worn outside the theatre. Shoe covers may be used.

- **Headgear** – hair, which may be a source of contamination, should be completely covered by a theatre hat. There are a variety of designs both washable and disposable. Men with sideburns should wear surgical bonnets.

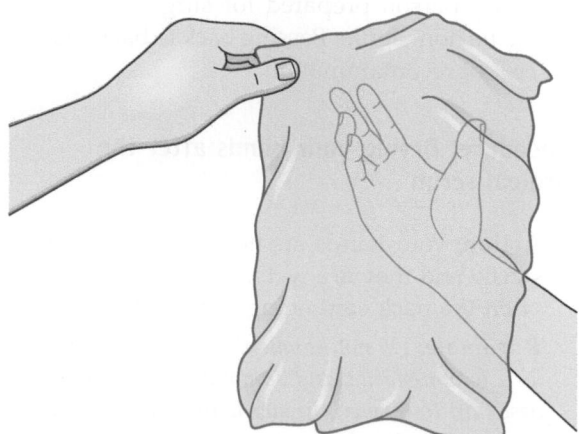

Figure 9.5 Drying hands after the surgical scrub.

- **Facemasks** – filter the air from the mouth and nose. They must be close fitting and should be changed between operations or if the procedure takes longer than 30 minutes.
- **Surgical gowns** – these are sterile and are worn over a scrub suit. They may be reusable or disposable and should have long cuffed sleeves. Fabric gowns may be prone to wicking of fluids, but the use of better quality thicker fabrics reduces this.
- **Surgical gloves** – these come in presterilized packs and in a variety of sizes. Some gloves have added maize starch as a powder, which helps in putting them on, but this type is not recommended as the powder may act as a foreign body and delay wound healing.

GOWNING

A sterile gown should be put on as soon as you have scrubbed up. Remember your hands are now sterile and you must not break asepsis by touching anything non-sterile. You will require assistance to put on your gown.

There are two main types of surgical gowns:

- Back-tying
- Side-tying.

Procedure: Putting on a back-tying gown

1. **Action:** Ask your unscrubbed assistant to open the pack containing the sterilized gown and present the open end to you.

   Rationale: The inside of the pack is sterile. Your assistant is non-sterile and must not touch the contents.

2. **Action:** Remove the sterile gown from its back, hold the shoulders and allow the gown to gently unfold (Fig. 9.6A).

   Rationale: Holding the gown correctly allows you to identify the sleeves. Gentle unfolding reduces air movement and the risk of

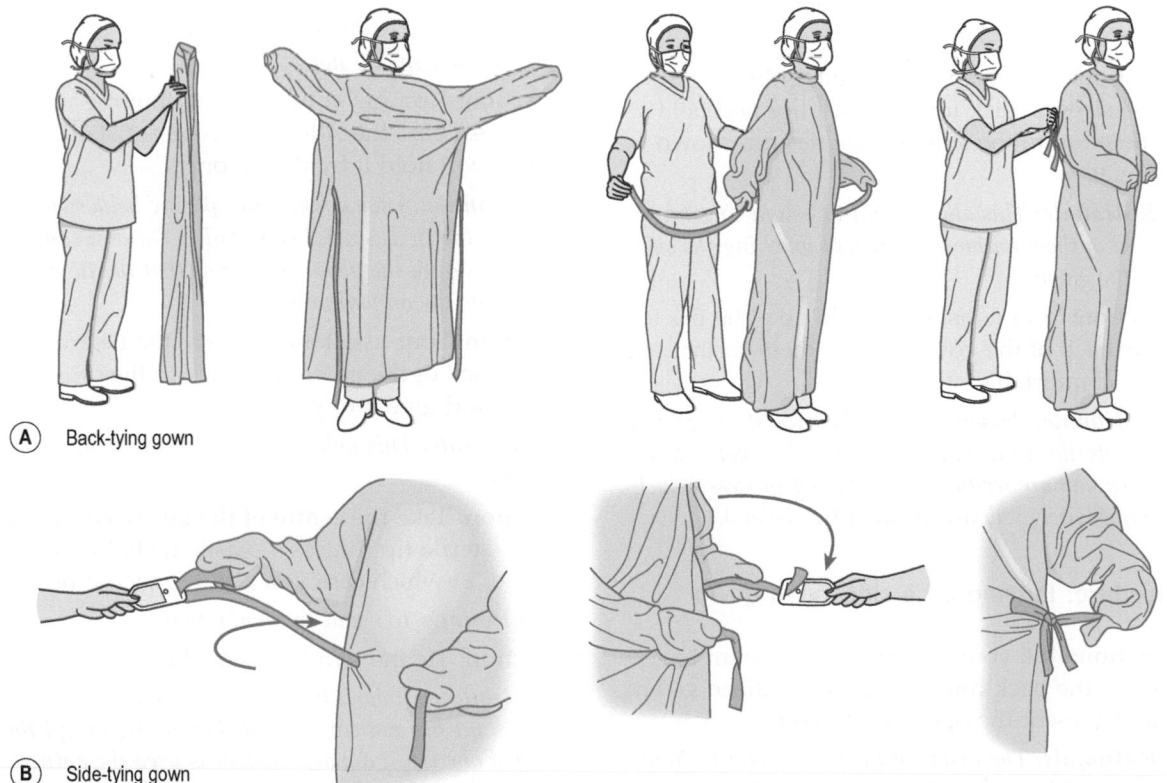

(A) Back-tying gown

(B) Side-tying gown

Figure 9.6 Gowning: (A) back-tying gown; (B) side-tying gown.

contaminating the gown. Make sure that you do not allow the gown to touch anything, including the floor.

3. **Action:** Slip one hand into each sleeve and push up to but not through the cuff. Open your arms wide, but do not attempt to adjust the gown over the shoulders.

   Rationale: Your hands should remain in the sleeves of your gown to avoid contamination. Efforts to pull the gown over your shoulders create a contamination risk.

4. **Action:** Ask your assistant to pull the gown over your shoulders, touching only the inside of the gown, and adjust it so that you are comfortable.

   Rationale: The inside of the gown is not considered to be sterile so your assistant can touch it, but you should not.

5. **Action:** Ask your assistant to tie the short ties along the back of the gown.

   Rationale: The back of the gown is now non-sterile.

6. **Action:** With your hands still within the sleeves, pick up the waist ties and hold them out to the sides (waist ties not shown Fig. 9.6).

   Rationale: This allows your assistant to grasp hold of them without the risk of touching the sides of the gown.

7. **Action:** Your assistant should take the ties to the back of the gown and tie them so that you are comfortable.

   Rationale: Remember that the back of the gown is not sterile. Your hands remain within your sleeves until you are ready for the gloving process, which immediately follows gowning (see below).

Procedure: Putting on a side–tying gown

1. **Action:** Ask your unscrubbed assistant to open the pack containing the sterilized gown and present the open end to you.

   Rationale: The inside of the pack is sterile. Your assistant is non-sterile and must not touch the contents.

2. **Action:** Remove the sterile gown from its back, hold the shoulders and allow the gown to gently unfold (Fig 9.6A).

   Rationale: Holding the gown correctly allows you to identify the sleeves. Gentle unfolding reduces air movement and the risk of contaminating the gown. Make sure that you do not allow the gown to touch anything including the floor.

3. **Action:** Slip one hand into each sleeve and push up to but not through the cuff. Open your arms wide, but do not attempt to adjust the gown over the shoulders.

   Rationale: Your hands should remain in the sleeves of your gown to avoid contamination. Efforts to pull the gown over your shoulders create a contamination risk.

4. **Action:** Ask your assistant to pull the gown over your shoulders, touching only the inside of the gown, and adjust it so that you are comfortable.

   Rationale: The inside of the gown is not considered to be sterile so your assistant can touch it, but you should not.

5. **Action:** Keeping your hands within the sleeves, pass the side tie to your assistant, who will hold it by the tip only.

   Rationale: Some gowns have plastic holders into which the tie is slotted (Fig 9.6B). The assistant touches only the plastic holder so that the tie itself remains uncontaminated.

6. **Action:** Your assistant will take the tie around the back of the gown and back to the original side and give it to you.

   Rationale: This will fix the gown into your waist.

7. **Action:** Take the centre of the tie, avoiding the non-sterile tip (unless a plastic tie holder is used, in which case you pull the tie out of it).

   Rationale: To avoid contamination.

8. **Action:** Tie the two ties into a bow.

   Rationale: To hold the gown together. Your assistant has not contaminated anything except the tip of one tie. If a plastic holder is used the entire gown is still sterile. Your hands remain within the sleeves until you have put on sterile gloves.

GLOVING

Sterile gloves should be worn for all surgical procedures. Gloves are available in a variety of sizes and practices should keep a range to meet the needs of all the surgical team. They are available with or without powder, which helps when putting them on.

There are three methods of donning surgical gloves:

- Open
- Closed
- Plunge.

Procedure: Open gloving

(This follows on from donning a sterile surgical gown.)

1. **Action:** Push both hands through the cuffs of the gown.
   Rationale: *A disadvantage of this method is that the gloves may become contaminated by skin contact.*
2. **Action:** Ask an assistant to open a pack of gloves and place them on a flat surface with the fingers pointing away from you (Fig. 9.7A).
   Rationale: *The right glove is on your right side.*
3. **Action:** Pick up the right glove with the thumb and forefinger of your left hand, touching only the inner folded-down surface of the glove (Fig. 9.7B).
   Rationale: *The inside may be touched freely by your ungloved hand because it will never come into contact with other sterile items such as gowns and drapes.*
4. **Action:** Pull the glove onto your right hand, leaving the cuff folded back, and hook it onto your thumb (Fig. 9.7C).
   Rationale: *This avoids touching the contaminated inner surface by the gloved left hand when unfolding it to cover the gown's right cuff.*
5. **Action:** Slide the fingers of your left hand between the palm and folded cuff of the left glove. Pick it up and pull it on to your left hand using your gloved right hand (Fig. 9.7D).

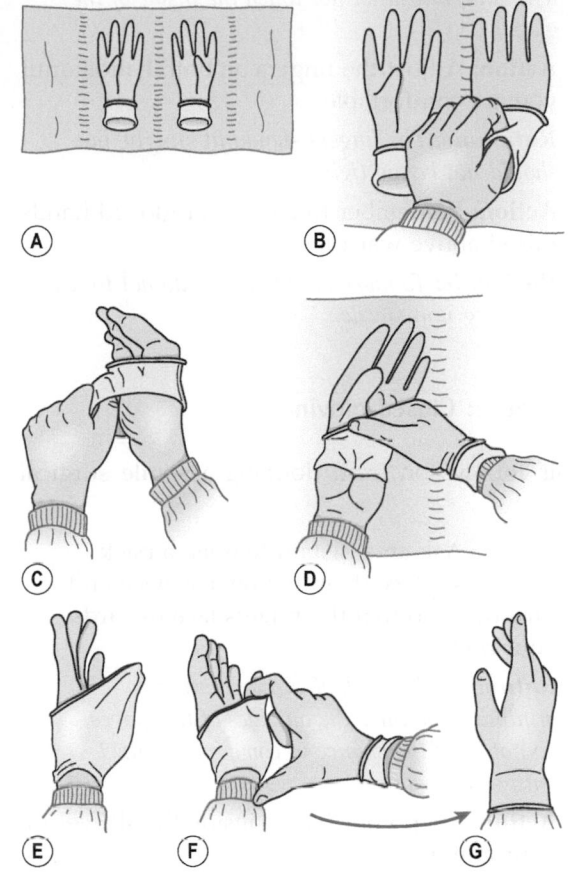

Figure 9.7 Open gloving.

Rationale: *The fingers of your gloved sterile right hand may touch only the outer sterile surface of the glove.*

6. **Action:** Pull the cuff of the glove over the cuff of the gown, making sure that the whole circumference is covered (Fig. 9.7E, F).
   Rationale: *Make sure that you touch only the outside of the glove and that there is no gap between the glove and the sleeve of the gown.*
7. **Action:** Using the gloved fingers of your left hand, slide them between the palm and cuff of the right hand glove and pull the cuff, which was hooked over your thumb, down and over the right cuff of the gown to include the whole circumference (Fig. 9.7G).
   Rationale: *Remember that you can touch the outside of the gloves with your sterile gloved*

left hand, but must not touch the inside of the glove.

8. **Action:** Adjust the fingers on both hands until you are comfortable

   Rationale: The fingers should fit snugly, but should not be too tight.

9. **Action:** Remember to keep your gloved hands raised above waist level.

   Rationale: To make sure that you do not touch anything non-sterile.

Procedure: Closed gloving

(This follows on from donning a sterile surgical gown.)

1. **Action:** Ask an assistant to open a pack of gloves, place them flat on a surface and turn them so that the fingers face towards your body.

   Rationale: The risk of contamination is minimized because the outsides of the gloves do not have the chance to come into contact with skin.

2. **Action:** Keep your hands inside the sleeves of your gown.

   Rationale: This ensures that your hands remain sterile inside the sterile gown, but it can make manipulation of the gloves more difficult. Practice makes perfect!

3. **Action:** Pick up the right glove (which is on the left) by the rim of the glove with your right hand (Fig. 9.8A).

   Rationale: Having turned the glove packet around, the right glove is on the left side and vice versa.

4. **Action:** Turn the hand of the glove over so that the palm is facing upwards with the fingers facing towards your elbow (Fig. 9.8B, C).

   Rationale: The glove is now in the correct position to be pulled on.

5. **Action:** Using your left hand, grasp the rim of the glove and pull it over your right hand until it covers the right cuff of the gown (Fig. 9.8D).

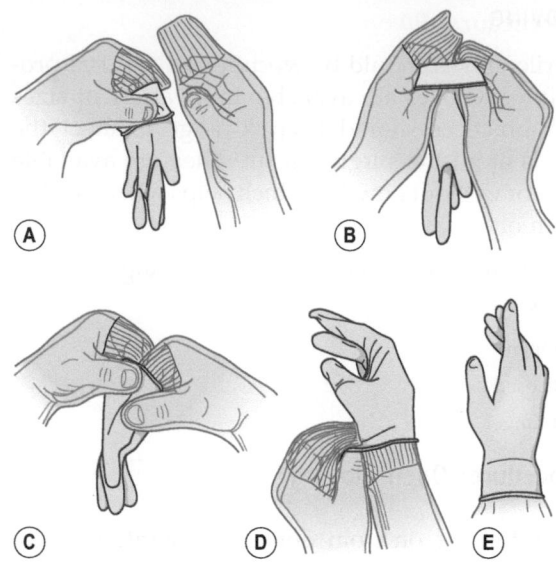

Figure 9.8 Closed gloving.

   Rationale: Your right hand still remains within the cuff, which prevents contamination of the outside of the glove.

6. **Action:** Allow your right hand to emerge from the cuff of the gown into the glove by carefully pulling the sleeve away from the glove (Fig 9.8E). Be careful not to pull the cuff out of the glove leaving a gap.

   Rationale: Your sterile hand has now passed into the sterile glove with no outside contamination.

7. **Action:** Use your left hand, still within its sleeve, to adjust the fingers of your right hand until you are comfortable.

   Rationale: The glove should fit snugly but not too tightly.

8. **Action:** Pick up the left glove with the left hand and repeat the process.

   Rationale: This is usually easier as your right hand is no longer within the sleeve. Contamination is minimized because the skin of your hands never touches the outside of the gloves.

9. **Action:** Remember to keep your gloved hands raised above waist level.

   Rationale: To make sure that you do not touch anything non-sterile.

Procedure: Plunge method

This method is sometimes used during a surgical procedure when a glove has become torn, punctured or contaminated. It involves the use of a scrubbed assistant and, as there are two people involved, there is a greater risk of contamination and it is rarely used.

1. **Action:** Ask an assistant to scrub up.

   Rationale: The assistant's hands must be sterile if your asepsis is to be maintained.

2. **Action:** Ask the scrubbed assistant to open a pair of sterile gloves and place them flat on a table.

   Rationale: This provides easy access to the gloves. Make sure that they are the correct size.

3. **Action:** The assistant will pick up one glove and, holding it by the cuff, open it using two hands.

   Rationale: This means that you can put your hand into the glove quickly.

4. **Action:** If you are wearing a pair of gloves that have become damaged you should have removed them first.

Rationale: There is no need to wear two pairs of gloves, but be careful not to touch anything while you are ungloved.

5. **Action:** Plunge your hand down into the appropriate glove and ask your assistant to repeat the process with the other glove.

   Rationale: As you push into the glove your fingers will slide into the appropriate position.

6. **Action:** Remember to keep your gloved hands raised above waist level.

   Rationale: To make sure that you do not touch anything non-sterile.

NB If you are using this method straight from scrubbing up, you should keep your hands within the sleeves of the gown as described in closed gloving. When the glove is presented to you, plunge your sleeved hand into the glove and then allow your fingers to emerge from the cuff into the glove.

Double gloving – this is sometimes recommended for contaminated or dirty operations (see Table 9.1). The most contaminated part of the procedure should be completed and then the first layer of gloves is removed leaving the fresh pair underneath. This would coincide with the introduction of fresh sterile instruments and redraping as necessary.

CHAPTER 10

Suturing techniques and common surgical procedures

CHAPTER CONTENTS

The aim of this chapter is to provide information about the basic surgical techniques that you should be able to do upon qualification and within the first couple of years of being in small animal practice. What it does not cover is the specialist or advanced techniques (e.g. recent developments in cranial cruciate repair, bowel surgery or orthopaedic surgery), knowledge of which may be gained by attendance on training courses, tuition by more experienced members of the veterinary profession both within your practice and in other practices, reading up-to-date journals and research via the internet. Another excellent way to learn and become practically proficient is the use of cadavers, although you should consider the moral and ethical issues associated with this.

SUTURING TECHNIQUES

Wounds heal by:

- **First intention** – occurs in surgical incisions and clean cuts. There is no loss of tissue and healing should occur within 5–10 days, although it may be speeded up by the use of sutures or other materials that hold the edges together (e.g. tissue glue or staples). There should be very little evidence of scarring.

- **Second intention** – occurs where the edges are widely separated and / or where there is tissue loss. This will take place if first intention is impossible or has failed (e.g. due to infection, movement between the edges or patient interference). Healing by this method may take days, weeks or even months depending on the wound. Evidence of scarring is inevitable and variable.

In any wound you should always consider trying to bring the edges together to promote rapid healing and this requires the use of suture material and needles and knowledge of an appropriate suturing technique.

SUTURE MATERIALS

Suture materials are required for a variety of purposes during surgery including:

- Apposing tissues to facilitate rapid healing
- Ligation of blood vessels
- Securing drains and tubes.

There are many types of suture material; the correct choice depends on the properties of the material, the nature of the wound, including the presence or absence of infection, the rate of healing of the tissue and the intended use of the suture.

The types of material (Table 10.1) can be broadly divided into:

1. **Absorbable / non-absorbable** – this refers to whether the material remains in the tissue and has to be removed manually or whether it will lose its strength and subsequently be removed by phagocytosis or hydrolysis over a predestined period of time.

2. **Monofilament / multifilament** – refers to the number of filaments that are twisted together to form a single strand. Multifilament materials may cause 'wicking' of bacteria and fluids through the tissues by capillary action; however, they are more pliable, and have a higher tensile strength and better handling and knot security than monofilament materials.

3. **Synthetic / non-synthetic or natural** – natural materials tend to cause a considerable tissue reaction and catgut in particular cannot be depended upon to produce reliable knots so these materials are no longer recommended. Synthetic materials produce little tissue reaction.

Size of suture material – there are two systems in use: the metric system and the United States Pharmacopoeia / European Pharmacopoeia system (USP / PhEur). Both systems are usually displayed on the packaging.

- In the **USP / PhEur** system, larger numbers represent suture material of a larger diameter while numbers followed by zero represent smaller sizes (i.e. material with the number 3 is much thicker than 3/0; 3/0 is thicker than 7/0).

- In the **metric system,** each unit represents 0.1 mm – so 4 metric is 0.4 mm in diameter.

- Use 3 metric for dogs and 2 metric for cats.

- Reduce by one size for delicate tissue and increase by one size for tough tissue.

Table 10.1 Suture materials commonly used in practice*

Suture material	Type	Trade name	Properties
Glycomer 631	Synthetic Absorbable Monofilament	Biosyn®	Initially 30% stronger than PDS®, but loses $2/3$ of its tensile strength within 21 days. Very strong, low memory so easy to handle. Very good knot security
Lactomer 9-1	Synthetic Absorbable Multifilament	Polysorb®	Loses $2/3$ of its tensile strength within 21 days. Completely absorbed by 56–70 days. Very good handling characteristics and excellent knot security
Poliglecaprone	Synthetic Absorbable Monofilament	Monocryl®	Loses $1/2$ of its tensile strength within 7 days. Excellent handling and reasonable knot security
Polydioxonone	Synthetic Absorbable Monofilament	PDS®, PDS II®	Lose $1/8$ of its tensile strength within 14 days. Lasts at least 180 days. Quite springy and has high memory so can be difficult to handle. Good knot security, but take care when tying the knot
Polyglactin 910	Synthetic Absorbable Multifilament	Vicryl® Vicryl rapide® (VR)	Loses $1/2$ of its tensile strength within 14 days and complete absorption within 60 days. VR undergoes quick hydrolysis and complete absorption within 42 days
Polyglycolic acid	Synthetic Absorbable Multifilament	Dexon®	Loses $1/3$ of its tensile strength within 14 days. Coated form is available that lasts longer and reduces 'wicking'
Polyglyconate	Synthetic Absorbable Monofilament	Maxon®	Loses $1/3$ of its tensile strength within 14 days
Polyglytone 6211	Synthetic Absorbable Monofilament	Caprosyn®	Loses all tensile strength by 21 days and is completely absorbed by 56 days. Excellent handling and knot security. Ideal for use in the oral cavity
Polyamide	Synthetic Non-absorbable Multi- or monofilament	Monosof® (monofilament nylon) Ethilon® (monofilament nylon) Surgilon® (braided multifilament nylon) Bralon® (braided multifilament nylon)	Relatively poor knot security and poor handling (Monosof® is the best). Little or no tissue reaction
Polybutester	Synthetic Non-absorbable Monofilament	Novafil®	Good handling and secure knots

Table 10.1 *Continued*

Suture material	Type	Trade name	Properties
Polyester	Synthetic Non-absorbable Multifilament	Mersiline® Dacron®	Poor handling and poor knot characteristics. Causes a moderate tissue reaction
Polypropylene	Synthetic Non-absorbable Monofilament	Prolene® Fluorofil® Surgilene®	Very good handling and knot characteristics
Stainless steel	Synthetic Non-absorbable Multi- or monofilament	Flexon®	Very strong. Excellent knot security, but prone to metal fatigue. Poor handling characteristics
Catgut / chromic catgut	Non-synthetic Absorbable Multifilament	–	Loses $\frac{1}{3}$ of its tensile strength within 7 days. Made from the intestinal mucosa of sheep or cattle – 90% collagen. Chromic catgut is pretreated with chromium salts to prolong absorption for up to 90 days, depending on type
Silk	Non-synthetic Non-absorbable Multifilament	Mersilk®	Loses $\frac{1}{3}$ of its tensile strength within 14 days

*After Hoad 2006, p 106, Minor Veterinary Surgery with permission of Elsevier Butterworth-Heinemann.

Choice of suture material – choose the smallest size of suture material that will provide adequate support. Smaller sizes will result in less tissue trauma and smaller knots with greater knot security. There is also a lower viability of any bacteria that may stick to the material. Table 10.2 suggests suitable choices of suture material for different tissues.

As a general rule when selecting suture material, consider the following:

- Avoid multifilament material in contaminated wounds – there is a risk of 'wicking' and the spaces between the strands may harbour blood, which will become a medium for bacterial growth.
- Avoid non-absorbable materials in hollow organs (e.g. in the bladder the suture may become a focus for deposition of crystals forming calculi).

- Avoid burying any suture material from a multi-use cassette – there may be a risk of contamination from previous use.
- Avoid using catgut in inflamed, infected or acidic wounds – absorption is more rapid in these wounds.
- Avoid reactive materials in the creation of stoma.
- Use slowly absorbable materials in fascia or tendons – the rate of healing is slow and the tissue requires the support of the sutures for some time.
- Use inert material in the skin.

SUTURE NEEDLES

There are many different types of suture needle and the choice depends on:

- Type of tissue to be sutured
- Size of the wound

Table 10.2 Choice of suture material for different tissues*

Tissue	Comment	Type
Skin	Non-absorbable	Monofilament/multifilament
Subcuticulis	Absorbable of short duration. Tissue heals quickly as it is not reliant on suture for much more than 14–21 days	Monofilament/multifilament
Fascia	Absorbable of long duration/non-absorbable. Tissue heals slowly and may rely on the strength of a suture for up to 9 months	Monofilament
Muscle	Absorbable of long duration/non-absorbable	Monofilament/multifilament
Hernia repair	Absorbable of long duration/non-absorbable	Monofilament
Viscera	Absorbable of short duration. Tissue heals quickly as it is not reliant on suture for much more than 14–21 days	Monofilament
Tendon	Non-absorbable	Monofilament
Vessel ligation	Absorbable of short duration. A non-absorbable multifilament (e.g. silk) may be used for large vessels (e.g. renal artery or vein)	Multifilament/monofilament
Vessel repair	Non-absorbable	Monofilament
Nerve	Non-absorbable	Monofilament

Adapted from Manual of Canine and Feline Surgical Principles. BSAVA. Gloucester.

- Suture pattern
- Type of suture material
- Surgeon's preference.

Table 10.3 and Figure 10.1 describe the basic components of suture needles.

Examples of **needle holders** (Fig. 10.2) include Gillies (which also provides a scissor action but no ratchet), Olsen-Hegar (which has a ratchet and scissor action) and McPhails (which has a spring ratchet). All needles, with the exception of straight ones, should be held in needle holders, which will provide control as the needle is pushed through the tissue and, when using cutting needles, will protect your gloves or fingers.

The needle should be grasped by the tips of the needle holder at a point on the needle that is one-third to half of the way along the needle from the suture material end. If the tissue is delicate you hold the needle closer to the suture material end, and closer to the point for tougher tissues.

SUTURE PATTERNS

There is an enormous range of suture patterns; if a wound is to heal satisfactorily it is important to choose a pattern that will both close an incision and provide maximum mechanical support with minimal tissue reaction. The choice of suture is also likely to affect the lengths of the surgical procedure and the healing process.

It is better to be proficient at a small range of suture patterns than to be bad at performing all of them. Suture patterns can be classified as to:

- Whether each suture is individually placed (i.e. **interrupted**) or linked to the one on either side of it (i.e. **continuous**)
- The way in which the tissues are apposed:
  - simple **interrupted** sutures restore and align the anatomical surface of the tissue (e.g. the skin), creating a smooth surface
  - **everting** sutures turn the tissue edges outwards (e.g. continuous mattress sutures)

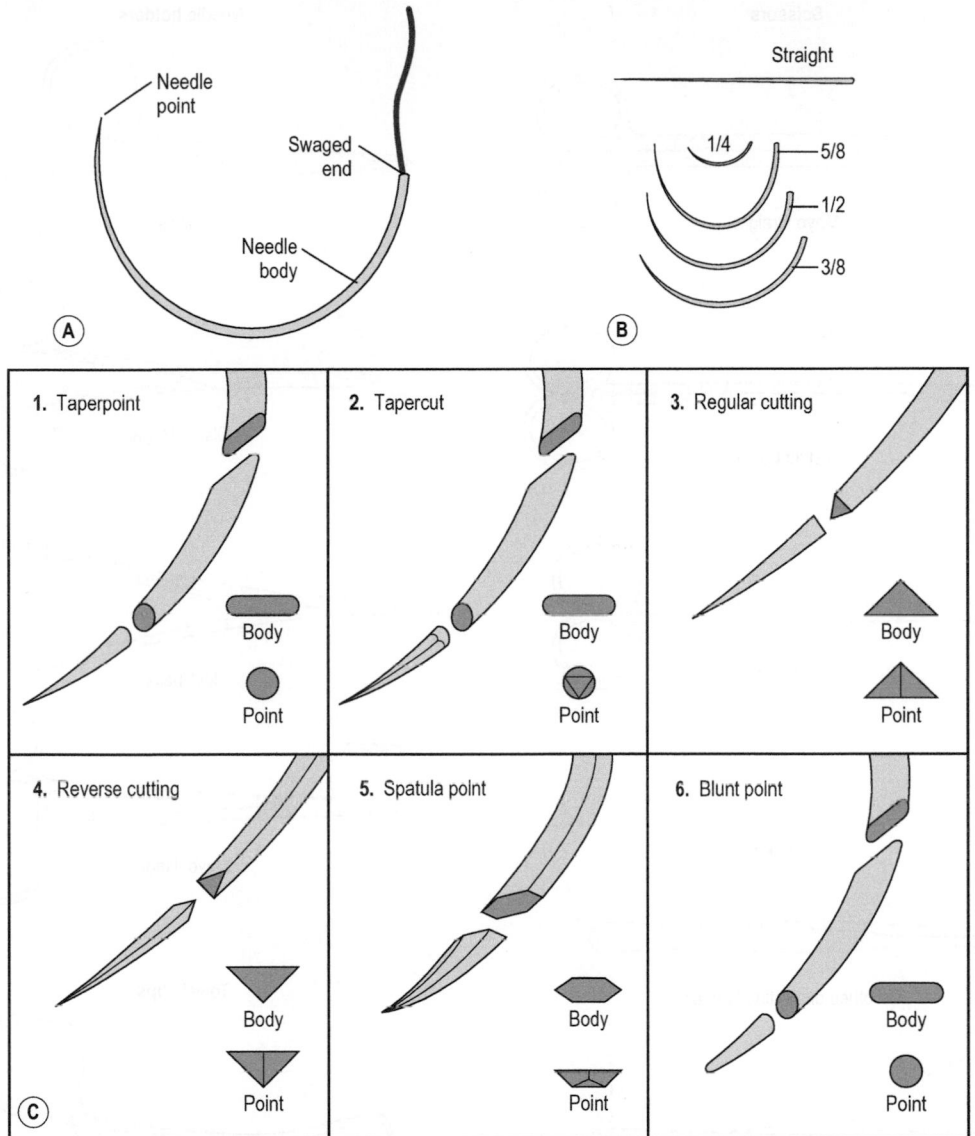

Figure 10.1 (A) Basic components of a needle. (B, C) Needle body shapes and sizes.

- **inverting** sutures turn the tissue edges inwards towards the lumen of an organ (e.g. Lembert sutures).

INTERRUPTED SUTURE PATTERNS

This type is often easier to do and may be the pattern of choice for the novice. Each individual suture is placed separately with its own knot so failure of one suture does not result in failure of the entire line. One disadvantage is that there are more knots and more suture material within the wound, which may result in an increased inflammatory response and an increased risk of infection. Interrupted sutures take longer to do, but they are the most common type.

Suture patterns will be described from the point of view of a right-handed surgeon.

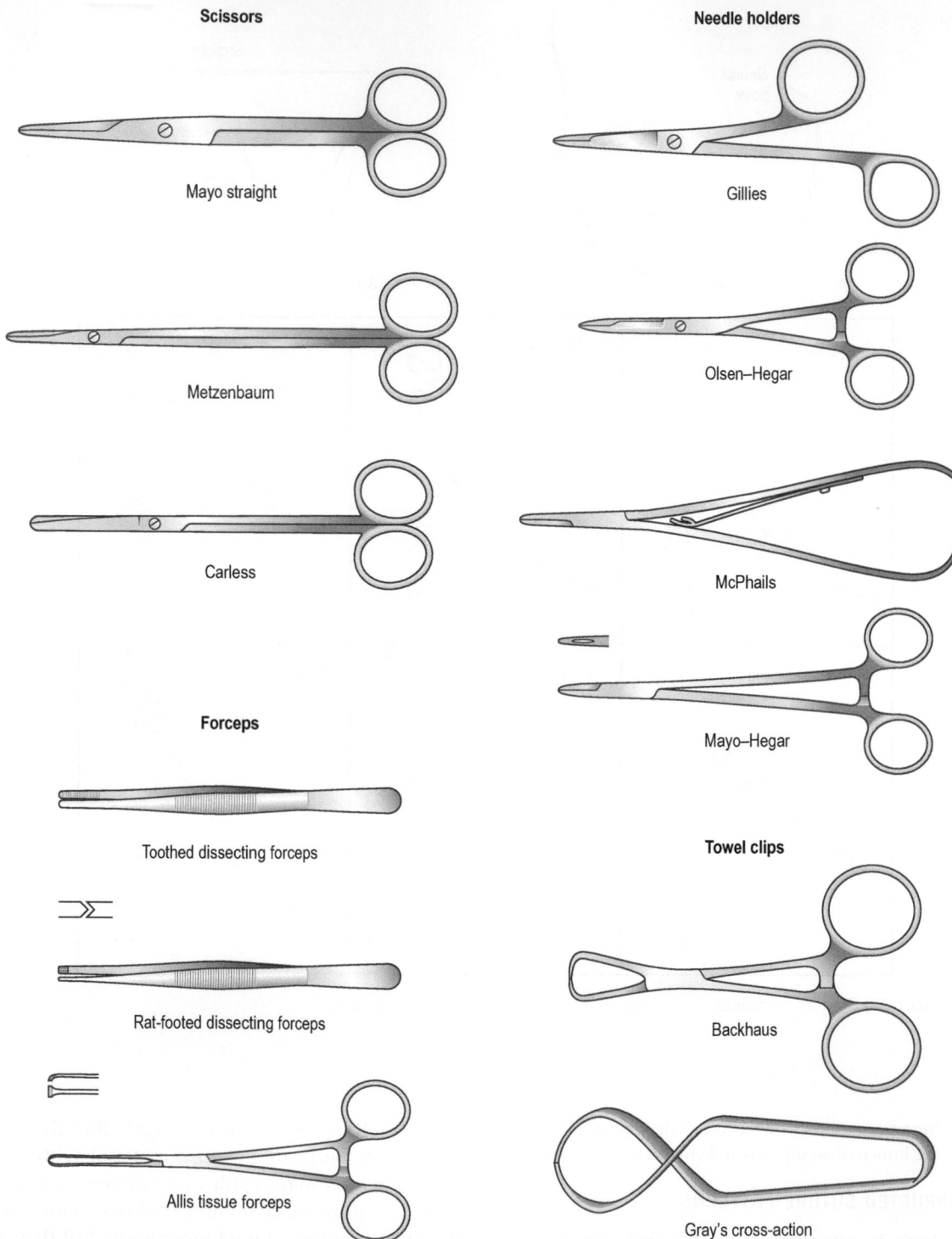

Figure 10.2 Examples of scissors, needle holders and forceps.

Table 10.3 Basic components of suture needles

Component of needle	Type	Comment
Attachment to suture material	Swaged (Fig. 10.1)	Suture material is fused to needle – presented in presterilized packs ready for immediate use; less trauma to the tissues; less risk of material fraying; needle is often sharper
	Eyed	Needle must be loaded with suture material – can be reused, cheaper than swaged; risk of trauma to the tissues from double layer of suture material at the eye – never knot the material to the eye
Gauge – refers to the thickness of the metal	Heavy gauged	Thicker metal prevents bending as the needle is pushed through tougher tissues
	Vascular-type	Thin. Diameter should be the same as that of the suture material to ensure that the hole left by the needle is filled by the suture material. Used to prevent leaks in vascular structures
Shape (Fig. 10.1) – use curved needles in the depths of a body cavity and progressively more straight needles as you pass up through the tissues towards the outer surface of the body	Curved	Used in deep wounds with restricted access
	Half curved	Straight shaft with a curve towards the point. More difficult to handle
	Compound curved	Have a different radius of curvature at the tip and along the shaft. These are used for anterior segment ophthalmic surgery and for blood vessel anastomoses
	Straight	Used in the skin where access is easy. These are not usually held by needle holders
Needle points (Fig. 10.1)	Non-cutting needles – round in cross section	Round-bodied	May be described as atraumatic as they do not cut the tissues as they pass through. If used in tough tissues, they may cause trauma by being pushed through
		Taperpoint	Have a sharp tip which broadens out spreading the tissues as it passes through. Used in easily penetrated tissues (e.g. intestine)
		Blunt point	Have a rounded blunt point that pushes through the tissues without cutting. Used for suturing friable soft tissues (e.g. liver or kidney)
	Cutting needles – often triangular in cross section and usually have two or three cutting edges. Used in tougher tissues (e.g. skin)	Tapercut	Compromise between round-bodied and a cutting needle. Has reverse cutting edge tip and a taperpoint body. Used for suturing dense fibrous tissue such as tendon
		Regular cutting	Has a third cutting edge along the concave edge of a curved needle
		Reverse cutting	Has a third cutting edge along the convex edge of a curved needle, which makes the needle stronger. Less likely to create cuts along the tension line of the suture.
		Spatula point	Have a flat top and bottom. Allows easy tissue penetration and is used in ophthalmic surgery

Procedure: Simple interrupted suture

1. **Action:** Sutures should be placed horizontally from right to left.

    Rationale: Left-handed surgeons should work in the opposite direction.

2. **Action:** Holding the needle with needle holders as described above, introduce the needle through the tissue on the far side (or right side) of the wound 2–5 mm away from the tissue edge (Fig. 10.3).

    Rationale: If sutures are placed too close to the edge, there is a risk that they will pull through. If they are too far away from the edge, too great a thickness of tissue will be pulled up and may invert. This will create an unsightly suture line, which may take longer to heal or may scar.

3. **Action:** Bring the needle up on the opposite side 2–5 mm away from the tissue edge (Fig. 10.3A).

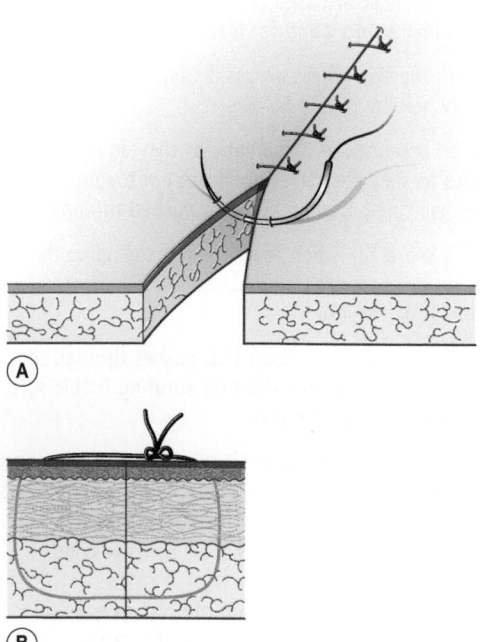

(A)

(B)

Figure 10.3 (A) Simple interrupted sutures. (B) The position of the knot in relation to the incision. (Reproduced with permission from Stephen Baines, Vicky Lipscomb and Tim Hutchinson: BSAVA Canine and Feline Surgical Principles, 2012, originally illustrated by Samantha J Elmhurst.)

Rationale: This is easiest to do using a curved needle.

4. **Action:** Pull the suture material through leaving about 3 cm sticking out of the far side.

    Rationale: The suture material will be used to form the knot. Be careful not to pull the suture right through the wound as you will then have to repeat it. If you leave a long piece of suture material it will be wasted when you cut it off. Over time this wastage becomes very expensive!

5. **Action:** Knot the two ends together as described below. The knot must be left offset from the wound and not resting in the incision (Fig. 10.3B).

    Rationale: To prevent it interfering with the healing process and then being difficult to remove from the tissue.

6. **Action:** Cut the suture material on either side, leaving the ends about 2–3 mm long.

    Rationale: The ends must be long enough to grasp with forceps during removal of the suture. If they are too long they may invite interference by the patient; if they are too short the knot may unravel.

7. **Action:** The resulting suture should be tight enough to result in apposition of the tissues but loose enough to avoid inversion of the edges.

    Rationale: Excessive tension and inversion of the suture line may delay healing and cause pain, which could lead to patient interference.

8. **Action:** Place the next suture about 5 mm along the wound.

    Rationale: The distance apart depends on the site and tissue of the wound.

Interrupted cruciate suture – this is currently a popular type of suture formed by two linked simple sutures arranged as a figure-of-eight and tied with one knot (Fig. 10.4). The advantages are that there are fewer knots, making it quicker to place, and the tension is spread better over a larger area than it is with a simple suture. Remove by cutting both loops so that you avoid dragging pieces of the suture that have been exposed to the external environment through the tissues.

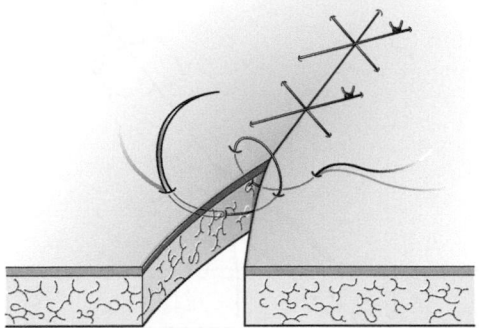

Figure 10.4 Interrupted cruciate suture pattern. (Reproduced with permission from Stephen Baines, Vicky Lipscomb and Tim Hutchinson: BSAVA Canine and Feline Surgical Principles, 2012, originally illustrated by Samantha J Elmhurst.)

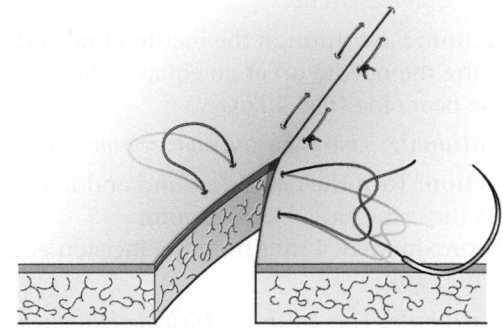

Figure 10.5 Horizontal mattress suture pattern. (Reproduced with permission from Stephen Baines, Vicky Lipscomb and Tim Hutchinson: BSAVA Canine and Feline Surgical Principles, 2012, originally illustrated by Samantha J Elmhurst.)

Procedure: Horizontal mattress suture

This is an everting suture.

1. **Action:** Holding the needle with needle holders, insert it into the tissue on the far side of the incision about 2–5 mm away from the edge. Pass across the incision and bring the needle up on the near side (Fig. 10.5).

   Rationale: This is the same as for a simple suture. The suture should be placed just below the dermis.

2. **Action:** Move about 6–8 mm along the incision and reinsert the needle into the tissue on the near side.

   Rationale: The suture material has made a horizontal line parallel to the edge of the wound (Fig. 10.5).

3. **Action:** Pass across the incision and bring the needle up on the far side.

   The suture material has described a rectangle across the incision (Fig. 10.5).

4. **Action:** Draw the suture material moderately tight so that the edges appose and then tie a knot.

   Rationale: Do not pull so tight that the edges evert.

5. **Action:** Repeat the process for the next suture, which should be about 4–5 mm away.

   Rationale: This type of suture can be used in areas of tension as the pressure exerted by the

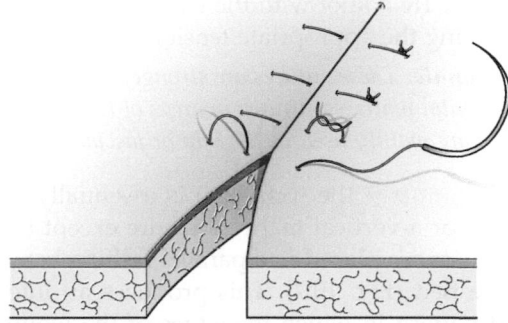

Figure 10.6 Vertical mattress suture pattern. (Reproduced with permission from Stephen Baines, Vicky Lipscomb and Tim Hutchinson: BSAVA Canine and Feline Surgical Principles, 2012, originally illustrated by Samantha J Elmhurst.)

horizontal sutures is spread evenly over a broad area, which reduces the likelihood of tearing through the tissue edges.

Procedure: Vertical mattress suture

This is a tension-relieving suture.

1. **Action:** Holding the needle with needle holders, insert the needle approximately 8–10 mm away from the edge of the incision on the far side (Fig. 10.6).

   Rationale: This will leave enough space to complete a stitch that is at right angles to the incision line. If you insert the needle too close there will not be enough room to complete the manoeuvre correctly.

2. **Action:** Pass through the incision line and bring the needle up at an equal distance on the near side (Fig. 10.6).

   Rationale: This is for the same reason as in 1.

3. **Action:** Turn the needle around and insert it on the same side, but at a point approximately 4 mm from the incision edge (Fig. 10.6).

   Rationale: This creates a stitch at right angles to the incision.

4. **Action:** Pass through the incision and bring the needle up at a point 4 mm from the incision.

   Rationale: The path described by the suture material is a line at right angles to the incision.

5. **Action:** Tie a knot with the two ends after applying the appropriate tension.

   Rationale: These sutures are stronger than horizontal mattress sutures in areas of tension. They are mainly used in the skin or fascia.

Halsted suture – the technique is essentially the same as for a vertical mattress suture except that two sutures are placed in a parallel fashion before they are tied (Fig. 10.7). This produces an interrupted pattern in which the edges of the wound are inverted.

Lembert suture – this is similar to the vertical mattress suture and is used to repair hollow organs. As the holding layer of an organ is the submucosa, the needle should penetrate only to this depth and *never* into the lumen. As the suture is tightened it inverts the tissues (Fig. 10.8).

Procedure: Gambee suture (Fig. 10.9)

This is a specialized suture used in the repair of the intestine.

1. **Action:** Holding the needle in needle holders, insert the needle through the serosa of the intestine on one side of the incision.

   Rationale: This is the outer layer of the area to be closed.

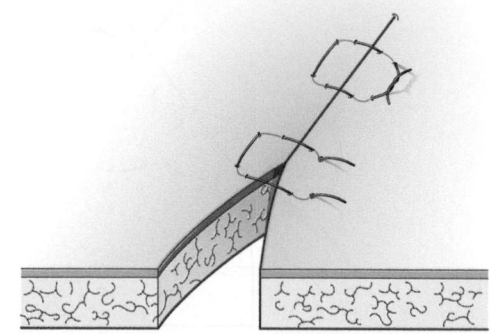

Figure 10.7 Halsted suture pattern. (Reproduced with permission from Stephen Baines, Vicky Lipscomb and Tim Hutchinson: BSAVA Canine and Feline Surgical Principles, 2012, originally illustrated by Samantha J Elmhurst.)

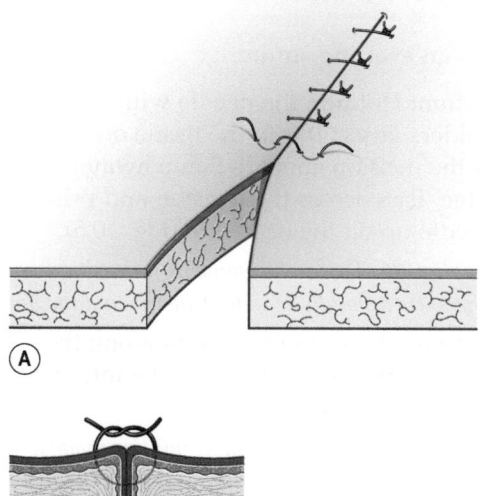

(A)

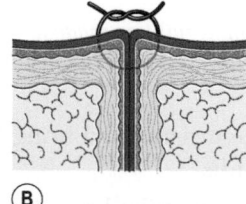

(B)

Figure 10.8 (A) Lembert suture pattern. (B) Note how this inverts the tissues. (Reproduced with permission from Stephen Baines, Vicky Lipscomb and Tim Hutchinson: BSAVA Canine and Feline Surgical Principles, 2012, originally illustrated by Samantha J Elmhurst.)

2. **Action:** Push the needle through the wall of the intestine right through to the mucosa and into the lumen and then return it through all the layers up to the serosal surface again (Fig. 10.9).

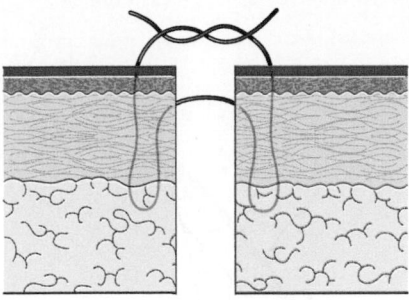

Figure 10.9 Gambee suture. (Reproduced with permission from Stephen Baines, Vicky Lipscomb and Tim Hutchinson: BSAVA Canine and Feline Surgical Principles, 2012, originally illustrated by Samantha J Elmhurst.)

Rationale: When this is repeated on the other side, the suture will help to prevent excessive eversion of the mucosal surface.

3. **Action:** Now cross the incision and insert the needle down through the tissue layers on the other side; then bring the needle back up to the serosal surface again (Fig 10.9).

Rationale: This completes the suture.

4. **Action:** Tie a knot with the two ends of the suture material.

Rationale: The aim of the suture is to reduce eversion of the mucosa and reduce wicking of intestinal contents to the serosal surface.

A modified Gambee is placed in the same way, but does not penetrate the lumen of the intestine.

CONTINUOUS SUTURE PATTERNS

A line of continuous sutures starts and ends with a knot, which decreases the amount of foreign material in the wound. Continuous sutures are much quicker to do, but if one of the knots comes undone the entire line unravels. Tension forces are distributed more evenly and a continuous suture line has been shown to have no more leakage than a line of interrupted sutures.

Procedure: Simple continuous suture (Fig. 10.10)

1. **Action:** Holding the needle with needle holders, place a simple interrupted suture and knot it, but only cut the end of the suture material that is not attached to the needle.

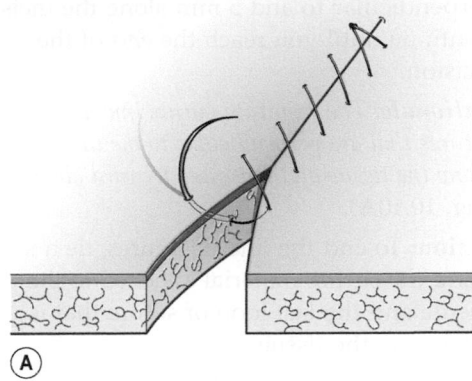

(A)

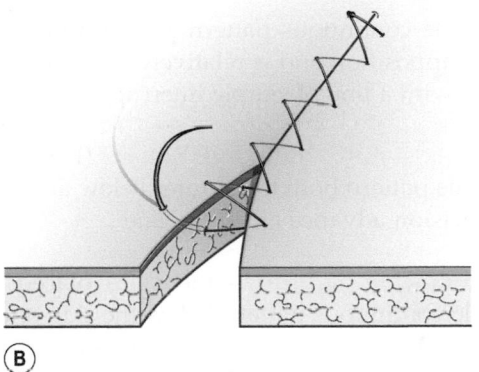

(B)

Figure 10.10 (A) Standard simple continuous suture pattern. (B) Running simple continuous suture pattern. (Reproduced with permission from Stephen Baines, Vicky Lipscomb and Tim Hutchinson: BSAVA Canine and Feline Surgical Principles, 2012, originally illustrated by Samantha J Elmhurst.)

Rationale: The knot should be positioned away from the incision (see simple interrupted above). This suture will be the anchor for the rest of the suture line.

2. **Action:** Insert the needle into the skin perpendicular to the incision and at an appropriate distance from the first suture.

Rationale: Sutures are usually placed at about 5 mm apart.

3. **Action:** Take the needle across to the other side and bring it up through the tissue directly opposite the entry point (Fig. 10.10A).

Rationale: Do not knot the suture.

4. **Action:** Insert the needle on the opposite side perpendicular to and 5 mm along the incision. Continue until you reach the end of the incision.

   Rationale: The resulting suture line has sutures that are perpendicular to the incision below the tissue and advances forward above it (Fig. 10.10A).

5. **Action:** To end the line of sutures, tie a knot using the suture material attached to the needle and the last loop of suture that is exterior to the tissue.

   Rationale: The knot must be secure to ensure that the whole line does not come undone.

A simple continuous pattern provides maximum tissue apposition and is relatively leak proof compared with a line of simple interrupted sutures.

Running simple continuous sutures (Fig. 10.10B) – in this pattern both the sutures below and above the incision advance along the line.

Subcutaneous sutures – these are placed in a simple continuous pattern below the skin and the bites of the suture lie vertical to the incision (Fig. 10.11A). They are used to eliminate dead space and to relieve tension on the skin sutures. This pattern should be used in conjunction with a buried knot(s). (See later description.)

Intradermal sutures – these are often used to replace skin sutures and to reduce scarring. They are useful to reduce patient interference and to eliminate the need for suture removal in sensitive areas (e.g. post castration or in fractious patients). The suture is started by burying the knot in the dermis (see later description) and the suture line lies intradermally. The bites of the suture lie parallel to the line of the incision (Fig. 10.11B) and the suture line is completed with another buried knot. Absorbable suture material should be used.

Procedure: Ford interlocking suture (Fig. 10.12)

1. **Action:** Holding the needle with needle holders, place a simple interrupted suture and

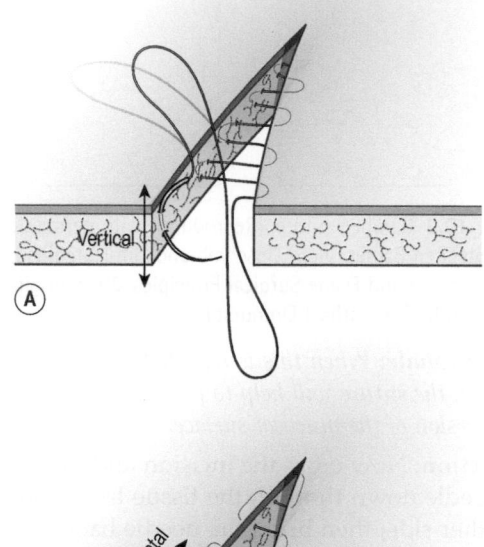

Figure 10.11 Suture patterns: (A) subcutaneous; (B) intradermal.

knot it, but cut only the end of the suture material that is not attached to the needle.

Rationale: The knot should be positioned away from the incision (see simple interrupted above). This suture will be the anchor for the rest of the suture line.

2. **Action:** Bring the needle up through the loop of the suture and then cross the incision and insert it into the tissue on the opposite side as you would for a simple continuous pattern (Fig. 10.12).

   Rationale: This action locks the simple suture in place.

3. **Action:** Take the needle across the incision and bring it up through the tissue on the opposite side. As the needle exits the tissue, bring it up through the loop of the previous suture.

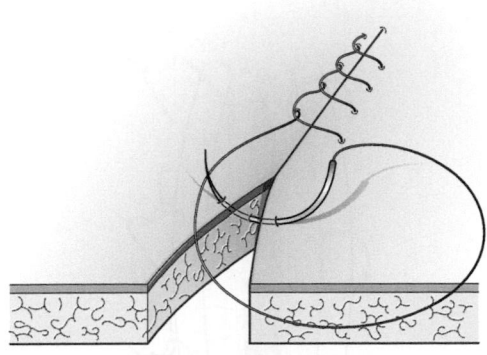

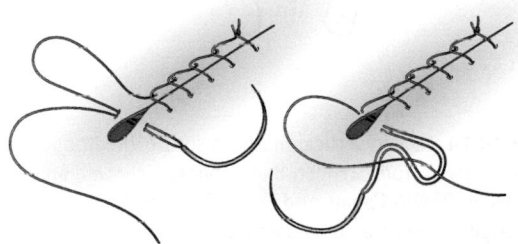

Figure 10.12 Ford interlocking sutures. (Reproduced with permission from Stephen Baines, Vicky Lipscomb and Tim Hutchinson: BSAVA Canine and Feline Surgical Principles, 2012, originally illustrated by Samantha J Elmhurst.)

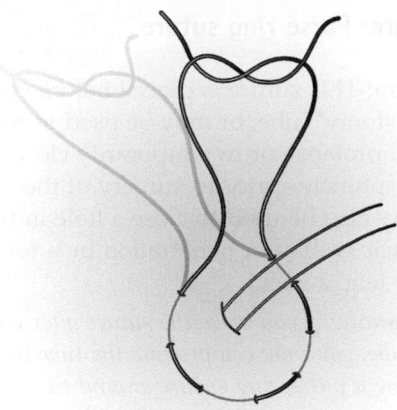

Figure 10.13 Purse ring suture. (Reproduced with permission from Stephen Baines, Vicky Lipscomb and Tim Hutchinson: BSAVA Canine and Feline Surgical Principles, 2012, originally illustrated by Samantha J Flmhurst.)

Rationale: This locks the previous suture in place.

4. **Action:** Repeat as you go along the incision (Fig. 10.12).

   Rationale: This interlocking suture is a form of 'blanket stitch' and can be placed quite quickly. It apposes the tissue more effectively than a simple interrupted pattern and distributes the tension better.

5. **Action:** To finish the line, insert the needle back down into the tissue on the same side as it has just been brought out from and pass it across the incision to exit on the other side. Retain the single end of the suture material on the first side. Tie the loop of material close to the needle to the single end. (Fig 10.12).

   Rationale: The locking effect means that the line is less likely to unravel as a result of patient interference.

This pattern uses up more suture material than other patterns. It can be time consuming to remove as each loop must be cut individually to avoid pulling suture material that has been exposed to the external environment through the inner tissues of the wound.

Continuous Lembert sutures – these are interrupted sutures (Fig. 10.8) placed as a continuous line and are inverting sutures used to close hollow organs. The needle must *not* penetrate into the lumen and the suture bites are placed perpendicular to the incision as in the vertical mattress suture pattern.

Continuous horizontal mattress sutures – start with a simple interrupted suture and then continue with linked sutures as described above (Fig. 10.5). The suture bites are parallel to the line of the incision. More tension on the suture line will produce greater tissue eversion.

SPECIALIZED SUTURE TECHNIQUES

A. Purse ring suture (Fig. 10.13) – This technique may be used to close visceral stumps and to secure percutaneous tubes into a viscus such as may be seen in gastrostomy and cystostomy procedures.

Procedure: Purse ring suture

1. **Action:** This suture is placed before you insert an 'ostomy' tube, or may be used to reduce a rectal prolapse or to temporarily close the anal sphincter prior to surgery of the rectum. It may also be used to close a hole in the thoracic wall after penetration by a foreign body (e.g. a stick).

   Rationale: If you place the suture after you insert the tube, you may compromise the tube lumen. Placing a purse ring suture around the anal sphincter prevents the passage of faeces, which may contaminate the surgical site – do not forget to remove it!

2. **Action:** Place a line of running sutures around the stump or – 'ostomy' tube so that the suture needle ends up at the same point as it started.

   Rationale: When this is pulled tight it will gather up the tissue like the top of a cloth purse.

3. **Action:** Leave a length of suture material free from each end.

   Rationale: This will allow you to pull the suture tight and will be used to tie the knot.

4. **Action:** Pull up the ends of the suture around the tube and tie the ends together (Fig. 10.13).

   Rationale: This will create a seal around the tube.

5. **Action:** If the purse ring suture is around a penetrating foreign body, slowly withdraw the foreign body as you tighten the suture.

   Rationale: This will create a seal as the hole is vacated. It may be necessary to roll the edges inwards with an instrument to achieve mucosal inversion and a tight seal.

B. Quilled suture (Fig. 10.14) – A quill is material such as a piece of rolled gauze or a piece of tubing from an old giving set that is used to distribute the tension of a suture over a greater surface area. You can use either vertical or horizontal mattress sutures.

Procedure: Quilled sutures

This uses vertical mattress sutures and tubing from a giving set.

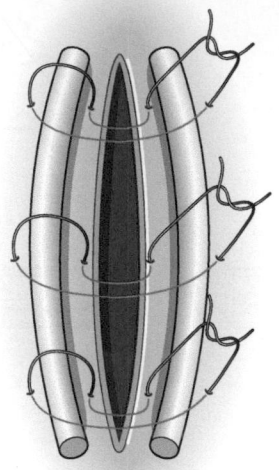

Figure 10.14 Quilled vertical mattress suture. (Reproduced with permission from Stephen Baines, Vicky Lipscomb and Tim Hutchinson: BSAVA Canine and Feline Surgical Principles, 2012, originally illustrated by Samantha J Elmhurst.)

1. **Action:** Cut two pieces of intravenous drip tubing to the approximate length of the incision.

   Rationale: You can use two pieces of rolled up gauze instead of tubing.

2. **Action:** Insert the needle approximately 8–10 mm away from the edge of the incision on the far side.

   Rationale: This will allow sufficient space to place the mattress suture at right angles to the line of the incision (Fig. 10.6).

3. **Action:** Pass through the incision line and bring the needle up through the tissue at an equal distance from the edge on the near side of the incision.

   Rationale: This is the same reason as no. 1.

4. **Action:** Turn the needle around and insert it on the same side, but at a point approximately 4 mm from the edge.

   Rationale: This creates a stitch at right angles to the line of the incision.

5. **Action:** Pass back through the incision and bring the needle up at a point 4 mm from the far edge.

   Rationale: This has now created a loop on the near side of the incision through which you place the piece of tubing.

6. **Action:** Before you pull the suture material completely through, place a short length of the tubing under the suture on the near side and then pull the suture tight (Fig. 10.14).

   Rationale: The tubing should lie parallel to the line of the incision. Pulling the suture tight will hold the tubing in place.

7. **Action:** On the far side of the incision, place the other piece of tubing parallel to the incision and between the two entry points of the suture. Secure the suture with a knot, which should lie on top of the tubing.

   Rationale: This will hold the tubing in place on the far side (Fig. 10.14).

8. **Action:** Continue to place a line of interrupted vertical mattress sutures along the incision line so that each one helps to hold the piece of tubing in place (Fig. 10.14).

   Rationale: The two lines of tubing help to spread the tension from the suture over a greater surface area.

C. **Chinese finger-trap suture** (Fig. 10.15) – This is a technique consisting of a series of knots that is used to secure a tube such as a suction drain to the

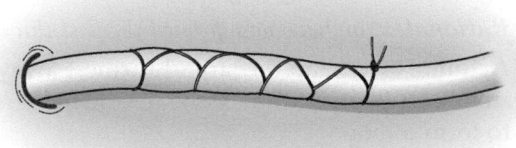

Figure 10.15 A Chinese finger-trap suture used to secure an active suction drain. (With permission from Baines S, Lipscomb V and Hutchinson T (2012) Manual of Canine and Feline Surgical Principles. BSAVA Gloucester, p 289.)

skin. Tension on the tube increases as the tube is pulled, thus preventing its removal.

Procedure: To tie a Chinese finger–trap suture

1. **Action:** Place a simple interrupted suture in the skin at a point close to the exit of the tube.

   Rationale: This will form a firm attachment of the tube to the body.

2. **Action:** Leave both ends of the suture material long.

   Rationale: These ends will allow you to wind them along the length of the tube.

3. **Action:** Take one end between the thumb and forefinger of your left hand and the other end in your right hand and pass them over each in the front of the tube and form the first throw of a simple knot.

   Rationale: You can tie a full surgical knot if you want, but one throw is usually sufficient to anchor the tube. The tension on the throw should slightly indent the tube, but must not be so tight that it occludes the lumen of the tube.

4. **Action:** Cross them over each other behind the tube and perform a throw again.

   Rationale: The suture will have moved along the tube.

5. **Action:** Cross them over each other in front of the tube and perform another throw.

   Rationale: The gap between each knot should be about 0.5–1 cm.

6. **Action:** Repeat this at least 5–6 times and terminate with a secure knot consisting of several throws.

   Rationale: The suture material will have entwined the tube in a net-like structure, which will hold it firmly in place (Fig. 10.15).

Suture removal – sutures should be removed once there is sufficient healing to prevent the wound reopening. This is usually at 10–14 days, but healing may take longer in debilitated patients or if there has been patient interference. If sutures are left in for too long then granulation tissue may cover the knots, making removal both difficult and painful.

KNOTS

A knot may be defined as two throws laid one on top of the other and tightened. It is the weakest point in a line of sutures and if it is incorrectly tied it will come undone and lead to reopening of the wound, which at the very least will delay healing but most severely could lead to evisceration and other complications.

Knot security depends on:

- The type of suture material – multifilament suture materials tend to have better knot-holding ability than monofilament suture materials (Table 10.1).
- The length of the cut ends – if they are too short the knot may unravel.
- The structure of the knot.

The tension applied to the knot is also important. The knot should not be too tight unless it is used as part of a ligature for haemostasis. Excessive tension may strangulate the tissue and will cause the patient some discomfort, which may lead to patient interference.

Knots may be tied:

- **Using instruments** – this is easier and more common than using hand tying and the advantage is that there is less wastage of suture material. There may be a loss of feeling when using instruments, but once you are proficient you will learn to gauge the tension of each throw.
- **By hand** – this technique is useful in confined or hard-to-reach spaces or when sutures have been preplaced (e.g. in closure of a thoracotomy). It is usually necessary to leave the ends of the suture material longer than when using instruments, which can lead to wastage. The technique may be one handed, which is useful in small spaces, or two handed, which allows better control.

TYPES OF KNOT

The type of knot (Fig. 10.16) formed tends to depend on the surgeon's technique.

Procedure: Tying a square knot using instruments

1. **Action:** Place a simple interrupted suture and leave the two ends of suture material free.

   Rationale: One end attached to the needle will be longer than the other end, which should be about 2–3 cm long.

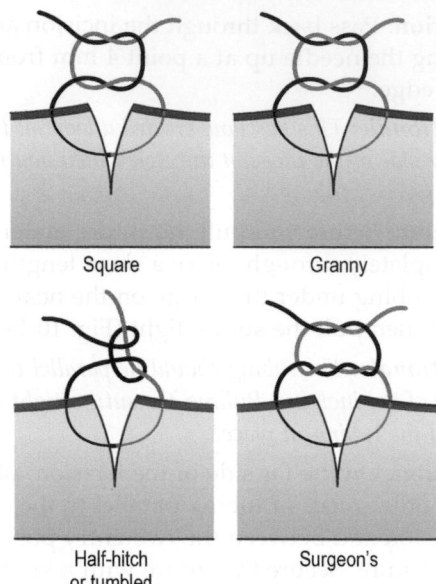

Figure 10.16 Types of knot.

2. **Action:** Holding the needle holders in your right hand, place the tips between the two strands of suture material and wrap the strand nearest to you (long end) around the needle holders to form a loop.

   Rationale: The long end is attached to the needle.

3. **Action:** Open the tips of the needle holders a little and grasp the short end of the suture material.

   Rationale: The short end is the end without the needle.

4. **Action:** Bring the short end through the loop towards you by reversing your hands and tighten the suture gently.

   Rationale: You have now formed the first throw.

5. **Action:** Now wrap the strand furthest away from you (long end) over the needle holders to form a loop.

   Rationale: This is the beginning of the second throw.

6. **Action:** Open the tips of the needle holder a little and grasp the short end of the suture material and pull it through the loop.

   Rationale: Gently allow this throw to form the knot to prevent the suture tightening excessively.

7. **Action:** Keep your hands low and parallel to prevent the knot tumbling.

   Rationale: Each throw should be directly on top of the other if it is not to become a half-hitch (Fig. 10.16).

NB Even pressure must be applied to each end; if one end is pulled with greater tension than the other a half-hitch will form. Hands should be on the same level – if one hand is lifted the suture will tumble and form a sliding two-half-hitch knot. If the ends are crossed incorrectly a granny knot will form (Fig. 10.16). Tumbled knots, half-hitches and granny knots are incorrect and may come undone.

Square knot – this is the most common type of knot and is used to anchor most suture patterns.

Slip knot – this is the same as a square knot except that the tension is uneven. One strand is held with more upwards pressure, resulting in a knot that can slide easily to tighten or to loosen.

Surgeon's knot (Fig. 10.16) – this is similar to the square knot except that the first throw has the strand of suture material thrown over the needle holders twice before the short strand is pulled through. This has the advantage of creating more friction so that the first throw is kept snug while the second standard throw is placed on top. A surgeon's knot is asymmetrical so must be followed by a square knot on top to ensure security.

Buried knots – this technique is used to start a line of subcutaneous or intradermal sutures to reduce the irritation that may be caused by the knots rubbing against superficial tissues. To bury the knot, introduce the needle deep in the far subcutaneous or intradermal tissue passing it up into the tissue, across the incision and then down into the tissue on the near side (Fig. 10.17), exiting deep in the incision line. Now form a knot, which will be buried within the incision line.

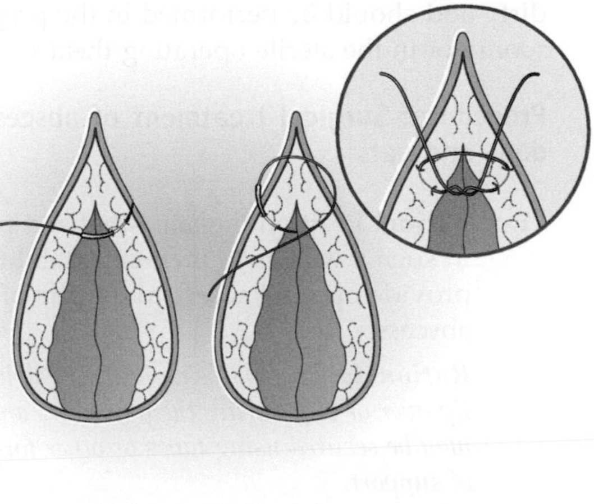

OTHER METHODS OF TISSUE REPAIR

1. **Surgical staples** – these cause little or no tissue reaction and they provide excellent tissue apposition and haemostasis. They may be used in a variety of situations both internally and externally and have the following advantages:

   a. Reduction in surgical time, which is of benefit to critically ill patients

   b. Reduction in tissue handling and trauma

   c. Reduction or elimination of contamination by intestinal contents

   d. Provide an easy and secure method of closing tissues such as the lung, liver and gastrointestinal tract, large vessels and vascular pedicles.

There are various types of stapler designed for internal use and for repairing skin wounds and the staples themselves come in different sizes. Removal is simple, but does require a removal device. The disadvantages are the additional expense and the time taken to

Figure 10.17 To bury a knot to start subcutaneous or intradermal sutures.

master the technique. The use of surgical staples does not compensate for poor surgical technique and may bring its own problems.

Box 10.1 outlines the factors to be considered in the use of surgical staples.

2. **Tissue adhesives** – these are cyanoacrylate monomers that become strong insoluble polymers on contact with the water on tissue surfaces. Setting time varies between 2 and 60 seconds depending on the thickness of the glue layer, the amount of moisture and the chemical makeup of the adhesive.

Tissue adhesives have been available for some time, but the original ones had many problems so they were not widely used. The more modern ones are much improved, but hand-sutured or stapled wound closure is still the method of choice.

The use of tissue glue has proved to be effective in:

a. Cutaneous wounds and incisions

b. Closing biopsy wounds

c. Repair and treatment of corneal ulcers – requires experience as the consequences of accidental misapplication could be disastrous

---

Box 10.1 Basic considerations in the use of surgical staples*

- Never use staples in tissues that are inflamed, oedematous or necrotic.
- Each staple must penetrate all the layers of the tissue.
- Select the correct size of staple – the staple must be able to close the tissue securely.
- Do not place too much tissue within the stapler.
- Check that the tissue is correctly aligned within the stapler and that no other tissues are caught up before firing the stapler.
- Carefully remove the stapler after firing to prevent disruption of the staple or the staple line.
- Check the staple or staple line for signs of haemorrhage, leakage or loose staples before leaving the site.

*Adapted from Manual of Canine and Feline Surgical Principles. BSAVA. Gloucester.

d. Closure of oral wounds following dental work

e. Surgical incisions where patient interference is likely and where the patient will not tolerate an Elizabethan collar.

f. Useful in small species (e.g. rodents) where the wound is very small.

Do not use tissue adhesive on infected wounds, deep puncture wounds or if the edges are under tension. Do not apply the adhesive too thickly or over a pool of blood or fluid and avoid burying the adhesive in deeper layers of tissue.

COMMON SURGICAL PROCEDURES

This section describes surgical procedures that are considered to be the essential requirements for the new veterinary graduate; by the end of your first year in practice you should be fully competent at them.

The list of procedures has been arranged in alphabetical order. It should be assumed that all are carried out under a general anaesthetic and that the surgical site has been prepared aseptically and draped appropriately. For details of these procedures see Chapters 8 and 9.

ABSCESSES

The most common type of abscess is that seen in cats resulting from bites and scratches. Abscesses are relatively rare in dogs, but do occur in rabbits.

Surgical treatment of an abscess is classified as dirty and should be performed in the preparation room not in the sterile operating theatre.

Procedure: Surgical treatment of abscesses in dogs and cats

1. **Action:** Position the anaesthetized patient in such a way as to maintain stability and provide optimal access to the site of the abscess.

   Rationale: The body should not be able to tip over or slip during the procedure and may be secured using tapes or other forms of support.

2. **Action:** The site should be clipped and prepared aseptically and sterile drapes should be placed over the patient and around the abscess.

    Rationale: This will prevent the introduction of new pathogens into the site. The drapes will help to absorb fluid, thus preventing the patient becoming excessively wet during the flushing of the abscess.

3. **Action:** Full aseptic technique must be observed. Gloves and safety glasses are recommended.

    Rationale: This will reduce the risk of introducing pathogens into the wound and the risk of acquiring infection from the patient. Safety glasses will prevent pathogens being splashed into the eyes.

4. **Action:** Using a sterile scalpel blade, make a stab incision into the skin overlying the abscess. The incision may be enlarged if necessary and the flow of exudate can be accelerated by the use of gentle pressure over the surrounding area.

    Rationale: This should result in the immediate release of purulent exudates, which may smell and may be blood-stained.

5. **Action:** Using a 20 ml syringe and a large gauge needle, flush out the abscess with warmed saline. You may add dilute chlorhexidine in a dilution of 1:40 if necessary.

    Rationale: Use at least 500 ml of fluid to achieve total irrigation and cleaning. Warming the fluid reduces cold shock. Chlorhexidine is an antiseptic, which will reduce the numbers of pathogens.

6. **Action:** Chronic abscesses may have a thick fibrous lining that should be debrided and then reflushed.

    Rationale: If the lining is not debrided there is a risk that the abscess will reform.

7. **Action:** Clean and dry the surrounding area and leave the wound open to drain.

    Rationale: Closure of the wound might trap remaining infection within the cavity and lead to reformation of the abscess.

8. **Action:** Abscesses with a large dead space may be partially closed with a Penrose drain in place (see below).

    Rationale: This will enable the purulent material to drain out more easily.

9. **Action:** If partial closure is performed, use absorbable monofilament suture material. The knot should have a minimum number of throws.

    Rationale: Monofilament suture material will not 'wick' up the infection. Using a knot with a minimum number of throws will reduce bacterial resistance.

10. **Action:** In most cases the wound is left open to drain and to heal by second intention, but in some cases it may be necessary to place a suitable dressing (see Ch. 4).

    Rationale: The dressing should be of a type that will absorb the exudate.

11. **Action:** The patient should be sent home with antibiotics, NSAID analgesics and, if necessary, an Elizabethan collar. The owner should be instructed to bathe the area gently with saline or cooled boiled water for the first 1–2 days if the abscess is still draining.

    Rationale: An Elizabethan collar may be necessary to prevent patient interference, but be careful if the abscess is around the neck area as the collar will rub. Gentle bathing will clean away the exudates, but should not be necessary after the second day as the wound dries and heals.

12. **Action:** The wound should dry up and heal within a few days.

    Rationale: A small percentage of abscesses return and will have to be redrained.

Procedure: Surgical treatment of abscesses in rabbits

The most common causative organisms are *Pasteurella multocida* and *Staphylococcus aureus*. Abscesses in rabbits are more difficult to treat than they are in cats and dogs because:

- The exudate is very often thick and 'cheesy' and does not drain easily from the abscess. It is not recommended to try and squeeze the pus out before instigating proper surgical treatment as this may seed abscesses to other areas, and may disperse the toxins subsequently killing the rabbit.

- Abscesses often occur on the face and may be associated with dental disease, which is difficult to resolve.
- The abscess may have several pockets of infection and a persistent lining membrane, which makes draining and treatment of the abscess less likely to be successful.
- The causative bacteria have a propensity for bone resulting in inflammation and bone abscessation, which is extremely difficult to treat.

The prognosis for rabbits suffering with abscesses must always be guarded.

1. **Action:** Before anaesthetizing the rabbit, perform a full clinical examination including taking blood for haematology and biochemistry, and taking radiographs to check for lung abscessation and for dental disease.

    Rationale: *Some abscesses may not be able to be treated and euthanasia should be considered.*

2. **Action:** After induction of anaesthesia, position the animal in such a way as to maintain stability and to provide optimal access to the site of the abscess.

    Rationale: *The body should not be able to tip over or slip during the procedure and may be secured using tapes or other forms of support.*

3. **Action:** The site should be clipped and prepared aseptically and sterile drapes should be placed over the patient and around the abscess.

    Rationale: *This will prevent the introduction of new pathogens into the site. The drapes will help to absorb fluid, thus preventing the patient becoming excessively wet during the flushing of the abscess.*

4. **Action:** Full aseptic technique must be observed. Gloves and safety glasses are recommended.

    Rationale: *This will reduce the risk of introducing pathogens into the wound and of acquiring infection from the patient. Safety glasses will prevent pathogens being splashed into the eyes.*

5. **Action:** Using a sterile scalpel, make a stab incision through the skin over the abscess

and very gently ease the exudate out through the wound.

Rationale: *The exudate will be thick and 'cheesy' and will not run out as it does in cat abscesses.*

6. **Action:** Take a swab for bacterial culture and sensitivity testing (see Ch. 5).

    Rationale: *The choice of antibiotics is limited in rabbits and it is important to choose the correct one.*

7. **Action:** Using a syringe and a nasolacrimal duct cannula, irrigate the abscess with warm saline. The use of proteolytic enzymes, such as trypsin, to liquefy the exudate has been suggested.

    Rationale: *If the exudate is liquefied it will be easier to flush out of the abscess. Draining the abscess does not guarantee that it will not recur.*

8. **Action:** If it possible to obtain a clear margin around the abscess, incise around the whole lesion to remove it intact.

    Rationale: *This will guarantee that the outer lining membrane has been removed thus reducing the chances of the abscess reforming. This is very difficult to do with dental abscesses.*

9. **Action:** Once the abscess has been drained, pack the cavity with calcium hydroxide or antibiotic-impregnated beads.

    Rationale: *These materials will absorb the exudate and promote healing.*

10. **Action:** Clean and dry the surrounding area and leave the wound to heal by second intention.

    Rationale: *Closing the wound might trap any residual infection in the cavity.*

11. **Action:** Send the rabbit home with the antibiotics indicated by the sensitivity test and ask the owner to bathe the wound gently with saline or cooled boiled water for the first 1–2 days.

    Rationale: *The most common antibiotic is enrofloxacin but, whichever one is used, antibiosis must be continued for 2–3 months to ensure resolution of the condition.*

12. **Action:** The rabbit should be placed in thoroughly cleaned hutch lined only with newspaper for a few days.

Rationale: To prevent the reintroduction of infection and contamination of the wound by bedding material.

Procedure: Placing a Penrose drain in an abscess

The Penrose drain is an example of a passive open drain and consists of a soft latex tube placed in the dead space after a surgical procedure. The technique may be used in a variety of surgical procedures including the draining of abscesses and aural haematomata.

1. **Action:** After draining the abscess, use a sterile scalpel blade to make a small incision above the opening of the abscess working from the inside to the outside. Leave the tip of the blade protruding through the small incision (Fig. 10.18A, B).

   Rationale: The incision should be no wider than the width of the Penrose drain tube.

2. **Action:** Using a pair of artery forceps, grasp the tip of the blade and retract it back into the cavity until the tips of the forceps can be seen within the cavity (Fig. 10.18B).

   Rationale: This makes an incision at the top of the abscess and reduces tissue damage by pushing the artery forceps through only once.

3. **Action:** Retrieve the scalpel blade from the abscess cavity.

   Rationale: It is no longer needed.

4. **Action:** Place the drain tube in the cavity and use the artery forceps to pick up one end and pull it through the incision until 4–5 cm of it protrudes (Fig. 10.18C).

   Rationale: This forms the top end of the drain.

5. **Action:** Using the scalpel blade and working from the inside outwards, make a small incision at the lowest point of the abscess. Leave the point of the blade protruding.

   Rationale: This will be the point from which the exudate drains.

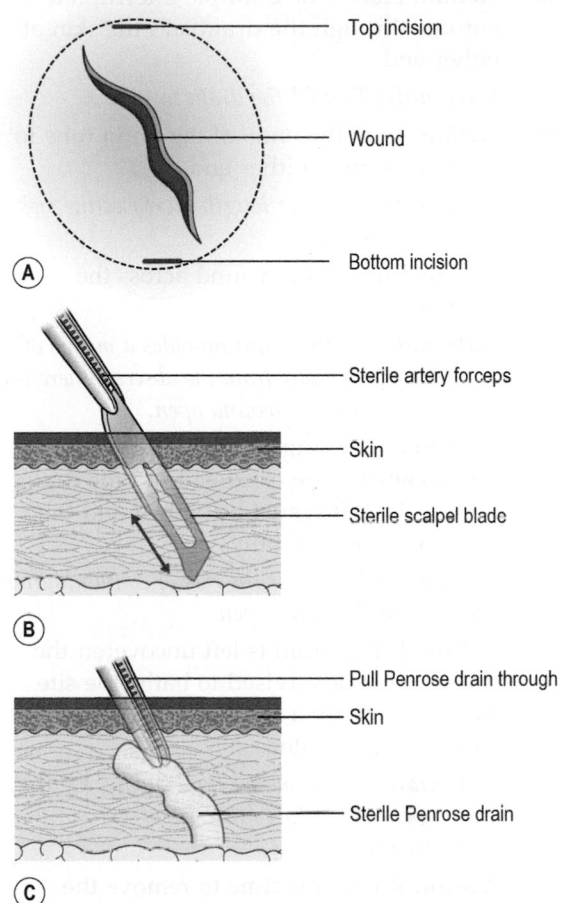

Figure 10.18 The Penrose drain: (A) Make an incision at the top of the wound. (B) Incise from inside to outside. (C) Pull the drain through.

6. **Action:** Using a pair of artery forceps, retract the blade back into the cavity until the tips of the forceps can be seen within the cavity.

   Rationale: The incision has not been made at the base of the wound.

7. **Action:** Retrieve the scalpel blade from the cavity. Manipulate the forceps to pick up the other end of the drain tube and pull it out through the bottom incision.

   Rationale: The drain tube is now lying inside the abscess with one end protruding from each incision.

8. **Action:** Place 1 or 2 simple interrupted sutures through the drain and the skin at either end.

   Rationale: To hold the drain in place.

9. **Action:** Trim the ends of the drain tube to about 2–3 cm at either end.

   Rationale: A longer length increases the risk of contamination.

10. **Action:** Suture the wound across the abscess.

    Rationale: As the drain provides a means of draining the exudate from the abscess, there is no need to leave the wound open.

11. **Action:** A dressing can be placed over the area to absorb the exudate from the drain tubing. The site must be bathed and the dressing changed daily.

    Rationale: To reduce the risk of contamination and to keep the drain open.

12. **Action:** If the drain is left uncovered the owner must be advised to bathe the site twice daily with a weak solution of salt in cooled boiled water.

    Rationale: This removes the exudate, keeps the drain open and reduces the risk of contamination.

13. **Action:** When it is time to remove the drain, prepare the area aseptically.

    Rationale: There is a risk of contamination.

14. **Action:** Remove the sutures from the top of the drain and pull the drain upwards until 'clean' drain is showing.

    Rationale: About a 5 mm length of clean drain is necessary.

15. **Action:** Cut the drain horizontally at this point.

    Rationale: This ensures that only clean drain enters the top incision, which helps to maintain asepsis.

16. **Action:** Remove the sutures from the bottom site and pull the rest of the drain through the incision.

    Rationale: This ensures that only clean drain enters the bottom incision, which helps to maintain asepsis.

17. **Action:** Clean the area and leave to heal.

    Rationale: The two small incisions will heal by second intention.

AURAL HAEMATOMATA

Aural haematomata may be seen in both dogs and cats and usually occur as a result of self-trauma following otitis externa or, in the case of cats, may be a result of fighting. The blood-filled swelling on the inner side of the ear pinna results from haemorrhage from the blood vessels supplying the cartilage. If left, the haematoma organizes and fibrosis and wound contracture result in a typical 'cauliflower ear'. Although this may be considered merely unattractive, it may also lead to an increased incidence of otitis externa and so the vicious circle continues.

Treatment is aimed at draining the haematoma and restoring the shape of the ear pinna by preventing contraction of the cartilage.

Procedure: Treatment of an aural haematoma

1. **Action:** Place the anaesthetized patient in lateral recumbency so that the affected ear is uppermost, and prepare the area aseptically.

   Rationale: To prevent the introduction of infection into the wound.

2. **Action:** Make an incision on the inner side of the ear pinna over the area of the haematoma.

   Rationale: An S-shaped incision is said to prevent twisting of the ear pinna during healing.

3. **Action:** Drain the serum and clot from the cavity formed between the outer skin and the cartilage of the pinna.

   Rationale: When blood is left to clot naturally it forms a clot with a layer of serum above it.

4. **Action:** Flush out the cavity with sterile saline and remove all traces of fibrin.

   Rationale: To clean the area and promote normal healing.

5. **Action:** Leave the wound slightly gaping and take steps to obliterate the dead space and prevent contracture of the pinna. There are several ways of doing this.

Rationale: Drainage of the haematoma is facilitated by the slightly open wound. Obliterating the dead space will prevent the haematoma reforming.

- Use of two staggered lines of interrupted mattress sutures arranged parallel to the ear canal.

  Rationale: To avoid reduction in the blood flow to the pinna. There must be sufficient sutures to prevent the formation of pockets in which fluid may accumulate. The sutures may be placed without involving the outer skin of the ear or they may be full thickness (Fig. 10.19).

- Use of sterilized buttons sutured to each other through the full thickness of the ear pinna.

  Rationale: These exert pressure through the cartilage and obliterate the dead space.

- Use of X-ray film cut to ear shape. This is sutured to the ear through the cartilage.

  Rationale: Used in cat's ears, which are too small for buttons.

- Use of a Penrose drain (see above and Fig 10.20).

  Rationale: This drains the haematoma, but does not address the problem of contracture of the ear pinna. It may not occur if the haematoma does not reform.

6. **Action:** Apply a non-adherent head bandage by placing the affected ear on top of the head and using the unaffected ear as an anchor (see Ch. 4).

Rationale: This will keep the ear clean and prevent self-trauma.

7. **Action:** Send the animal home with an Elizabethan collar and NSAID analgesia for at least 5 days. Antibiotics should not be necessary if the technique has been aseptic.

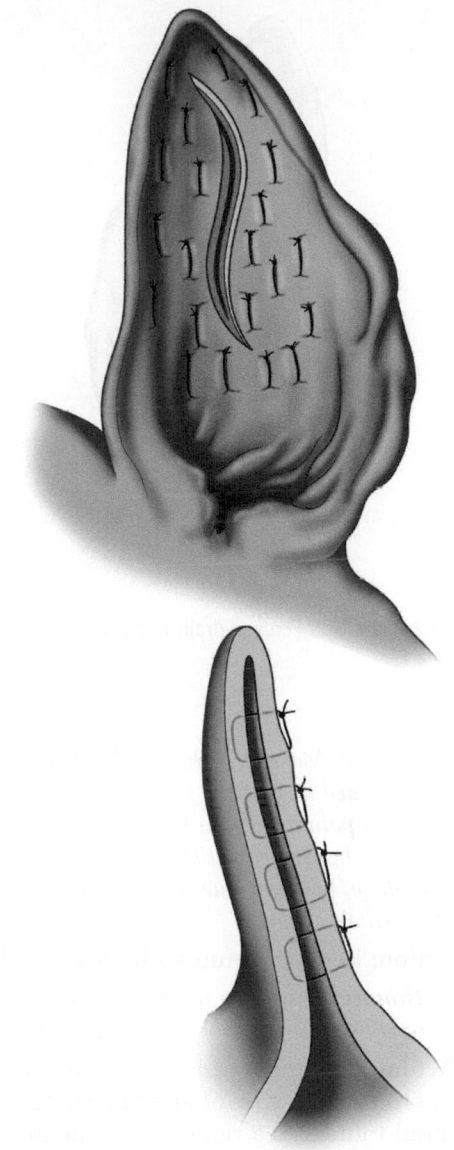

Figure 10.19 Sutures should be placed vertically rather than horizontally for aural haematoma repair. They may be placed through the cartilage without incorporating the skin on the convex surface of the ear, or they may be full thickness.

Rationale: Surgery involving the cartilage of the pinna is painful and this may lead to self-trauma.

8. **Action:** Check the ear within 2–3 days and rebandage if necessary.

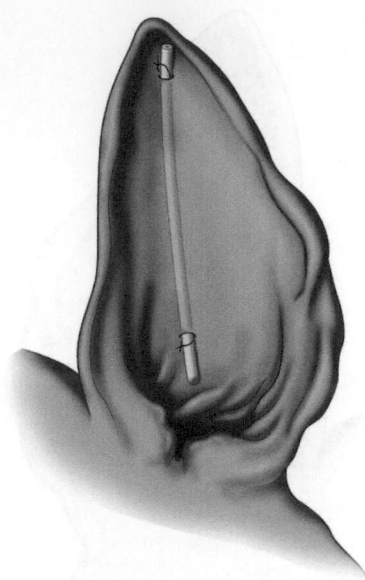

Figure 10.20 Use of a Penrose drain to treat an aural haematoma.

Rationale: Make sure that the haematoma has not reformed or that the sutures are not causing swelling, pain or wound breakdown. If the wound is healing well there may be no need to rebandage, but continue the use of the Elizabethan collar.

9. **Action:** Remove sutures within 10–14 days.

   Rationale: Assuming healing has occurred and there is no recurrence of the haematoma.

10. **Action:** The initial cause is probably otitis externa so any case of aural haematoma should undergo a rigorous examination of the ear canal.

    Rationale: This should be repeated at intervals to prevent recurrence.

NB Aural haematomata can also be treated medically by draining the haematoma and then injecting corticosteroids into the cavity. This has been reported to produce satisfactory results.

CYSTOTOMY

A cystotomy is an incision into the urinary bladder and may be performed to remove cystic or urethral calculi, identify or biopsy cystic masses or to repair ectopic ureters. The approach may also be used to repair a ruptured bladder (e.g. following a road traffic accident or an abdominal kick).

Procedure: Cystotomy for the removal of cystic calculi

1. **Action:** Prior to surgery the bladder should be radiographed to establish the presence of cystic calculi.

   Rationale: Depending on their type, some calculi are radiodense and will show up on a plain radiograph whereas others are radio-opaque and will require the use of positive- or double-contrast techniques (see Ch. 6). Ultrasonography may also be used.

2. **Action:** Position the anaesthetized patient in dorsal recumbency on a stable operating table and secure with ties or sandbags.

   Rationale: The patient's body should not be able to tilt to either side.

3. **Action:** Clip and prepare aseptically an area from about 5–10 cm above the xiphoid to 5–10 cm below the pubis and about 10 cm either side of the midline.

   It is important to prepare a large enough area to prevent the risk of breaking asepsis.
   Rationale: The exact size depends on the size of the patient.

4. **Action:** Make a midline incision from the xiphoid to the pubis – laparotomy.

   The incision should allow adequate access to the bladder.

5. **Action:** Use retractors to retract the abdominal wall.

   Rationale: To provide adequate exposure of the bladder.

6. **Action:** Identify and isolate the bladder from the remainder of the abdominal cavity using wet sterile swabs.

   Rationale: To prevent contamination of the other abdominal organs. Remember to count the swabs and make sure that you remove all of them before closing the abdomen.

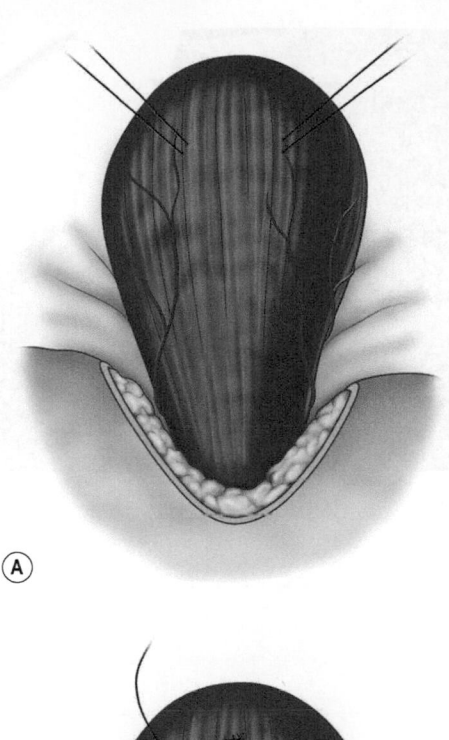

(A)

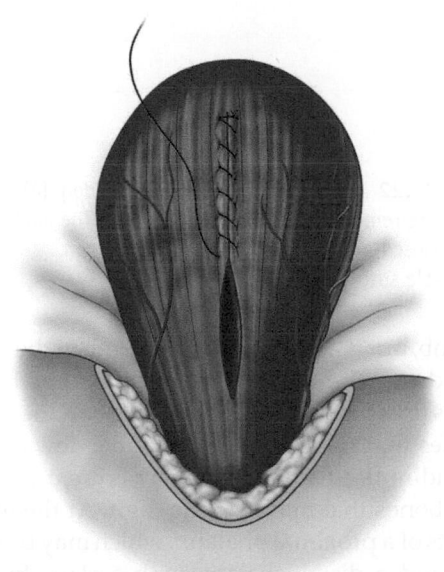

(B)

Figure 10.21 Cystotomy is indicated to remove calculi, repair trauma, resect or biopsy neoplasms, or correct congenital abnormalities. (A) Isolate the bladder and place stay sutures in it to facilitate manipulation. Make the incision in the dorsal or ventral aspect of the bladder. (B) Use a simple continuous suture to close the incision. If the bladder is thin and if leakage occurs, a two-layer closure can be used, but this is seldom necessary.

7. **Action:** Place a couple of stay sutures on the apex of the bladder (Fig. 10.21A).

   Rationale: To aid manipulation of the bladder.

8. **Action:** Drain urine from the bladder by cystocentesis.

   Rationale: To prevent urinary contamination of the surrounding tissues.

9. **Action:** Make an incision on the dorsal or ventral side of the bladder. This should be away from the ureters and urethra and between the major blood vessels.

   Rationale: To prevent any permanent or functional damage.

10. **Action:** Drain the urine from the bladder by suction if this has not already been done by cystocentesis.

    Rationale: Urine can be drained by either method, but it is necessary to do this to prevent contamination.

11. **Action:** Wash out the calculi, taking care to ensure that you remove all of them. Make sure that you do not contaminate the surrounding tissues. You can also insert a finger into the bladder to feel for any remaining calculi (Fig. 10.22A).

    Rationale: Urinary contamination may lead to peritonitis. Do not leave any calculi in the bladder as the clinical signs will return very quickly.

12. **Action:** Close the bladder using absorbable monofilament suture material and a continuous appositional suture pattern (Figs 10.21B and 10.22B,C).

    Rationale: The aim is to create a water-tight seal that will not promote the formation of calculi. A single layer of sutures should be sufficient if the bladder wall is thick. If the bladder is thin walled the lumen may be penetrated, but if absorbable monofilament material is used this should not lead to calculus formation.

13. **Action:** Lavage the surrounding tissues with sterile saline.

    Rationale: To remove any contamination.

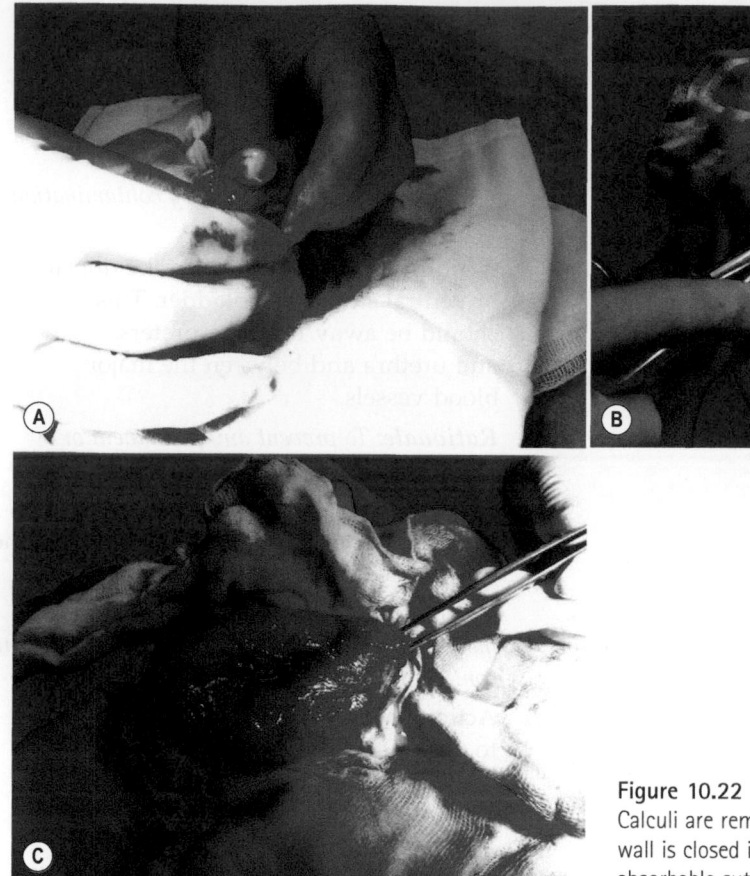

Figure 10.22 Performing a cystotomy in a dog: (A) Calculi are removed from the bladder. (B, C) The bladder wall is closed in two layers using monofilament absorbable suture material.

14. **Action:** Remove all swabs and count them to make sure that none are left behind.

    Rationale: One swab left in the peritoneal cavity can quickly cause a potentially fatal peritonitis.

15. **Action:** Before closing the abdominal wound replace the instruments, gloves and drapes with a fresh sterile set.

    Rationale: To remove the risk of contamination.

16. **Action:** Close the skin incision appropriately.

    Rationale: See previous descriptions.

DEW CLAWS

The dew claw is the first digit on the medial side of each distal limb. It is usually present on the forelimb, but is absent on the hindlimb in the majority of dogs. The breed standard for some breeds, such as the Pyrenean Mountain dog and the Briard, specifies that there must be a double dew claw on the hindlimb. Anatomically there is great variation in the bones that make up the digit. At the most it consists of a proximal phalanx, which may be shortened, and a distal phalanx with a claw. In other individuals it consists of little more than a rudimentary distal phalanx and claw that is attached by skin to the medial side of the tarsus or carpus.

Dew claws are removed because they may catch and tear, resulting in pain and haemorrhage. Removal is also recommended because, as the digit is not weight bearing, the nail may grow and curl around to penetrate the accompanying digital pad.

Removal may be done:

A. In the **first few days after birth** – under the Veterinary Surgeons Act 1966, the dew claws may be removed by a lay person without an anaesthetic providing that that person is over 16 years of age and the eyes of the puppy have not opened. It is preferable for a veterinary surgeon to perform this task, but many breeders remove the dew claws themselves.

Procedure: Dew claw removal in neonatal puppies

1. **Action:** Separate the bitch from her litter by putting her in a separate room and closing the door.

   Rationale: Inevitably the puppies will cry out as a result of handling and the pain of the procedure, and this may distress the bitch, which may get in the way.

2. **Action:** Check the puppy to identify where there are dew claws and which of these the owner wants removed.

   Rationale: Dew claws are usually present on the forelimb, but may not be on the hindlimb. There may be individual variation within the litter. Always check with the owner what they want to be done.

3. **Action:** Prepare the area around each dew claw aseptically.

   Rationale: It may be difficult to clip the hair, but steps should be taken to ensure asepsis as much as possible.

4. **Action:** Inject a small amount of local anaesthetic into the area.

   Rationale: To aid analgesia.

5. **Action:** Ask an assistant to restrain the puppy in his / her hands, then extend a paw and abduct the dew claw.

   Rationale: The puppy will naturally wriggle, which makes the procedure more difficult.

6. **Action:** Using a pair of sterile Mayo scissors, cut through the metatarso / carpophalangeal joint (Fig. 10. 23A).

   Rationale: As the puppy is very young this does not usually require much force. A scalpel blade can be used if necessary.

7. **Action:** Apply pressure to the wound using a sterile gauze swab.

   Rationale: To control haemorrhage, which is usually minimal.

8. **Action:** Appose the skin edges using a simple interrupted suture and non-absorbable suture material, tissue glue or allow healing to take place by second intention.

   Rationale: There are few problems associated with this procedure at this age.

9. **Action:** Repeat with the other dew claws.

   Rationale: You may have to remove claws from all four limbs.

10. **Action:** Put the puppy into a warm box and repeat with the rest of the litter.

    Rationale: As the puppy is very young it must be kept warm.

11. **Action:** When the whole litter has been done, check each puppy for signs of haemorrhage; if all is well then allow the bitch to return to them.

    Rationale: Both the bitch and puppies will be happier once they are reunited.

12. **Action:** Ask the owner to check the puppies regularly for signs of haemorrhage, pain, infection or poor healing and to call you if there are any problems.

    Rationale: A puppy that is crying out, failing to suckle or failing to grow would be a cause for concern.

B. In **puppies over 1 week of age (adults)** – as, by law, the procedure requires a general anaesthetic – it is recommended that the puppy is left until it is at least 3 months old and the procedure is often carried out at the same time as neutering (Fig.10.23B, C).

Procedure: Dew claw removal in adult dogs

1. **Action:** The anaesthetized patient is positioned in lateral recumbency.

   Rationale: This provides easy access to the surgical site on all limbs.

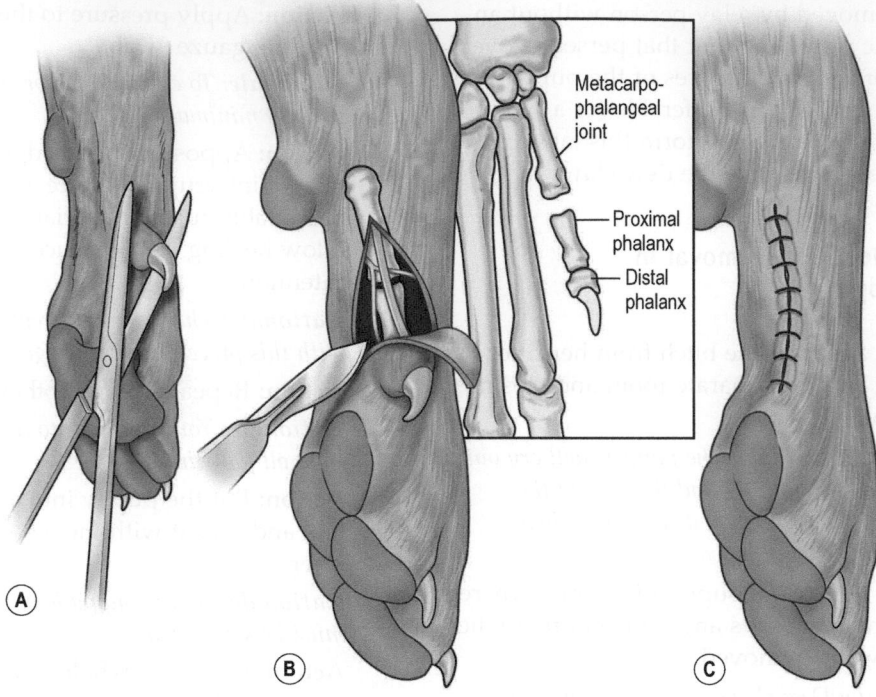

Metacarpo-
phalangeal
joint

Proximal
phalanx

Distal
phalanx

A

B

C

Figure 10.23 Dew claw removal in: (A) puppies under 1 week; (B) puppies over 1 week; (C) finished wound in puppies over 1 week.

2.   **Action:** Clip and prepare aseptically the area around each dew claw to be removed.
     Rationale: As described in Chapter 9.

3.   **Action:** Make an elliptical incision around the base of the digit at the point where it articulates with the metacarpal or metatarsal bone (Fig. 10.23B).
     Rationale: In some cases, particularly in the hindlimb, this attachment may be little more than skin.

4.   **Action:** Abduct the digit and dissect the subcutaneous tissues around the joint.
     Rationale: To free the digit from its attachments – this will vary between individuals.

5.   **Action:** Ligate the blood vessels supplying the digit (Fig 10.23B).

     Rationale: These are the dorsal common and axial palmar digital arteries.

6.   **Action:** Disarticulate the metacarpo- or metatarsophalangeal joint with a scalpel blade.
     Rationale: If you use bone cutters to cut through the joint the result is much less neat and tidy.

7.   **Action:** Appose the subcutaneous tissues as described previously.
     Rationale: To obliterate the dead space and prevent the likelihood of haemorrhage and infection.

8.   **Action:** Place a row of simple interrupted sutures in the skin (Fig. 10.23C).
     Rationale: To appose the skin edges and promote rapid healing.

9. **Action:** Cover with a soft padded bandage, which should remain in place for 3–5 days (see Ch. 4).

   Rationale: To prevent infection and patient interference.

10. **Action:** The patient should be sent home with NSAID analgesia and if necessary an Elizabethan collar.

    Rationale: There will be a degree of pain from the procedure. An Elizabethan collar will prevent interference with the wound or the bandage. Antibiotics should not be necessary if asepsis has been observed during the procedure.

11. **Action:** Remove the bandage in 3 days and rebandage if necessary.

    Rationale: This depends on the appearance of the wound and the degree of healing.

12. **Action:** Remove the sutures in 7–10 days.

    Rationale: Depending on the degree of healing.

GASTROINTESTINAL FOREIGN BODIES

A foreign body may be defined as anything that can be ingested but cannot be digested and it includes bones, which are slowly digested. Foreign bodies are rare in cats but relatively common in dogs, particularly in some breeds such as Labradors and Springer Spaniels.

Foreign bodies can be classified as:

- Discrete – nuts, balls, bones, plastic toys all of which result in a distinct area of blockage or damage
- Linear – tights, string, knickers. These may be carried through the intestine and if one end becomes fixed in one place (e.g. in the stomach), the remainder passes down the intestine resulting in corrugation and damage to the intestinal wall.

Table 10.4 describes the location and clinical signs associated with a range of foreign bodies.

Procedure: Gastrotomy

This is an incision through the stomach wall. The main use is in the removal of gastric foreign bodies and it is preceded by a laparotomy.

1. **Action:** Position the anaesthetized patient in dorsal recumbency on a stable operating table and secure with ties or sandbags.

   Rationale: The patient's body should not be able to tilt to either side.

2. **Action:** Clip and prepare aseptically an area from about 5–10 cm above the xiphoid

Table 10.4 Location and treatment of alimentary foreign bodies

Location	Examples	Clinical signs	Treatment
Oral cavity	Fish hooks, salmon vertebrae on cats' teeth, tin lids, bones across the hard palate	Sudden onset of distress, rubbing face on the ground, pawing at the mouth, bleeding from the mouth, excessive salivation, foreign body may be visible protruding from the mouth but should be easily seen on close examination	Sedation. Open mouth and remove. In some cases a rapid-acting anaesthetic may be necessary (e.g. fish hooks especially if there is tissue trauma and bleeding)
Pharynx	Balls, bones, large lumps of cheese or other solid food, fish hooks	Sudden onset of choking, gagging, coughing, retching, salivation. If the airway is blocked there will be difficulty in breathing leading to respiratory arrest	Rapid acting anaesthetic. Object must be removed as soon as possible to prevent asphyxia – remember ABC. If animal is unconscious once foreign body has been removed, intubate and provide oxygen

Table 10.4 *Continued*

Location	Examples	Clinical signs	Treatment
Oesophagus	Chop bones, hide chews	Regurgitation of food soon after eating, signs of discomfort, risk of aspiration pneumonia, history of eating bones Foreign body often becomes stuck over the heart base where there is a risk of erosion into the major vessels	Under general anaesthetic and following radiography, +/− contrast, either: 1. Grasp with crocodile forceps or use forceps on an endoscope and slowly bring up through the mouth. Risk of tearing the mucosa 2. Gently push down into the stomach from where it can more easily be removed by gastrotomy. Bones may be digested 3. Remove by thoracotomy
Stomach	Balls, stones, nuts, toys, tights, cloth, string, wool, etc.	May be a history of eating foreign bodies. Intermittent vomiting usually occurs within 30 minutes of eating. Vomiting occurs when the pylorus is obstructed. May persist for some time until owner notices loss of weight and dehydration	Under general anaesthetic and after radiography +/− contrast to confirm the diagnosis, perform a gastrotomy
Small intestine	Any foreign body that is small enough to pass through the pylorus, particularly linear foreign bodies	Persistent vomiting not related to feeding, dehydration, loss of electrolytes, abdominal pain	Under general anaesthetic and after radiography +/− contrast to confirm the diagnosis, perform an enterotomy. Section of damaged gut may have to be resected followed by an end-to-end anastomosis of the two ends **NB** Linear foreign bodies may be difficult to detect and an exploratory laparotomy may be necessary to confirm the diagnosis
Rectum	Needles still attached to thread may become wedged across the sphincter. Faecoliths – balls of bone fragments dehydrated by passage through the colon	Discomfort on defaecation, fresh blood in faeces, constant licking of anus and dragging anus along the ground	Under sedation or general anaesthesia gently ease out of the rectum. Needles may be pushed out through the side of the anal sphincter. Use of liquid paraffin to soothe rectum and to help passage of any smaller particles (e.g. of bone)

to 5–10 cm below the pubis and about 10 cm either side of the midline.

Rationale: It is important to prepare a large enough area to prevent the risk of breaking asepsis. The exact size depends on the size of the patient.

3. **Action:** Make a midline incision from the xiphoid to the pubis – laparotomy.

Rationale: The incision should allow adequate exteriorization of the stomach and intestine.

4. **Action:** Use retractors to retract the abdominal wall.

Rationale: To provide adequate exposure of the gastrointestinal tract.

5. **Action:** Inspect the entire gastrointestinal tract.

Rationale: To check for evidence of material that may cause obstruction or perforation.

6. **Action:** If there is no evidence of intestinal damage, exteriorize the stomach and isolate it from the remainder of the abdominal contents by using moistened sterile swabs.

    Rationale: To reduce contamination by stomach contents. Remember to count the swabs and make sure that you have removed them all before closing the abdomen. Exteriorization of the stomach is relatively difficult.

7. **Action:** Place a couple of stay sutures in the wall of the stomach or ask a scrubbed-in assistant to hold the stomach.

    Rationale: To assist in manipulation of the stomach and to prevent spillage of the stomach contents.

8. **Action:** Make a stab incision into the stomach wall in an area where there are fewer vessels and capillaries in the ventral aspect of the stomach between the greater and lesser curvatures.

    Rationale: To keep haemorrhage to a minimum. The incision should not be too close to the pylorus as this could result in the inversion of too much tissue into the lumen, which may cause an obstruction in outflow.

9. **Action:** Widen the incision with scissors.

    Rationale: To enable examination of the stomach lumen and removal of the foreign body without stretching the edges of the wound.

10. **Action:** Use suction to aspirate the stomach contents and then remove the foreign body.

    Rationale: To prevent spillage into the peritoneal cavity.

11. **Action:** If the foreign body is linear and is lying in both the stomach and the intestine, do not try to pull it out of the gastrotomy wound unless it moves easily. Instead you should make several incisions in the stomach wall and / or

intestine as appropriate and ease it out gently – you may need to cut it into pieces but be careful that you do not lose a piece.

Rationale: The foreign body may have become attached to the intestinal mucosa and pulling it may cause severe damage.

12. **Action:** Check the gastric lumen thoroughly. Look for areas of necrosis or perforation.

    Rationale: To make sure that everything has been removed. You have to remove necrotic or damaged areas.

13. **Action:** Close the stomach wall (and intestine if this has been incised) using an absorbable suture material and a double layer of inverting sutures (see previous descriptions).

    Rationale: To promote healing and prevent leakage.

14. **Action:** Check the entire intestinal tract for any additional foreign material.

    Rationale: To make sure that nothing that could cause an immediate recurrence has been left in the intestine.

15. **Action:** Lavage the surrounding abdominal organs.

    Rationale: To reduce the risk of contamination.

16. **Action:** Remove all swabs and count them to make sure that none are left behind.

    Rationale: One swab left in the peritoneal cavity can quickly cause a potentially fatal peritonitis.

17. **Action:** Before closing the abdominal wound, replace the instruments, gloves and drapes with a fresh sterile set.

    Rationale: To remove the risk of contamination with gastric contents.

18. **Action:** Close the skin incision appropriately.

    Rationale: See previous descriptions.

Procedure: Enterotomy

This is an incision through the intestinal wall; it may be used to remove foreign bodies, examine the intestinal tract or to take full thickness biopsies (Fig. 10.24). A laparotomy is performed to gain access to the intestine.

1. **Action:** Position the anaesthetized patient in dorsal recumbency on a stable operating table and secure with ties or sandbags.

    Rationale: *The patient's body should not be able to tilt to either side.*

2. **Action:** Clip and prepare aseptically an area from about 5–10 cm above the xiphoid to 5–10 cm below the pubis and about 10 cm either side of the midline.

    Rationale: *It is important to prepare a large enough area to prevent the risk of breaking asepsis. The exact size depends on the size of the patient.*

3. **Action:** Make a midline incision from the xiphoid to the pubis – laparotomy.

    Rationale: *The incision should allow adequate exteriorization of the stomach and intestine.*

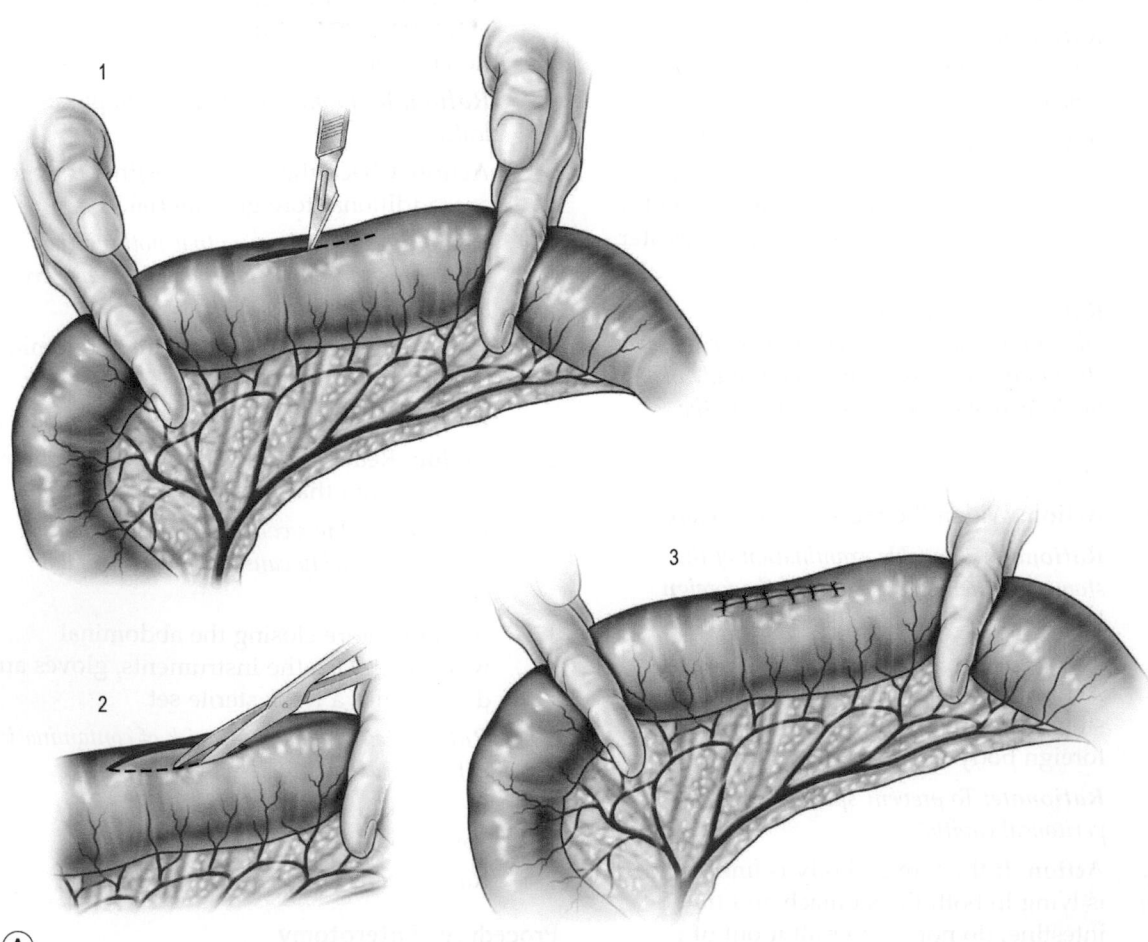

(A)

Figure 10.24 (A) Stages in an enterotomy: 1. Make an incision on the antimesenteric border of the intestine. 2. Enlarge the incision with scissors. 3. Close with simple interrupted sutures.

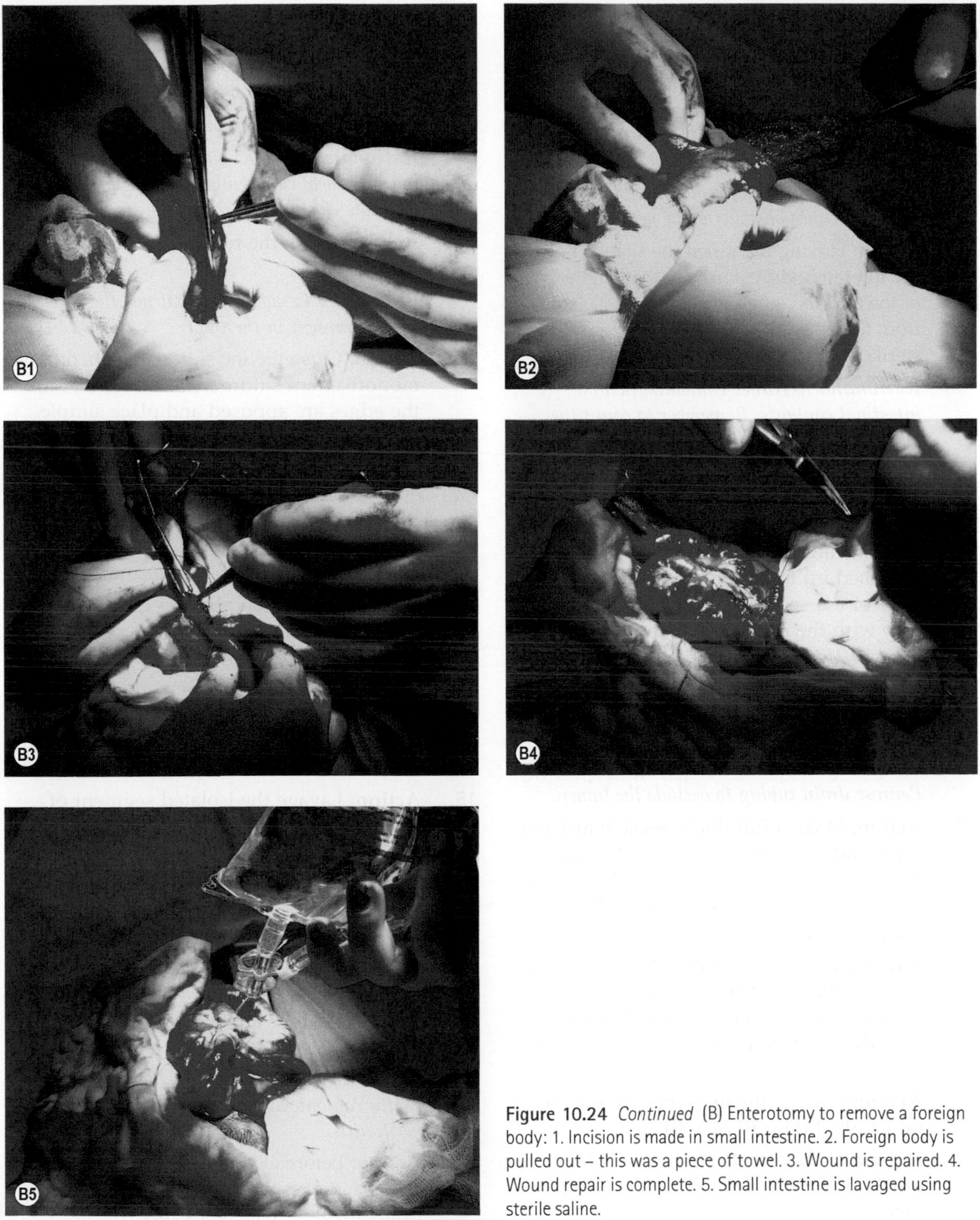

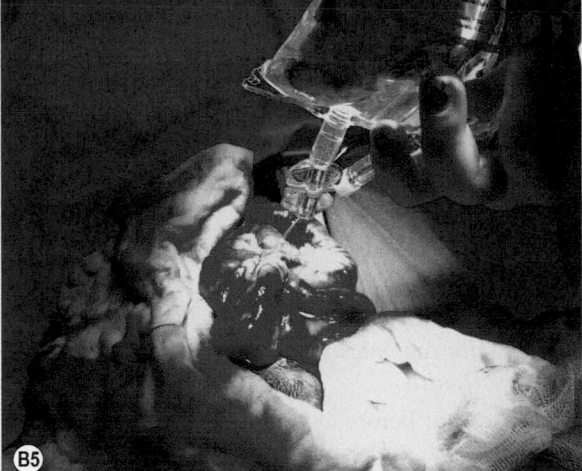

Figure 10.24 *Continued* (B) Enterotomy to remove a foreign body: 1. Incision is made in small intestine. 2. Foreign body is pulled out – this was a piece of towel. 3. Wound is repaired. 4. Wound repair is complete. 5. Small intestine is lavaged using sterile saline.

4. **Action:** Use retractors to retract the abdominal wall.

   Rationale: To provide adequate exposure of the gastrointestinal tract.

5. **Action:** Inspect the entire gastrointestinal tract.

   Rationale: To check for evidence of material that may cause obstruction or perforation.

6. **Action:** Having identified the site(s) of the foreign body, exteriorize the length of the affected small intestine and isolate it from the rest of the abdomen using wet sterile swabs.

   Rationale: To reduce contamination by intestinal contents. Remember to count the swabs and make sure that you have removed them all before closing the abdomen.

7. **Action:** Gently milk the intestinal contents away from the identified segment of intestine and ask an assistant (who has scrubbed in) to occlude the lumen at both ends of the segment using a scissor-like grip with the index and middle fingers (Fig. 10.24A, B).

   Rationale: This will reduce the chances of spillage of intestinal contents. If help is not available then use non-crushing intestinal forceps (e.g. Doyen) or make a ligature using Penrose drain tubing to occlude the lumen.

8. **Action:** Make a full thickness stab incision into healthy tissue distal to the foreign body and on the antimesenteric border of the intestine. The incision should be longitudinal.

   Rationale: Healthy tissue will heal better and more rapidly than damaged tissue, which may not heal at all. It is much easier to close the wound away from the area of mesenteric blood vessels.

9. **Action:** Enlarge the incision with scissors or a scalpel (Fig. 10.24A, B).

   Rationale: To allow the foreign body to be eased out of the wound without damaging the edges.

10. **Action:** Gently milk the foreign body through the wound (Fig. 10.24B).

    Rationale: Be careful not to damage the lining mucosa, especially if the foreign body has become stuck to it.

11. **Action:** Use suction to remove intestinal contents from the isolated segment.

    Rationale: To reduce the risk of contaminating the peritoneal cavity and other organs and to facilitate closure of the incision.

12. **Action:** Check the rest of the intestine and the stomach.

    Rationale: To make sure that no other foreign body is present in the tract.

13. **Action:** Close the incision using absorbable monofilament suture material. Make sure the edges are apposed and place simple interrupted sutures that penetrate the lumen 2–3 mm from the edge of the wound and 2–3 mm apart (Fig. 10.24A). Pull them tight so that the knot sinks down into the muscularis.

    Rationale: This will make a leak-proof seal.

14. **Action:** Moderately distend the intestinal lumen by injecting sterile saline and then apply gentle pressure over the area (Fig. 10.24B).

    Rationale: To check for leakage through the wound. If leakage occurs then place additional sutures.

15. **Action:** Lavage the isolated segment of intestine and place omentum over the suture line.

    Rationale: This will wash away any intestinal contents that may have been spilt. If there has been substantial contamination the entire abdomen must be lavaged. A layer of omentum will help to seal the incision.

16. **Action:** Remove all swabs and count them to make sure that none are left behind.

    Rationale: One swab left in the peritoneal cavity can quickly cause a potentially fatal peritonitis.

17. **Action:** Before closing the abdominal wound, replace the instruments, gloves and drapes with a fresh sterile set.

    Rationale: To remove the risk of contamination with intestinal contents.

18. **Action:** Close the skin incision appropriately.

    Rationale: See previous descriptions.

NB It is rarely, if ever, necessary to enter the large intestine to remove a foreign body. Once a foreign body enters the wider bore of the colon it will usually pass out naturally. If a foreign body is in the distal ileum it may be possible to milk it into the colon rather than performing an enterotomy.

LUMPECTOMY

Lumpectomy is a term used to describe the excision of a mass with an obvious margin so that it is clearly delineated. Strictly these are small benign masses (e.g. lipoma) that lie within the skin or subcutaneous tissues and are not on or close to delicate structures such as the eye or the anus. Closure of the resulting wound should be able to be done by routine methods.

Procedure: Lumpectomy

1. **Action:** Before proceeding with the lumpectomy and during a consultation, the patient should be thoroughly examined to ascertain the location and size of all masses.

   Rationale: The owner may have found several lumps and will not be pleased if you leave any behind.

2. **Action:** Take a fine needle aspirate from each one (see Ch. 5).

   Rationale: To check for type and malignancy, which may influence your technique.

3. **Action:** If possible, mark the location of each mass by clipping away a piece of hair or using a small amount of correction fluid around it.

   Rationale: This will save time once the patient is anaesthetized and will ensure that you remove all the masses identified by the owner.

4. **Action:** On the day of the operation, the patient is anaesthetized and placed in a position that gives optimal access to the mass.

Rationale: If several masses are to be removed the position may have to be changed.

5. **Action:** Clip and prepare the site aseptically.

   Rationale: To prevent the entry of infection into the surgical site.

6. **Action:** Apply a little tension on the skin around the mass with the finger and thumb of your left hand. Make an oval incision around the mass, leaving a clear margin of 0.5–1 cm (Fig. 10.25A, B).

   Rationale: Applying tension fixes the mass in place, making incision easier. Leaving a wide margin ensures any cells that may have migrated from the mass will also have been removed – this is particularly important if the mass is malignant.

7. **Action:** Extend the incision to the hypodermal tissues, at which point the skin edges should spring apart.

   Rationale: At this level it is easier to see the subcutaneous tissues.

8. **Action:** Clamp or ligate and then transect any blood vessels supplying the mass or those that are in the way.

   Rationale: To prevent excessive loss of blood, which will block your view of the area.

9. **Action:** Dissect down under the mass and cut it away from the tissues using scissors.

   Rationale: Use of scissors provides more control of the incision and there will be less likelihood of cutting something vital.

10. **Action:** Control haemorrhage with haemostats and sterile swabs.

    Rationale: To prevent excessive loss of blood, which will block your view of the area.

11. **Action:** When the lump has been removed (Fig. 10.25C), place it in a pot with 10% formalin ready to be sent to a lab for histopathology.

    Rationale: To identify the type and potential malignancy of the mass.

12. **Action:** Close the subcuticular layer and the skin using a routine technique

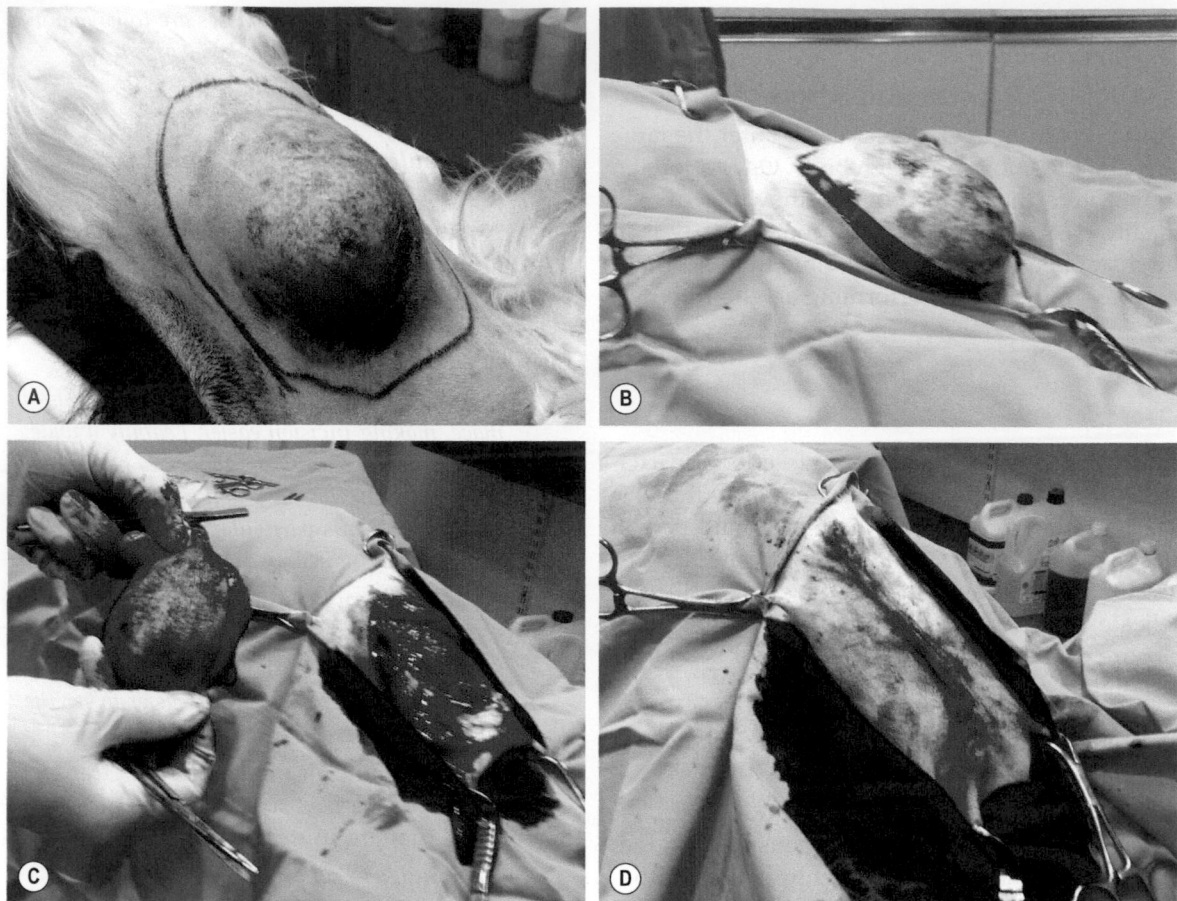

Figure 10.25 Stages in a lumpectomy: (A) The surrounding area is clipped and wide margin is delineated. (B) First incision is made. (C) Lump – a lipoma – is removed. (D) Surgical wound is closed.

and remembering to close the dead space (Fig. 10.25D).

Rationale: Pay attention to the tension of your sutures – if they are too tight they may affect the rate of healing and cause discomfort leading to patient interference.

13. **Action:** If there are several masses to be removed, use a fresh sterile kit and gloves for each one.

    Rationale: To reduce the chances of spread of tumour cells.

14. **Action:** If strict asepsis has been observed there is no need for postoperative antibiotics.

Rationale: There should be little chance of infection.

15. **Action:** Consider the use of an Elizabethan collar if there is any chance of patient interference.

    Rationale: To promote rapid healing.

An animal is neutered to prevent reproduction, and the surgical procedures involved in neutering make up a large proportion of the routine operations during a normal working day. As a newly qualified veterinary surgeon you should know

Table 10.5 Advantages and disadvantages of neutering an animal

	Ovariohysterectomy (spay)	Orchidectomy (castration)
Advantages	Prevents the birth of unwanted young	Prevents the birth of unwanted young
	No more seasons	Reduces aggression and territoriality*
	No false pregnancies	Reduces hypersexuality*
	Reduces the incidence of mammary tumours	Reduces the tendency to wander*
	Prevents development of pyometra in later life	Prevents the development of Sertoli cell tumours
		Prevents territorial urine spraying in tomcats (may not always work)
Disadvantages	May increase the likelihood of obesity	May increase the likelihood of obesity
	In some breeds the coat may become more coarse	Permanent so no chance of deciding to breed from the animal at a later date
	Permanent so no chance of deciding to breed from the animal at a later date	
	Slight risk of incontinence if a bitch is spayed very young	

*These effects depend on the age at which the animal is castrated. If done later there may be no reduction in the behavioural pattern.

how to perform these techniques, and by the end of your first year in practice you should have become proficient at them.

Table 10.5 describes the advantages and disadvantages of neutering an animal.

1. OVARIOHYSTERECTOMY

This procedure, colloquially known as 'spaying', involves the removal of both the uterus and the ovaries. The most common reason for performing an ovariohysterectomy is to prevent reproduction, but the technique is also used in the treatment of pyometritis or other conditions of the reproductive tract such as neoplasia.

When using the technique as a means of routine neutering, it is important to consider the age at which it is done:

- **Dog (bitch)** – this depends on practice protocols. Some practices recommend spaying the bitch when she is fully grown but may not have had her first season; however, this depends on the breed. Smaller breeds such as Jack

Russell Terriers mature earlier (by approximately 6 months old) than larger breeds such as Great Danes (by approximately 18 months old). Other practices recommend spaying after the bitch has had her first season. It is not recommended to spay a bitch while she is in season as blood vessels may be engorged, leading to potentially fatal loss of blood.

- **Cat (queen)** – it is usually done when the cat is about 4–5 months old and this is not dependent on the first season. In a young queen, the age at which the first season occurs will depend on the time of year she was born. Kittens born in the spring may not come into season until early spring the following year, whereas those born in late summer will also come into season in early spring but may be significantly younger. Queens may be spayed whilst they are in season, but extra care must be taken to prevent haemorrhage.

- **Rabbit (doe)** – it is usually recommended between 4 months and 2 years old. The rabbit is an induced ovulator and shows few overt signs of oestrus, either physical or behavioural, so sexual maturity is difficult to assess. During pregnancy or pseudopregnancy the blood vessels become engorged and friable so extra care must be taken to ensure haemostasis.

Procedure: Ovariohysterectomy in the bitch

1. **Action:** Place the anaesthetized bitch in dorsal recumbency on a stable operating table and secure with ties or sandbags.

   Rationale: The body must not be able to tilt or move during the procedure.

2. **Action:** Clip and prepare aseptically the ventral abdomen from the xiphoid to the pubis.

   Rationale: To prevent the entry of infection into the surgical site (see Ch. 9).

3. **Action:** Identify the umbilicus and visually divide the caudal abdomen into thirds. Make a 4–8 cm incision into the cranial third. In deep-chested breeds, be prepared to extend the incision caudally and / or cranially; in prepubertal young bitches, make an incision in the middle third of the caudal abdomen.

   Rationale: This site will allow exteriorization of the ovaries without using excessive traction. The exact position of the tract varies with size and maturity of the individual, and the site of the incision should facilitate ligation of the uterine body.

4. **Action:** With a scalpel, incise the skin and subcutaneous tissues longitudinally until you can grasp the linea alba. Tent it outwards and make a stab incision through it.

   Rationale: Tenting the linea alba prevents the risk of incising any of the underlying tissues. This enables you to enter the peritoneal cavity.

5. **Action:** Extend the stab incision through the linea alba with scissors.

   Rationale: To increase the view of the abdominal contents and to facilitate their exteriorization.

6. **Action:** Lift the left side of the abdominal wall with forceps and locate the left uterine horn with your index finger (Fig. 10.26A).

   Rationale: You can use a bitch spay hook if you want to.

7. **Action:** Gently run your fingers cranially along the inside of the abdominal wall to pick up the uterine horn and broad ligament (Fig. 10.26B).

   Rationale: This will allow you to see it and to identify it as the uterine tract. A full bladder may make exteriorization of the uterus more difficult.

8. **Action:** Run your fingers cranially up towards the ovary and digitally identify the suspensory ligament (which runs cranially towards the caudal pole of the kidney); pull it gently caudally and medially (Fig. 10.26C).

   Rationale: This is a taut fibrous band at the proximal edge of the ovarian pedicle. As you gently pull on it, it will become tauter.

9. **Action:** Place a finger under the ligament and, using blunt scissors, cut cranially about 1 cm from the ovary.

   Rationale: By cutting at this point you should avoid the ovarian blood vessels. The suspensory ligament can sometimes be broken using only your fingers. This is done to raise the ovary and its blood supply by about another 1 cm towards the outside.

10. **Action:** Push a pair of closed artery forceps through the broad ligament caudal to the blood vessels, then retract a little, open the jaws and clamp on the vascular pedicle proximal to the ovary (Fig. 10.26D).

    Rationale: This clamp will serve as a groove for placing a ligature.

11. **Action:** Release the artery forceps and reclamp 4–5 mm closer to the ovary. Leave the forceps in situ until the ligature has been placed.

    Rationale: This prevents backflow of blood after transection of the pedicle.

12. **Action:** Take a length of absorbable monofilament suture material and place a ligature around the pedicle into the crushed area. If necessary, use a figure-of-eight ligature (Fig. 10.26E).

    Rationale: In some cases it may be necessary to fix it in position by passing a needle through an avascular part of the suspensory

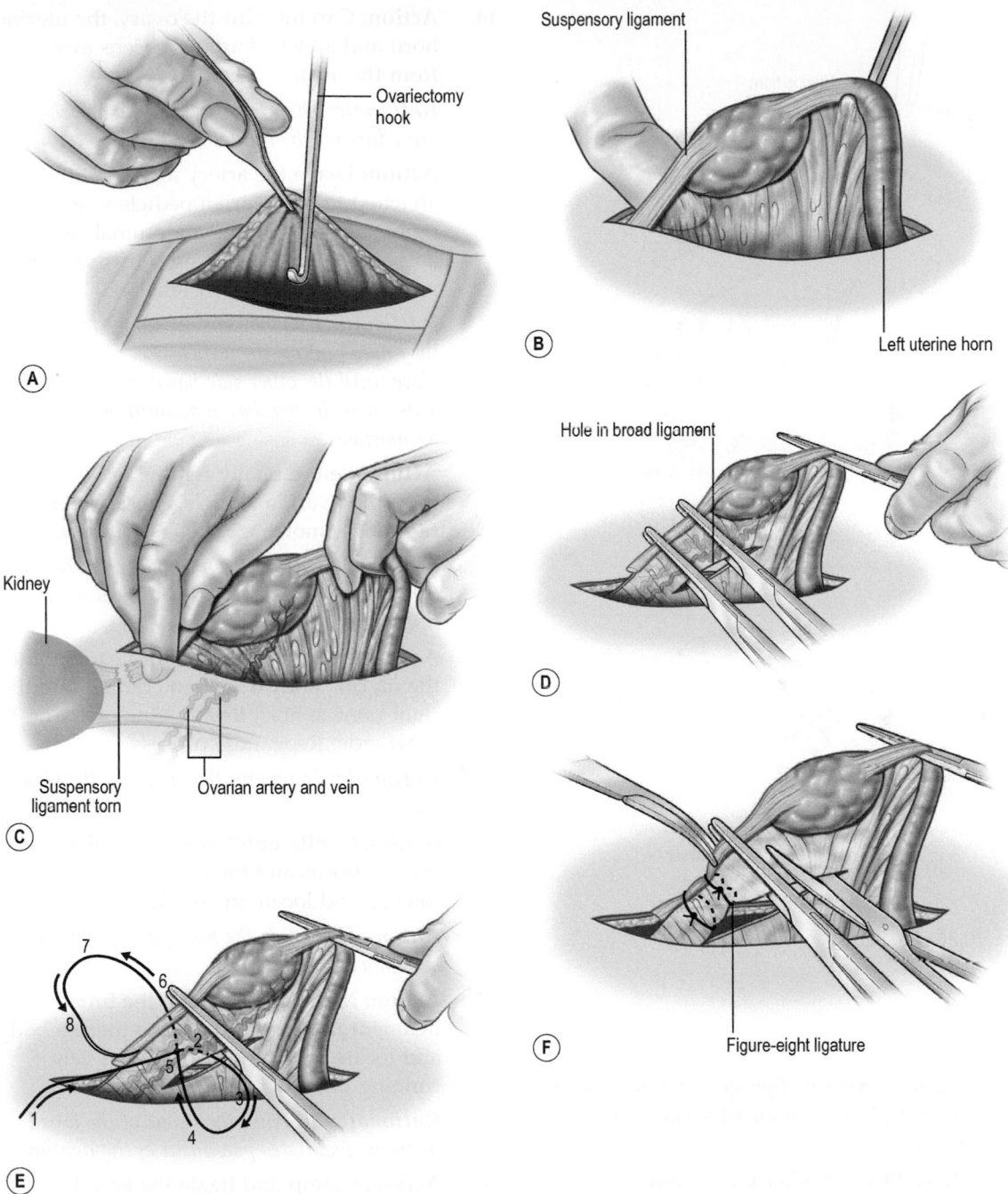

Figure 10.26 Stages in an ovariohysterectomy in a bitch: (A) Lift the abdominal wall and slide a spay hook or your fingers into the cavity (left side illustrated). (B, C) Lift the uterine wall up and identify the broad and suspensory ligaments. (D) Ligate the ovarian pedicle using artery forceps. (E) Place a figure-of-eight or single ligature around the ovarian pedicle. (F) Cut on the ovarian side of the ligature. (G) Separate the broad ligament from the uterine horn and ligate the broad ligament if it appears vascular. (H) Ligate the uterine body using a figure-of-eight suture or single sutures around the uterine vessels running on either side of cervix.

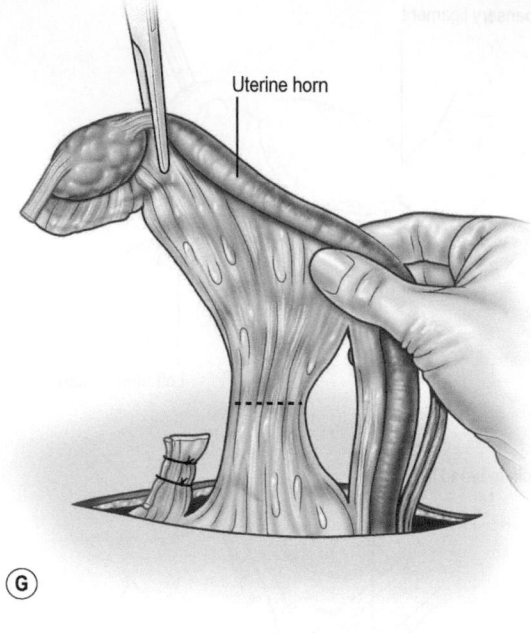

Uterine horn

(G)

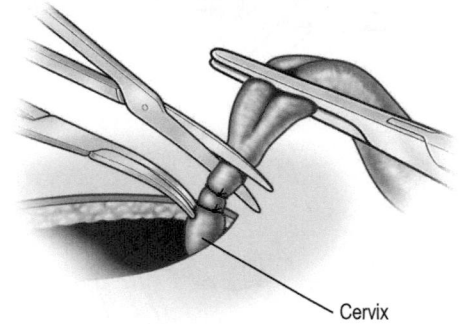

Cervix

(H)

Figure 10.26 *Continued*

ligament to prevent slippage. A figure-of-eight
ligature will ensure haemostasis and prevent
slippage.

13. **Action:** Place another pair of artery forceps
    across the pedicle closer to the ovary and
    cut between the two (Fig. 10.26F).

    *Rationale: One pair of forceps will remain on
    the ovarian pedicle and the other will be
    attached to the ovary as it is withdrawn from
    the abdomen – this stops residual blood leaking
    into the surgical site.*

14. **Action:** Carefully lift the ovary, the uterine
    horn and attached artery forceps away
    from the area.

    *Rationale: This clears the way to repeat the
    procedure on the right side.*

15. **Action:** Leave the artery forceps still
    attached to the ovarian pedicle with their
    points angled into the abdominal cavity
    and their handles sticking outwards. Make
    sure they are not under tension.

    *Rationale: If the forceps are under tension
    they may pull off the pedicle. Leave them in
    place until the other side has been dealt with.
    This gives the maximum amount of time for
    haemostasis.*

16. **Action:** Before finally removing the forceps
    from the ovarian pedicle, check for any
    sign of haemorrhage. Religate if necessary.

    *Rationale: Haemorrhage is relatively rare, but
    its source can be difficult to locate at a later
    time.*

17. **Action:** Trace the uterine horn caudally to
    the uterine body and then cranially up the
    right uterine horn towards the ovary on the
    other side. Repeat the process.

    *Rationale: To remove the ovary on the right
    side.*

18. **Action:** Gently apply traction to the two
    uterine horns and their attached artery
    forceps and locate the uterine body.

    *Rationale: This is the final part of the tract to
    be removed.*

19. **Action:** Make a window in the broad
    ligament on either side of the uterine body
    and locate the uterine artery and vein
    running on either side (Fig. 10.26G).

    *Rationale: Breaking the tissue of the broad
    ligament facilitates placement of the ligatures.*

20. **Action:** Clamp and ligate the broad
    ligament if the bitch is in season or
    pregnant, or if the ligament is infiltrated by
    an excessive amount of fat.

    *Rationale: During oestrus and pregnancy the
    blood vessels become engorged and, because of
    this, ovariohysterectomy is not recommended at
    these times. Excessive fat may impede*

tightening of the ligatures so there is a risk of slippage.

21. **Action:** Apply cranial traction on the uterus and place a pair of artery forceps across the uterine body cranial to the cervix (Fig. 10.26H).

    Rationale: To crush and close the uterine vessels. This will serve as a groove in which a ligature is placed.

22. **Action:** Release the artery forceps and place a figure-of-eight suture within the crushed area through the uterine body and encircling the blood vessels on either side.

    Rationale: This will ligate both sets of vessels in one suture. You can place an individual suture around each uterine vessel as it runs on either side of the cervix.

23. **Action:** Place another suture around the uterine body closer to the cervix.

    Rationale: This will further ligate the blood supply and close the cervix.

24. **Action:** Place a pair of artery forceps across the uterine body cranial to the figure-of-eight suture and transect the uterine body between the suture and the artery forceps. Gently tear away any remnants of broad ligament.

    Rationale: The entire uterine tract has now been surgically removed from the body.

25. **Action:** Lift the uterine tract away from the surgical incision, remove the attached artery forceps and dispose of the tissue correctly.

    Rationale: Under health and safety legislation, body parts are disposed of in the clinical waste.

26. **Action:** Observe for signs of haemorrhage on the uterine stump and religate if necessary.

    Rationale: Always check for signs of haemorrhage before closing the abdomen.

27. **Action:** Replace the uterine stump in the abdomen and release the artery forceps. Observe for signs of haemorrhage.

    Rationale: Allow a little time (seconds) for the tissues to return to their normal position.

28. **Action:** Close the abdomen in three layers: fascia / linea alba, subcutaneous tissue, skin.

    Rationale: To promote healing, close the dead space and reinstate the normal anatomy of the abdominal wall.

29. **Action:** Check the bitch after 3 days and remove sutures after 7–10 days.

    Rationale: Depending on practice policy.

NB It is also possible to perform an ovariohysterectomy in a cat using this technique.

Procedure: Ovariohysterectomy in the queen

1. **Action:** Once the cat is anaesthetized, check what sex it is.

    Rationale: There have been many cases of 'queens' being clipped ready for surgery only to find that they have two testes and vice versa!

2. **Action:** Place the cat in right lateral recumbency on a stable examination table and secure the front and back legs by tying them to the cleats on the table.

    Rationale: The body wall must be under a degree of tension to facilitate the surgical incision through the lateral abdominal wall.

3. **Action:** By palpation, locate the wing of the ilium and the greater trochanter of the femur. Imagine an equilateral triangle – these anatomical points will form two of the points of the triangle and your flank incision will be the third (i.e. the apex).

    Rationale: Make sure you know the skeletal anatomy of the area (Fig. 10.27).

4. **Action:** Clip and prepare aseptically an area that is larger than this triangle.

    Rationale: To prevent the entry of infection into the surgical site (see Ch. 9).

5. **Action:** Using a scalpel, make an incision approximately 1 cm long at a point 2–3 cm vertically below the wing of the ilium.

    Rationale: As you become more experienced your incision will become smaller; when you first start to spay cats your incision may be larger (e.g. 2 cm). Larger skin incisions may

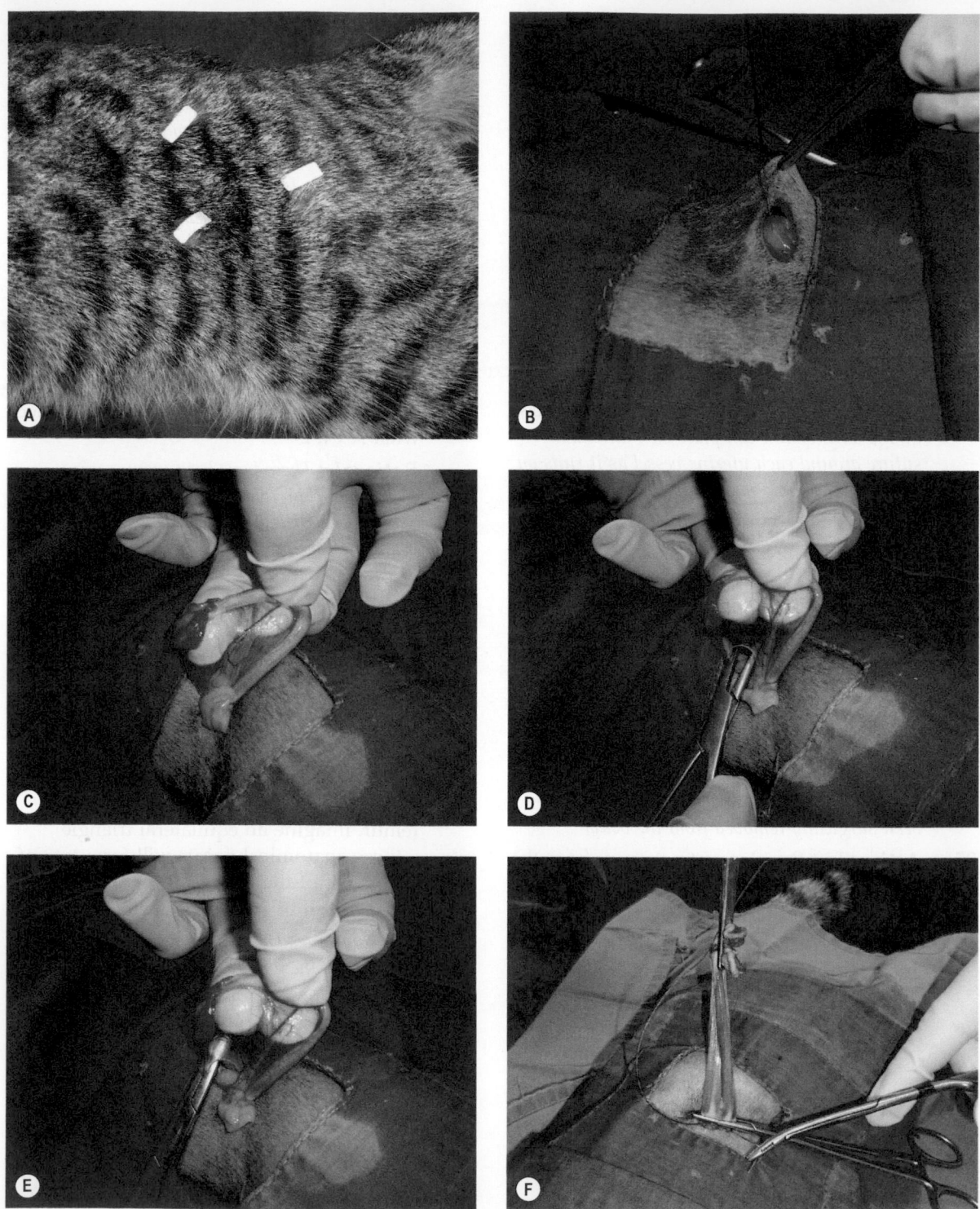

Figure 10.27 Ovariohysterectomy in the queen. (A) Markers placed to identify area to be clipped. (B) The fat pad under the skin is identified and removed. (C) The ovary and uterine horn are exteriorized. (D) A pair of artery forceps is used to create a window through the broad ligament. (E) The artery forceps are used to clamp the suspensory ligament. (F) Both suspensory ligaments have been transected, the ovaries and uterine horns exteriorized and the cervix is clamped using artery forceps.

lead to an increase in patient interference and the need to resuture.

6. **Action:** Immediately below the skin is a layer of fat that should be picked up with rat-toothed forceps. Cut away a small piece (Fig. 10.27B).

   Rationale: This allows you to see the surgical site more clearly.

7. **Action:** The two layers of abdominal muscle can now be seen. Pick up and tent the first layer using rat-toothed forceps and make a vertical incision. Repeat with the second layer.

   Rationale: Tenting the muscle to cut it ensures that you do not incise an underlying abdominal organ.

8. **Action:** You may also have punctured the peritoneum, in which case you are now in the peritoneal cavity. If not, the peritoneum will appear as a shiny or transparent layer of tissue that can be stabbed with spay forceps.

   Rationale: The peritoneum is sometimes quite tough and you must push through it positively. If you do not do this you will be searching for the uterus beneath the layer of abdominal muscle and not inside the cavity.

9. **Action:** Once in the peritoneal cavity, you may be able to see the uterine horns and pick them up using spay forceps or a spay hook. If the uterine tract is not visible introduce the spay forceps or spay hook to pick up one or both horns or the broad ligament (Fig. 10.27C, D).

   Rationale: The uterine horns run horizontally and lie dorsal to the bladder and just ventral to the hypaxial muscles of the vertebral column. In pregnant queens the uterine horns will lie much more ventral and may be masked by the parts of the alimentary tract.

10. **Action:** Taking the left side first, follow the left uterine horn cranially towards the left ovary. Gently apply traction caudally to bring the ovary into sight and identify the suspensory ligament (Fig. 10.27E).

Rationale: As you pull on the uterine horn you will feel the suspensory ligament become tauter.

11. **Action:** Place a pair of artery forceps across the ovarian pedicle as far cranially as possible.

    Rationale: This clamp will serve as a groove for placing a ligature.

12. **Action:** Place a second pair of artery forceps closer to the ovary.

    Rationale: This clamp prevents backflow of blood after transection of the pedicle.

13. **Action:** Loosen the first pair of artery forceps and replace them closer on the ovarian side of the second pair.

    Rationale: The crushed area will be used to place the ligament.

14. **Action:** Using absorbable / monofilament suture material or catgut, place a ligature in the site of the first pair of artery forceps and tie it as tight as possible.

    Rationale: This will prevent haemorrhage from the ovarian pedicle.

15. **Action:** Tear or cut between the two pairs of artery forceps and gently pull up the ovary and uterine horn.

    Rationale: Tearing the tissue of the ovarian pedicle will promote elastic recoil of the blood vessels; however, it is better to cut the tissue in larger cats. (Do not tear the tissue of bitches as the blood supply and tissue are more substantial.)

16. **Action:** Leave the artery forceps attached to the body side of the ovarian pedicle with the points angled into the abdominal cavity, making sure that they are not under any tension.

    Rationale: This gives the maximum time for haemostasis. If the forceps are under tension they may pull off the pedicle.

17. **Action:** Before finally removing the artery forceps from the pedicle, check for signs of haemorrhage.

    Rationale: Haemorrhage in this procedure is rare, but it can occur as a result of poor haemostatic technique.

18. **Action:** Trace the uterine horn to the uterine body and then cranially to the other uterine horn to locate the other ovary. Repeat the procedure.

    Rationale: To remove the ovary on the right side. It may be relatively difficult to locate the second uterine horn.

19. **Action:** Once both ovaries are removed from their attachments apply gentle traction on the uterine horns (Fig. 10.27F).

    Rationale: To bring the uterine body into view and exteriorize it.

20. **Action:** Place a pair of artery forceps across the caudal part of the uterine body close to the cervix (Fig. 10.27F).

    Rationale: The forceps should be large enough to crush the uterine blood vessels, which run on either side of the cervix within the broad ligament. This area of crushed tissue will be used to place the ligature.

21. **Action:** Place a second pair of artery forceps across the uterine body slightly more cranial than the first.

    Rationale: These will be just cranial to the point of transection of the uterine body.

22. **Action:** Remove the first pair of forceps and replace them cranial to the second pair.

    Rationale: This will further ensure haemostasis.

23. **Action:** Place a ligature around the uterine body in the area caudal to the two pairs of artery forceps and where the tissue was crushed by the first pair of artery forceps.

    Rationale: The ligature will prevent haemorrhage and close the cervix.

24. **Action:** Cut between the two pairs of artery forceps.

    Rationale: The uterine tract has now been surgically removed from the body.

25. **Action:** Lift the ovaries and uterine tract and the attached artery forceps away from the body. Detach the forceps and dispose of the tissue correctly.

    Rationale: Under health and safety legislation, body parts are disposed of in the clinical waste.

26. **Action:** Observe for signs of haemorrhage in the uterine stump. Remove the remaining pair of artery forceps and observe again.

    Rationale: Haemorrhage in the queen is quite rare, but you should always take a few seconds to check.

27. **Action:** Allow the uterine stump to return to the abdomen and observe for haemorrhage.

    Rationale: Haemorrhage may sometimes occur as the tissues relax into their normal position.

28. **Action:** Close the abdomen in three layers using continuous sutures and monofilament suture material – muscle (both layers together), fat and intradermal or skin.

    Rationale: The choice of absorbable or non-absorbable material in the skin depends on practice policy. Non-absorbable material is removed in 7–10 days, which provides a chance to check the patient. If intradermal sutures are used there is no need to use skin sutures and it may reduce patient interference.

Procedure: Ovariohysterectomy in the doe

The rabbit has a duplex uterus and each uterine horn is separate and leads to a separate cervix (Fig. 10.28) There is a single vagina and no uterine body. The uterus lies within the caudal abdomen dorsal to the bladder.

1. **Action:** Place the anaesthetized rabbit in dorsal recumbency on a stable operating table and restrain the hindlimbs in extension using ties attached to the cleats in the table.

    Rationale: The body must be supported and must not be able to tilt to one side or the other.

2. **Action:** Clip and aseptically prepare the ventral abdomen from the xiphoid to the pubis and about 5 cm on either side of the midline.

    Rationale: The lateral boundaries of the aseptic area will vary with the size of the rabbit.

3. **Action:** Make a 2–3 cm midline incision between the umbilicus and the pubis.

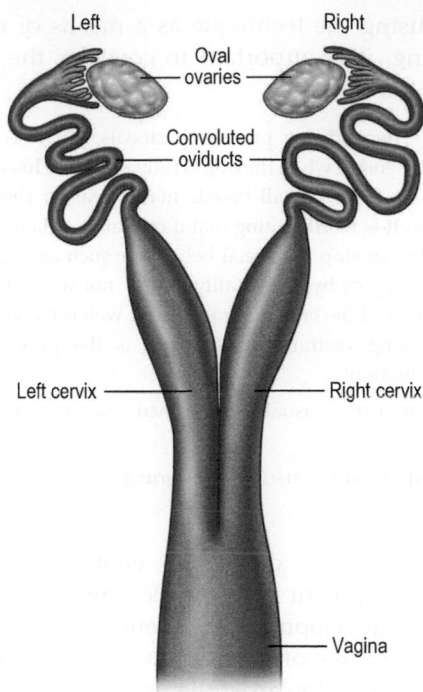

Figure 10.28 Duplex uterus of the rabbit.

Rationale: If necessary the length of the incision can be increased.

4. **Action:** Identify the rectus muscles and the linea alba. Tent the muscles and linea alba and make a stab incision using a scalpel or blunt scissors.

    Rationale: Tenting the tissues reduces the risk of incising the thin-walled caecum or bladder, which may be lying pressed close to the ventral body wall.

5. **Action:** Lift the sides of the abdominal wall and locate the uterine horns.

    Rationale: The uterus is pink and flat and can be distinguished from the intestine by the fact that the intestine is darker and more round.

6. **Action:** Selecting the left side first, follow the left uterine horn cranially until you locate the ovary.

    Rationale: The ovaries are often hidden in fat and may be difficult to see. They may be palpated as small pea-shaped structures within the fat.

7. **Action:** Locate the ovarian pedicle, consisting of the suspensory ligament and the ovarian blood vessels, and dissect away any fat.

    Rationale: There may be a significant amount of fat associated with the uterine tract. It varies with the age of the animal – older animals may be fatter – and the degree of overall obesity. The suspensory ligament is relatively long, which makes exteriorization of the ovaries quite easy.

8. **Action:** Apply two pairs of artery forceps across the ovarian pedicle and place a transfixing suture on the ovarian side.

    Rationale: There is not enough room along the ovarian pedicle to use a three-clamp method as described in the cat and dog.

9. **Action:** Cut between the two pairs of forceps.

    Rationale: The pedicle is easily torn and the tissue is friable – take care to ensure that haemostasis has been achieved.

10. **Action:** Observe the pedicle for signs of haemorrhage before and after releasing the artery forceps and replacing the stump in the peritoneal cavity.

    Rationale: There is a risk that suture material may lacerate the blood vessels. Electrocautery may assist in haemostasis.

11. **Action:** Identify any blood vessels within the broad ligament and ligate them individually down to the level of the cervix.

    Rationale: Vessels are often hidden in the fat of the broad ligament. The tissue is quite friable and bleeding may result from dissecting away the fat.

12. **Action:** Place two pairs of artery forceps across the uterus.

    Rationale: The uterus may be removed caudal or cranial to the two cervices. It is preferable to remove the uterus caudal to the cervices to prevent the development of uterine neoplasia. If this is done the stump should be sealed securely to prevent leakage of urine into the abdomen from the urethra, which opens into the vaginal vestibule at its proximal end.

13.   **Action:** Identify the uterine blood vessels running on either side of the cervices. Place a double ligature using transfixing sutures across the uterus or distal vagina and caudal to the artery forceps.

   Rationale: To prevent bleeding from the vessels and close the stump. Care must be taken to ensure that the ureters and the blood vessels supplying the bladder are not accidentally clamped and ligated. This may occur if the uterine clamps are placed too far caudally.

14.   **Action:** Cut the tissue between the artery forceps and observe for signs of haemorrhage before and after releasing them.

   Rationale: To ensure that blood loss is not occurring.

15.   **Action:** Allow the stump to return to a natural position and observe for signs of haemorrhage.

   Rationale: Haemorrhage may occur as the tissues relax.

16.   **Action:** Close the abdomen in three layers: muscle, fat and subcuticular tissues.

   Rationale: To promote healing and restore the anatomy of the body wall.

17.   **Action:** It is recommended to give one dose of metoclopramide postoperatively.

   Rationale: To prevent ileus. This is most likely if surgery has been prolonged or if the gastrointestinal tract has been handled.

2. ORCHIDECTOMY

This procedure, colloquially referred to as 'castration', involves the removal of both testes from the scrotal sac. Vasectomy, involving the removal of a length of the ductus deferens (vas deferens) but leaving the testes in the scrotal sac, retains the male's libido but prevents the delivery of sperm into the female tract and thus pregnancy. This technique is rarely performed in dogs, cats and rabbits, but is sometimes done in male ferrets (hobs).

Table 10.5 lists the advantages and disadvantages of castration.

When using the technique as a means of routine neutering, it is important to consider the age at which it is done:

- **Dog** – depends on practice protocols, but it is usually recommended when the dog is fully mature. This will vary with the breed: small breeds mature earlier than larger breeds. It is worth noting that if castration is being recommended to stop antisocial behaviour such as aggression, wandering or hypersexuality, it may not work if the dog is older and the behaviour pattern is well established. The only thing castration guarantees is the prevention of reproduction!
- **Cat (tomcat)** – usually performed after the age of 4–5 months.
- **Rabbit (buck)** – usually performed over the age of 4 months.

Retained testes – during the embryological and fetal development of the male animal, the testis begins its development in a similar position in the abdomen to that of the ovary and then travels retroperitoneally towards the inguinal ring. Each testis descends into the scrotum at an age that is characteristic of the species (e.g. in dogs the testes have descended by about 10–20 days after birth). It is therefore important for the animal to be checked prior to castration as the testes may not be present in the scrotum.

Failure of the testes to descend normally may be described as:

- **Monorchid** – if only one testis is present in the scrotum; such an animal will be normally fertile
- **Cryptorchid** – if both testes are retained in the abdomen; such an animal is likely to be infertile but will retain its libido.

Retained testes are more likely to develop Sertoli cell tumours and because of this they should be removed. When performing the operation to remove a retained testis it is important to remember the route taken by the normal fetal testis as it descends. The retained testis may be close to the inguinal canal, in which case it may be able to be manipulated into the scrotal sac and removed by normal castration techniques, or it may be lying within the abdomen and dorsal to the bladder. Removal will then require a laparotomy and the incision may have to be extended to enable you to locate the testis.

Procedure: Castration in the dog using the open method

1. **Action:** Place the anaesthetized dog in dorsal recumbency on a stable operating table and restrain the hindlegs using ties attached to the cleats under the table.

   Rationale: The body should not be able to tilt to one side or the other.

2. **Action:** Check that both testes are present in the scrotum.

   Rationale: The testes may not have descended into the scrotum, in which case the dog is cryptorchid.

3. **Action:** Clip and prepare aseptically the ventral part of the caudal abdomen and the medial aspect of the thighs.

   Rationale: To prevent the entry of infection into the surgical site. Try to avoid inducing 'clipper rash' in the skin – this area is very sensitive.

4. **Action:** Apply pressure on the scrotum to push one testis as far as you can into the prescrotal area (Fig. 10.29).

   Rationale: This area of skin will heal better than the skin of the scrotum.

5. **Action:** While maintaining pressure on the testis, incise the skin and subcutaneous tissue over the median raphe of the displaced testis and continue to incise until you are able to exteriorize the testis.

   Rationale: This part of the testis has the largest circumference so once it pops out through the incision everything else will follow easily.

6. **Action:** Incise the parietal tunic over the testis, but do not incise the tunica albuginea.

   Rationale: Cutting the tunica albuginea would expose the testicular parenchyma.

7. **Action:** Place a pair of artery forceps across the tunic at the point where it attaches to the epididymis (Fig. 10.29).

   Rationale: This will prevent bleeding from the spermatic blood vessels.

8. **Action:** Using your fingers, separate the ligament of the tail of the epididymis from the tunic. This is helped by applying traction using the artery forceps on the tunic. Continue until the testis is fully exteriorized from the tunic.

   Rationale: The testis will now be separated from the tunic and you will be able to see the structures of the spermatic cord (i.e. ductus deferens and blood supply).

9. **Action:** Identify the ductus deferens and the vascular cord within the spermatic cord and place a pair of artery forceps across the spermatic cord close to the reflected tunic (Fig. 10.29).

   Rationale: This crushed area will provide a groove into which the ligatures are placed.

10. **Action:** Place another pair of artery forceps across both structures slightly closer to the testis.

    Rationale: This will increase the amount of haemostasis.

11. **Action:** Release the first pair of artery forceps and reposition them caudal to the second pair (i.e. closer to the testis).

    Rationale: To make sure that haemostasis is complete.

12. **Action:** In the crushed area on the ductus deferens and the vascular cord, place a figure-of-eight suture around them.

    Rationale: To bring about complete haemostasis.

13. **Action:** Place another encircling ligature around both structures.

    Rationale: To make sure that haemostasis is complete.

14. **Action:** Cut between the two pairs of artery forceps. You will now have one pair of forceps attached to the spermatic cord and testis and the other pair attached to the spermatic cord leading towards the body.

    Rationale: To remove the testis.

15. **Action:** Observe for signs of haemorrhage before releasing the artery forceps and replacing the spermatic cord in the tunic.

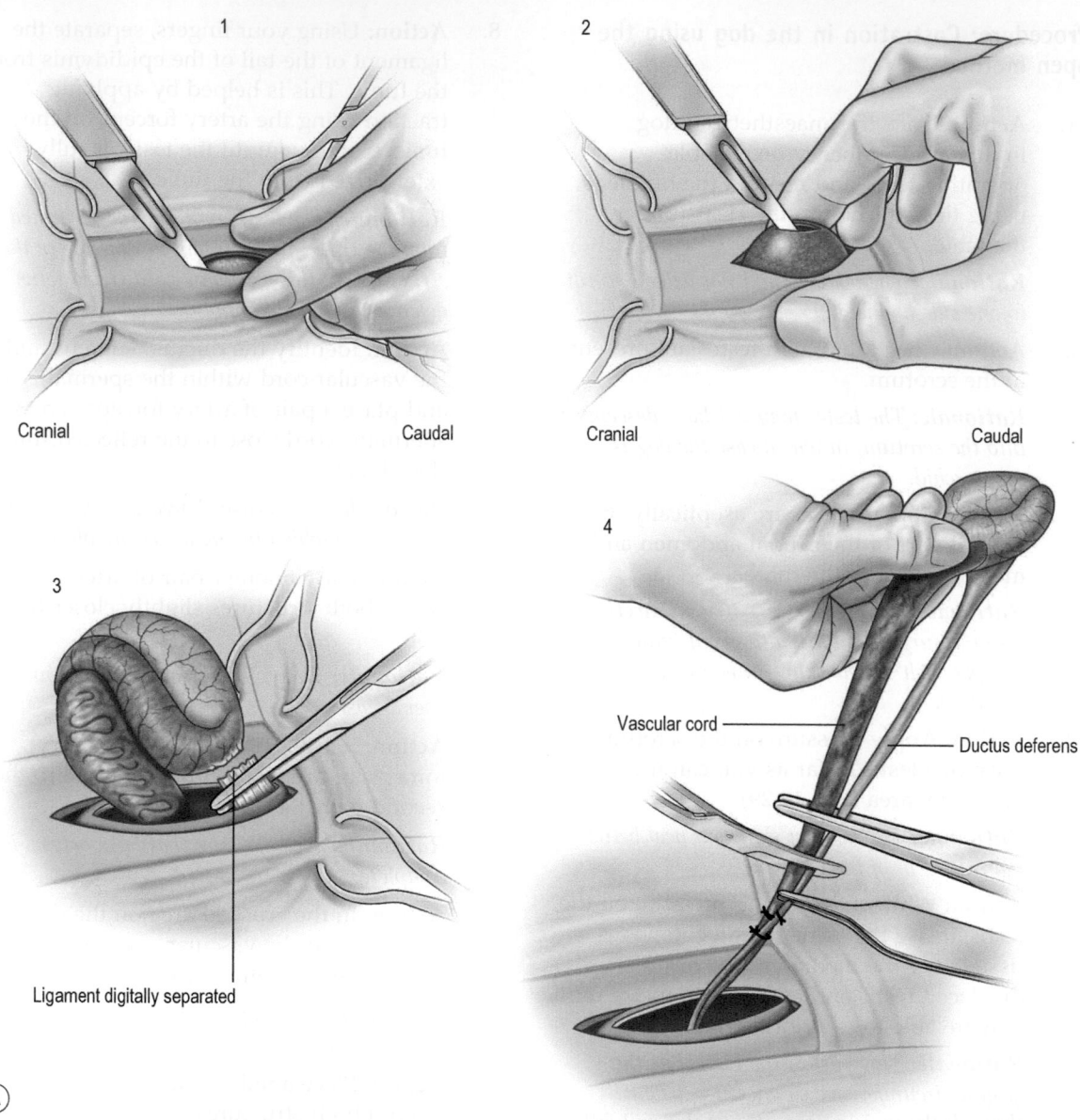

Cranial   Caudal

Cranial   Caudal

Ligament digitally separated

Vascular cord

Ductus deferens

(A)

Figure 10.29 (A) Stages in an open canine castration: 1. Advance one testicle into the prescrotal area by applying pressure over the scrotum. Make an incision over the testicle. 2. Incise the spermatic fascia and parietal vaginal tunic. 3. Place a pair of artery forceps across the tunic where it attaches to the epididymis and digitally separate the ligament of the tail of the epididymis from the tunic. 4. Ligate the ductus deferens and vascular cord individually, and then encircle both with a proximal circumferential ligature.

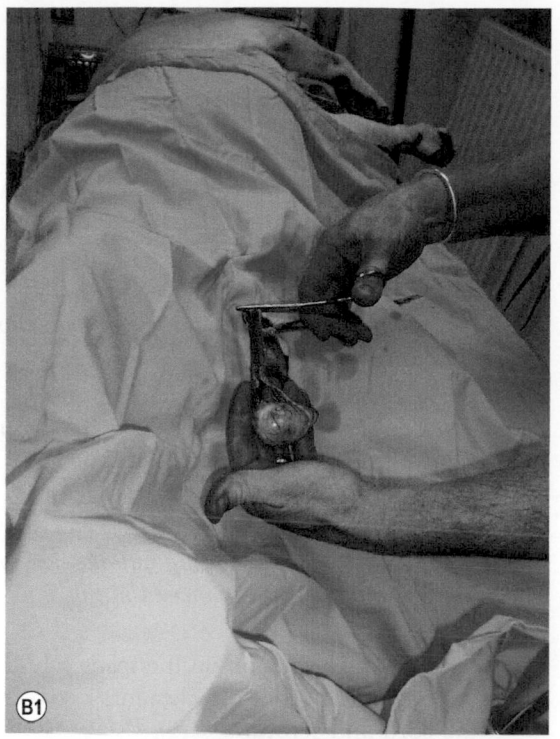

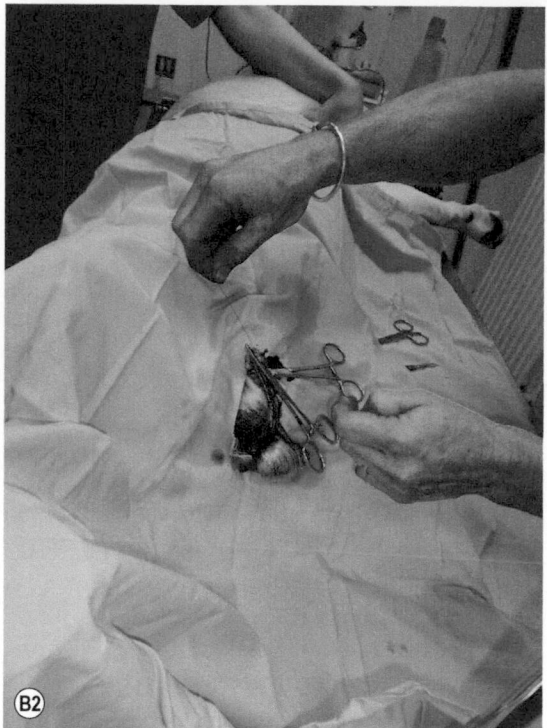

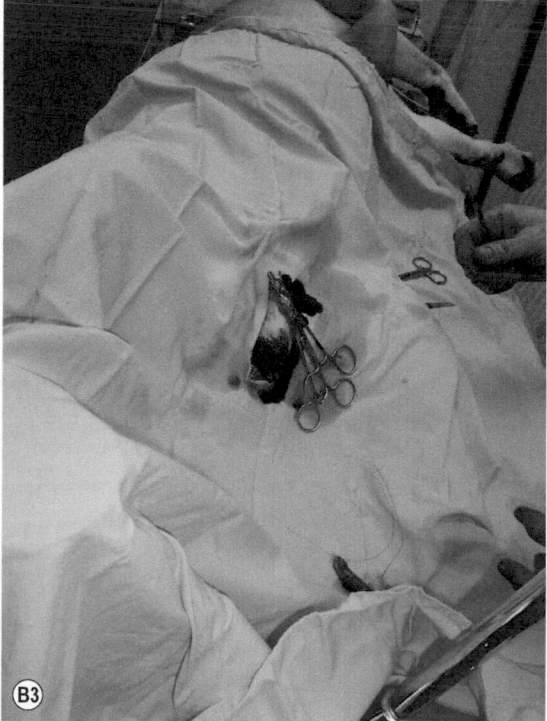

Figure 10.29 *Continued* (B) Open castration: 1. Tunic has been separated from the tail of the testis. A pair of artery forceps has been placed across the spermatic cord, which has been freed from the tunic. 2. A suture is being tied across the clamped area of the cord. 3. Testis has been removed leaving a pair of artery forceps around the remains of the spermatic cord and another around the end of the tunic.

Rationale: To restore the anatomy as much as possible.

16. **Action:** Place an encircling ligature around the cremaster muscle and the tunic.

    Rationale: To close off the tunic associated with this testis, which will prevent herniation from the peritoneal cavity.

17. **Action:** Advance the other testis into the prescrotal wound and remove as described.

    Rationale: To complete the castration.

18. **Action:** Close the incision in three layers: dense fascia, subcutaneous tissues and skin using an appropriate technique.

    Rationale: Removal of skin sutures in this area can be problematic in some individuals and it may be a good idea to use absorbable sutures.

19. **Action:** Check in 2–3 days for signs of swelling, haemorrhage or patient interference (e.g. excessive licking). Use an Elizabethan collar if necessary.

    Rationale: Depends on practice protocols.

Procedure: Castration in the dog using the closed method

1. **Action:** Place the anaesthetized dog in dorsal recumbency on a stable operating table and restrain the hindlegs using ties attached to the cleats under the table.

    Rationale: The body should not be able to tilt to one side or the other.

2. **Action:** Check that both testes are present in the scrotum.

    Rationale: The testes may not have descended into the scrotum, in which case the dog is cryptorchid.

3. **Action:** Clip and prepare aseptically the ventral part of the caudal abdomen and the medial aspect of the thighs.

    Rationale: To prevent the entry of infection into the surgical site. Try to avoid inducing 'clipper rash' in the skin – this area is very sensitive.

4. **Action:** Apply pressure on the scrotum to push one testis as far as you can into the prescrotal area.

Rationale: This area of skin will heal better than the skin of the scrotum.

5. **Action:** While maintaining pressure on the testis, incise the skin and subcutaneous tissue over the median raphe of the displaced testis and continue to incise until you are able to exteriorize the testis.

    Rationale: This part of the testis has the largest circumference so once it pops out through the incision everything else will follow easily.

6. **Action:** Bring the spermatic cord out through the skin incision as much as you can by reflecting fat and fascia from the parietal tunic using a damp gauze swab.

    Rationale: This will clear your view of the tissue and prevent fat getting into the ligature. The parietal tunic is not incised in this technique.

7. **Action:** Place traction on the testis while you tear the fibrous attachments between the cord and scrotum.

    Rationale: To aid the removal of the testis from the scrotal sac.

8. **Action:** Place a pair of artery forceps across the spermatic cord.

    Rationale: To crush the blood supply and achieve haemostasis.

9. **Action:** Release the artery forceps and reposition them approximately 5 mm closer to the testis.

    Rationale: The crushed area will be used to place the ligatures.

10. **Action:** Blunt dissect through the spermatic cord to create a window between the ductus deferens and the vascular cord.

    Rationale: This will be used to pass suture material through to form a ligature.

11. **Action:** Place a figure-of-eight suture around the ductus deferens and the spermatic cord within the crushed area and using the window in the tissue.

    Rationale: The two structures are still enclosed within the tunic of the spermatic cord. The figure-of-eight suture will ligate the blood supply and close off the ductus deferens.

12. **Action:** In a large dog you might place a second encircling ligature around the entire cord at the level of the previously replaced artery forceps.

    Rationale: *There is a greater risk of ligature slippage with a closed technique in large dogs and steps should be taken to ensure that this does not happen.*

13. **Action:** Place another pair of artery forceps across the entire cord and caudal to the first pair, i.e. closer to the testis.

    Rationale: *To bring about complete haemostasis.*

14. **Action:** Cut across the spermatic cord between the artery forceps and remove the testis.

    Rationale: *The first testis is removed and disposed of within the clinical waste.*

15. **Action:** Observe for signs of haemorrhage before releasing the artery forceps on the cord.

    Rationale: *If necessary, place another ligature across the spermatic cord.*

16. **Action:** Repeat with other testis.

    Rationale: *To complete the castration.*

17. **Action:** Close the incision in three layers: dense fascia, subcutaneous tissues and skin using an appropriate technique.

    Rationale: *Removal of skin sutures in this area can be problematic in some individuals and it may be a good idea to use absorbable sutures.*

18. **Action:** Check in 2–3 days for signs of swelling, haemorrhage or patient interference (e.g. excessive licking). Use an Elizabethan collar if necessary.

    Rationale: *Depending on practice protocols.*

Procedure: Castration in the young cat (i.e. 4–5 months old)

1. **Action:** Place the anaesthetized cat in lateral recumbency with the hindlegs pulled cranially.

    Rationale: *This position will expose the scrotum. There is no need to fix the body in position.*

2. **Action:** Check that the cat is male and that there are two testes present in the scrotum.

    Rationale: *It is always important to check the sex of the cat as sexual differentiation is not as easy as it is in the dog. Make sure that it is not a cryptorchid.*

3. **Action:** Pluck the hair from the scrotum and prepare the area aseptically.

    Rationale: *Clipping is not usually necessary unless the cat is very young and plucking is difficult.*

4. **Action:** Fix the position of one testis within the scrotum by applying pressure with your finger and thumb at the base of the scrotum.

    Rationale: *This will prevent the testis moving within the scrotum and make the incision easier.*

5. **Action:** Using a scalpel blade, make a small incision (approximately 1 cm) towards the end of the scrotum and, using pressure on the testis, exteriorize it.

    Rationale: *To gain access to the testis.*

6. **Action:** Apply traction to the testis and pull it out as far as possible.

    Rationale: *This will stretch the spermatic cord.*

7. **Action:** Ask an assistant to hold the testis using a pair of artery forceps clamped around the spermatic cord.

    Rationale: *The assistant need not be scrubbed in as the artery forceps will be removed with the testis and the procedure is very quick.*

8. **Action:** Place a tight ligature around the spermatic cord and as close to the incised scrotum as possible.

    Rationale: *To bring about haemostasis.*

9. **Action:** Place a pair of artery forceps across the cord close to the ligature and cut through the cord close to the testicular side of the forceps.

    Rationale: *The use of forceps prevents the cord springing back into the scrotum/body cavity before you have had time to check for haemostasis. Do not leave a long length of spermatic cord hanging from the scrotum as* *this can lead to a condition known as scirrhous cord in which the spermatic cord becomes swollen and infected.*

10. **Action:** Observe for signs of haemorrhage; if all is well then allow the cord to retract into the scrotum and release the artery forceps.

    Rationale: Haemorrhage is rare in young cats, but you must always check.

11. **Action:** Remove the other testis through a separate incision in the scrotum using the same procedure.

    Rationale: This surgical operation should take under 5 minutes to be completed.

12. **Action:** The two incisions in the scrotum are left to heal by second intention and the owner should be warned to watch out for evidence of infection or excessive patient interference.

    Rationale: There are rarely any complications associated with castration in young cats.

Procedure: Castration in the mature cat

Mature cats have bigger testes with a better-developed blood supply so haemostasis becomes more important.

1. **Action:** Place the anaesthetized cat in lateral recumbency with the hindlegs pulled cranially.

    Rationale: This position will expose the scrotum. There is no need to fix the body in position.

2. **Action:** Check that the cat is male and that there are two testes present in the scrotum.

    Rationale: It is always important to check the sex of the cat as sexual differentiation is not as easy as it is in the dog. Make sure that it is not a cryptorchid.

3. **Action:** Pluck the hair from the scrotum and prepare the area aseptically (Fig. 10.30).

    Rationale: Clipping is not usually necessary unless the cat is very young and plucking is difficult.

4. **Action:** Fix the position of one testis within the scrotum by applying pressure with your finger and thumb at the base of the scrotum.

    Rationale: This will prevent the testis moving within the scrotum and make the incision easier.

5. **Action:** Using a scalpel blade, make a small incision (approximately 1 cm) towards the end of the scrotum and, using pressure on the testis, exteriorize the testis within its tunic.

    Rationale: To gain access to the testis.

6. **Action:** Excise the tunic, bring the testis out of the surrounding tissue and using your fingers separate the attachment of the ligament of the tail of the testis from the tunic (Fig. 10.30).

    Rationale: The tunic can be pushed cranially providing access to the two structures within the spermatic cord.

7. **Action:** Identify the ductus deferens, separate it from the testis (Fig. 10.30) and, using the ligated vascular cord as one strand and the ductus deferens as another, tie 2–3 square knots (5–6 throws).

    Rationale: This will increase haemostasis and prevent the tissue of the spermatic cord prolapsing through the scrotum.

8. **Action:** Cut the vascular cord and ductus deferens distal to the knot (Fig. 10.30).

    Rationale: The testis has now been removed.

9. **Action:** Check for any signs of haemorrhage and allow the remaining tissues to retract into the scrotum.

    Rationale: Elastic recoil of the cord will pull it up towards the body cavity.

10. **Action:** Remove the testis on the other side using the same procedure.

    Rationale: The castration is now complete.

11. **Action:** The two incisions in the scrotum are left to heal by second intention and the owner should be warned to watch out for evidence of infection or excessive patient interference.

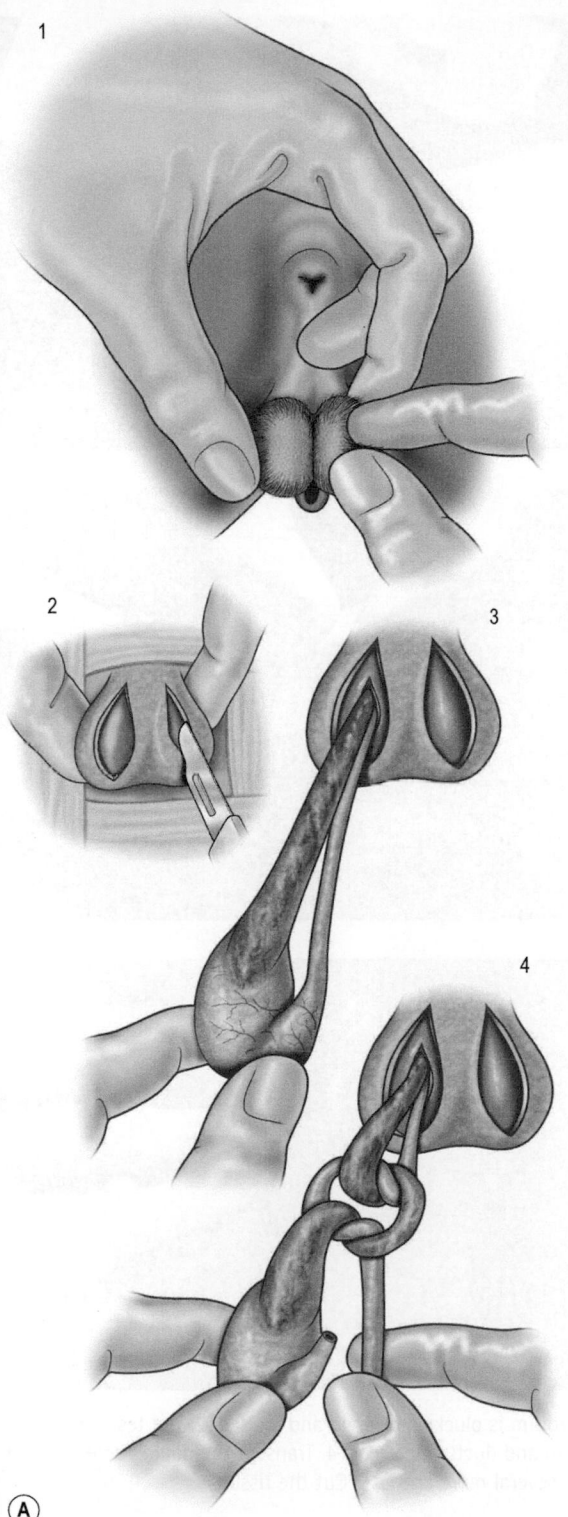

Figure 10.30 Castration in the mature cat: (A) 1. For feline castration, pluck hair from the scrotum and aseptically prepare the scrotum for surgery. 2. Make cranial to caudal skin incisions over each testicle. 3. Incise and separate the parietal tunic from the testicle, then transect the ductus deferens near the testicle. 4. Tie two to three square knots with the ductus deferens and the spermatic vessels.

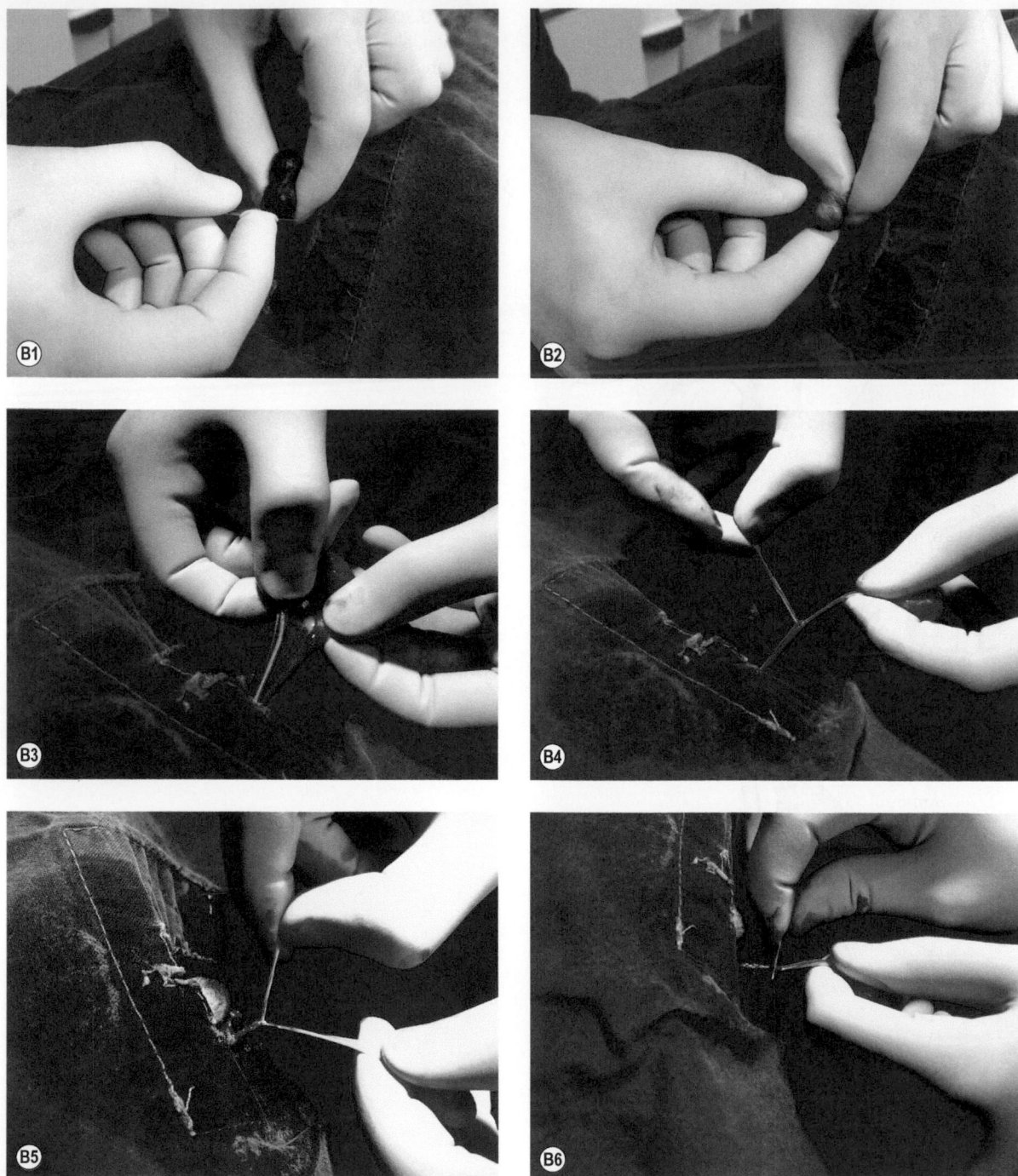

Figure 10.30 *Continued* (B) Castration in the mature cat. 1. The scrotum is plucked, cleaned and incised. 2. The testis is brought out of the scrotum. 3. Identify and separate the vascular cord and ductus deferens. 4. Transect the ductus deferens and tie a square knot using the ductus deferens and vascular cord. 5. Tie several more knots. 6. Cut the tissue.

Rationale: There are rarely any complications associated with castration even in more mature cats.

Procedure: Castration in the rabbit

1. **Action:** Before anaesthetizing the rabbit, check that both testes have descended into the scrotum.

   Rationale: Rabbits have two large testes that are easily visible in the adult but, as the inguinal ring remains open, they are able to be withdrawn into the abdominal cavity. This may happen if the level of anaesthesia is too light.

2. **Action:** Place the anaesthetized rabbit in dorsal recumbency and restrain the hindlegs using ties attached to the cleats under the table.

   Rationale: The body must not be able to tilt to one side or the other.

3. **Action:** Clip and aseptically prepare the abdomen caudal to the umbilicus, the medial aspect of the thighs and the scrotal sacs.

   Rationale: To prevent the entry of infection into the surgical wound. Take care to avoid damaging the delicate skin of the scrotal sacs with the clippers.

4. **Action:** Incise the skin of the scrotum and exteriorize the testis by blunt dissection.

   Rationale: The skin may be tightly adherent to the tunic of the testis and may have to be stripped away.

5. **Action:** Blunt dissect the ligament of the tail of the testis away from the tunic.

   Rationale: To release the testis from its attachments.

6. **Action:** Identify the structures within the spermatic cord (i.e. the ductus deferens and the vascular cord consisting of the spermatic artery and vein).

   Rationale: A closed technique is used in rabbits to decrease the risk of herniation through the inguinal ring. In older males there

may be a large amount of fat around the cord, which makes identification difficult.

7. **Action:** Close to the scrotal incision, place a pair of artery forceps across the ductus deferens and the vascular cord.

   Rationale: This crushed area will be used to place the ligature. The blood vessels are more friable than in the dog and cat so care must be taken at this stage.

8. **Action:** Place another pair of artery forceps across the spermatic cord caudal to the first pair (i.e. closer to the testis).

   Rationale: To ensure haemostasis.

9. **Action:** Release the first pair of artery forceps and reposition them caudal to the second pair across the spermatic cord.

   Rationale: To make sure that haemostasis is complete.

10. **Action:** Place a ligature around the ductus deferens and the vascular cord in the crushed area left by the first pair of artery forceps.

    Rationale: To ensure haemostasis.

11. **Action:** Cut the spermatic cord between the two pairs of artery forceps.

    Rationale: To remove the testis.

12. **Action:** Observe for signs of haemorrhage before releasing the artery forceps.

    Rationale: Religate if necessary. The presence of fat within the cord may mean that the ligatures are not tied tightly enough.

13. **Action:** If all is well then allow the remains of the spermatic to go back into the scrotum.

    Rationale: Elastic recoil will pull the remains of the tissue towards the inguinal ring.

14. **Action:** Remove the second testis using the same technique.

    Rationale: This may be done through the same skin incision or through a second one.

15. **Action:** Close the skin using intradermal sutures or tissue glue.

Rationale: Rabbits have a higher incidence of self-trauma than cats and dogs and it may be necessary to put in an extra layer of subcuticular sutures as a precaution.

NB Herniation of the abdominal contents is rare owing to the presence of a fat pad located over the internal inguinal ring. The inguinal canal remains open so closed castration is recommended; some surgeons also close the inguinal canal especially if an open technique is used.

Bibliography

Allen, W.E., 1992. Fertility and Obstetrics in the Dog. Blackwell Scientific Publications, London.

Aspinall, V., 2008a. Clinical Procedures in Veterinary Nursing. Butterworth-Heinemann, Oxford.

Aspinall, V., 2008b. Infectious diseases: how can we prevent their spread? CPD supplement in Veterinary Nursing Times vol 2, September 2008.

Aspinall, V., 2011. The Complete Textbook of Veterinary Nursing. Butterworth-Heinemann, Oxford.

Aspinall, V., Cappello, M., 2009. Introduction to Veterinary Anatomy and Physiology, second ed. Butterworth-Heinemann, Oxford.

Baines, S., Lipscomb, V., Hutchinson, T., 2012. Manual of Canine and Feline Surgical Principles. BSAVA, Gloucester.

Bexfield, N., Lee, K., 2010. BSAVA Guide to Clinical Procedures in Small Animal Practice. BSAVA, Gloucester.

Bowden, C., Masters, J., 2003. Textbook of Veterinary Medical Nursing. Butterworth-Heinemann, Oxford.

Bush, B.M., 1975. Veterinary Laboratory Manual. Heinemann, Oxford.

Bush, B.M., 1991. Interpretation of Laboratory Results for Small Animal Clinicians. Blackwell Scientific Publications, Oxford.

Evans, H.E., 1993. Miller's Anatomy of the Dog, third ed. Saunders, Philadelphia.

Flecknell, P. (Ed.), 2000. Manual of Rabbit Medicine and Surgery. BSAVA, Gloucester.

Fossum, T.W., 2007. Small Animal Surgery. Mosby, Missouri.

Guidance on the Operation of the Animals (Scientific Procedures) Act, 1986. HMSO, London.

Hall, L.W., Clarke, K.W., Trim, C.M., 2001. Veterinary Anaesthesia. Saunders, Oxford.

Hillyer, E.V., Quesenbury, K.E., 1997. Ferrets, Rabbits and Rodents: Clinical Medicine and Surgery. WB Saunders, Philadelphia.

Hoad, J., 2006. Minor Veterinary Surgery. Butterworth-Heinemann, Oxford.

How, K.L., Fleens, N., Stokhof, A.A., et al., 2001. Current concepts in resuscitation of dogs and cats. European Journal of Companion Animal Practice 11, 19–26. http://en.wikipaedia.org/wiki/Blood_type_(non-human).

Kerr Morag, G., 2002. Veterinary Laboratory Medicine. Blackwell Science, Oxford.

Lane, D.R., Cooper, B. (Eds), 2003. Veterinary Nursing, third ed. Butterworth-Heinemann, Oxford.

Lane, D., Cooper, B., Turner, L., 2003. Textbook of Veterinary Nursing. BSAVA, Gloucester.

Lee, R. (Ed.), 1995. Manual of Small Animal Diagnostic Imaging. BSAVA, Gloucester.

McKelvey, D., Hollingshead, K.W., 2000. Small Animal Anaesthesia, second ed. Mosby, London.

Martin, C., Masters, J., 2007. Textbook of Veterinary Surgical Nursing. Butterworth-Heinemann. Oxford.

Masters, J., Bowden, C. (Eds), 2001. BVNA Pre-Veterinary Nursing Textbook. Butterworth-Heinemann, Oxford.

O'Malley, B., 2005. Clinical Anatomy and Physiology of Exotic Species. Elsevier Saunders, Oxford.

Pace, C., 2007. ECG interpretation and basic arrhythmias. CPD supplement in Veterinary Nursing Times vol 1, September 2007.

Ramsey, I. (Ed.), 2011. BSAVA Small Animal Formulary. BSAVA, Gloucester.

RCVS, 2011. RCVS Guide to Professional Conduct 2011. RCVS, Belgravia House, 62-64 Horseferry Road, London SW1 2AF.

Samuelson, D.A., 2006. Textbook of Veterinary Histology. WB Saunders, Philadelphia, p. 142.

Simpson, J.W., Hall, E.J. (Eds), 1996. Manual of Canine and Feline Gastroenterology. BSAVA, Gloucester.

Slatter, D., 2003. Textbook of Small Animal Surgery. WB Saunders, Philadelphia.

Spencer, C., 2009. Feeding hospitalised patients for a speedy recovery. Veterinary Nursing Journal 24(7).

Taylor, S.M., 2010. Small Animal Clinical Techniques. WB Saunders, Missouri.

Tilley, L.P., 1992. Essentials of Canine and Feline Electrocardiography. Lea & Febiger, Philadelphia.

Torrance, A.G., Mooney, C.T. (Eds), 1998. Manual of Small Animal Endocrinology. BSAVA, Gloucester.

Wheeler, S.J. (Ed.), 1995. Manual of Small Animal Neurology, second ed. BSAVA, Gloucester.

World Health Organization, 2009. WHO guidelines on hand hygiene in health care. WHO Press, Geneva.

www.biology.ed.ac.uk. The Microbial World – Penicillin and other antibiotics.

www.merckvetmanual.com.

www.rcvs.org.uk. Royal College of Veterinary Surgeons – advice on blood transfusions.

www.vpisuk.co.uk/CommonPoisons/tabid/119/default. aspx.

Index

Printed and bound by CPI Group (UK) Ltd, Croydon, CR0 4YY

03/10/2024

01040349-0016